HEALTH CARE POLITICS, POLICY, AND SERVICES

Health Care Politics, Policy, and Services

A Social Justice Analysis

Gunnar Almgren, M.S.W., Ph.D.

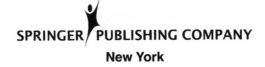

SPRINGER PUBLISHING COMPANY
New York

Springer Publishing Company, LLC
11 West 42nd Street
New York, NY 10036

Acquisitions Editor: Lauren Docket
Production Editor: Matthew Byrd
Cover Design: Mimi Flow
Typeset by Techbooks

07 08 09 10/5 4 3 2 1

Library of Congress Cataloging-in-Publication Data

Almgren, Gunnar Robert, 1951-Health care politics, policy, and services: a social justice analysis/Gunnar Almgren.
   p. ; cm.
   Includes bibliographical references and index.
   ISBN 0-8261-0236-0
1. Medical policy—United States. 2. Medical policy—United States—History. 3. Social justice—United States.
   I. Title.
   [DNLM: 1. Delivery of Health Care—United States. 2. Health
   Services—economics—United States. 3. Health Services—history—United States.
   4. Social Justice—United States. 5. Socioeconomic Factors—United States.
   W 84 AA1 A448h 2007]

RA395.A3A4795 2007
362.10973—dc22

                                                                    2006027538

Printed in the United States of America by Bang Printing

Contents

Foreword

Health care policy is challenging, complex, and dynamic in nature. During the beginning of the 21st century, tremendous changes have taken place including documentation of increased disparities in health care to poor and disabled individuals and families, inhumane managed care cost-cutting and restrictions, changing demographic characteristics and social determinants, advanced developments in medical technology, new medications that increase life expectancy, inequalities in access to health care, and growing recognition of the importance of increased public and private financing of the health care system.

This is the first comprehensive book focusing on infusing a social justice perspective that frames universal entitlement to adequate health care as one of the foundations and essential preconditions of a democratic government. Dr. Gunnar Almgren is to be applauded for this significant contribution to interdisciplinary knowledge-building in health policies and trends, with special attention to their effects on the poor, the elderly, and other at-risk populations. Health care policies and programs are discussed in terms of their underlying values and ethical dilemmas, their development and implementation, and their outcomes and effectiveness.

This important book provides up-to-date information on the progressive social policies, programs, and service delivery systems relevant to the health care field. Professor Almgren does an admirable job of helping the reader to understand the ever-changing organizational structure and functions of today's health care field. The reader is aptly introduced to social justice-oriented policies that can authorize and support federal, state, and local health care service delivery systems, while maximizing accessibility, acceptability, accountability, ethics, evidence-based practices, and multidisciplinary care. Professor Almgren's premise is that all citizens in American society have the right to preventative, curative, and restorative health care policies and services. This calls for an equal distribution of limited health care resources to all citizens in need, regardless of their income status, or physical or mental disabilities.

This is an outstanding book which examines the ecology, organization, and financing of health care policies and practices. The social justice perspective provides an original framework for incorporating the consequences of discrimination, oppression, economic injustice, empowerment, and reconciliation into health care policies and practices. The author is to be commended for doing an excellent job of focusing on the needs of all citizens, with emphasis on the at-risk and low-income populations in order to advocate for policy reforms and action strategies that may well result in positive changes to the health care system.

Throughout the book, the author integrates organizational, social, epidemiological, and ethical context with health care policies and practices. There is an ongoing critical need for health care restructuring and reform, and this book provides a well-organized and very informative synthesis by critically analyzing the theoretical and evidence-based paradigms for improving health care planning, administration, service delivery, and quality assurance and evaluation. This book is a gem. It offers a huge amount of information on health care policy. Each topic is presented in a highly readable, timely, and comprehensive manner. *This indispensable and essential text belongs on the desk of every graduate student and professor teaching public health policy, health care policy, social work in health settings, health care policy for nurses, health care for the poor, health care issues and policies, and social policy in health care settings.*

Albert R. Roberts, D.S.W., Ph.D.
Professor of Social Work and Criminal Justice
Rutgers, the State University of New Jersey

Preface

Students entering the health professions usually take at least one health care policy course, one that typically acquaints future health care professionals with the basics of health care organization, finance, politics, and some of the most pressing health care policy challenges. While there are a number of excellent health care policy texts available that offer this essential policy background, something more is needed.

Students in the health professions of Nursing, Pharmacy, Medicine, Dentistry, Public Health, and Social Work are entering practice at a time when the U.S. health care system is widely acknowledged to be in dire need of fundamental reform. Health care inflation has reached an unsustainable level, there are significant worries about health care access even among the middle class, and some of the most promising advancements in health care are overshadowed by large disparities in the burden of disease and the probability of reaching old age.

Health care policy, even at the introductory level, now requires a richer dialog that frames the evaluation of the health care system by what is known about the prevalence of disparities in health and health care, the implications of findings from social epidemiology for the organization of the health care system, and how different perspectives on social justice might lead to very different conclusions about the optimal direction of health care reform. The health care practitioners who have committed their lives and their careers to the health of others should not be the objects of this dialog, they should instead be at the forefront of it. This book offers the background needed to do so.

The genesis of the book is a series of health care policy courses, taught over many years, to students in the health professions and in public policy both at the University of Chicago and the University of Washington. Although I always wanted a textbook that applied a social justice perspective to the requisite content of introductory health care policy, I was never able to find one. In the end, the only solution was to produce the book I believed my students should have. Thus, this book provides its readers with a comprehensive description and analysis of the historical evolvement of the U.S. health care system that is framed by an explicit social justice critique. The book then provides the extensive coverage of health care system structure, finance, and performance that is essential to a solid introduction to health care policy. The policies and politics of alternative approaches to health care reform are introduced and considered, but not before the discussion is contextualized by some preceding background chapters on the prevalence and origins of disparities in health and in health care. The book concludes with a perspective on health care reform that is informed by the social justice theory of the late John Rawls—a theory that frames universal entitlement to adequate health care as one of the basic and essential preconditions of democratic governance.

In order to accomplish all this, the book is organized into eight chapters, beginning with a chapter that brings different theories of social justice to bear on the question of basic entitlement to health care. The second chapter provides a narrative of the evolvement of the U.S. health care system, a perspective that is essential to understanding the system's organization and financing—the task taken up in the third and fourth chapters. The fifth chapter provides the essential background in long-term care policy, including the considerations and prospects for adapting the nation's long-term care system to the unprecedented demands of the immediate decades. Chapters 6 and 7 examine in sequence patterns of disparity in health and in health care, and the explanations forthcoming from the emerging discipline of social epidemiology. The final chapter illuminates the political economy of health care reform and considers the reasons why health care reform has remained politically stalemated despite broad public support for the notion of universal access to health care. It culminates with a proposed health care system model that reconciles the preservation of individual preferences for health care with the imperative of universal entitlement that is based on the principles of social justice formulated by John Rawls.

Although this book is written with careful attention to the facts pertaining to the demography of health care and disparities in health, it is not written to be neutral or dispassionate. The book is framed by a particular theory of social justice that provides the philosophical foundations of the progressive social policy movement—otherwise known as political liberalism. To the many readers who may disagree with the particular theory of justice that frames much of the book's analysis of health care policy, I hope the book nonetheless engages you in an examination of health care policy *as a problem of social justice*. If that indeed occurs, I will happily call the book a success.

Acknowledgments

For the perspective on social justice that frames the analysis of this book I am actually more indebted to my parents, Gayle and Peter, than I am to John Rawls. Like many of their generation, my parents were determined that each of their children understand the structural nature of poverty and privilege—sans the sociological jargon. I have many things to thank my parents for, among them the conviction that endemic despair cannot coexist with claims to just governance.

For the writing of the book itself I am most indebted to my wife, Linda. She encouraged me to write the book in the first place, supported me at every turn as the manuscript progressed, and at various other critical junctures lovingly made the big and little sacrifices needed to get the work completed. Linda is my partner and my soulmate in all things that truly matter to me, including whatever contributions this book might make to the classroom discourse on health care.

Much of my gratitude also goes to my colleagues and students both at the University of Chicago and the University of Washington. The book is in large part inspired by their intellectual energy and collective commitment to social justice, albeit from very diverse points of view.

Finally, there is a significant share of gratitude to others who provided generous and essential editorial assistance: Al Roberts at Rutgers University, Jennifer Perillo at Springer Publishing Company, and at the University of Washington, Julie Miller, Gioia Rizzo, and Michele Hutchinson. Thank you all.

CHAPTER ONE

A Primer on Theories of Social Justice and Defining the Problem of Health Care

The premise of this chapter is that relatively few students in public health, medicine, nursing, and social work have more than a superficial acquaintance with specific theories of social justice. Although this text employs a very specific (Rawlsian) social justice framework in its analysis of health care policy, the text's chosen perspective will be contextualized and highlighted by contrasting it with other dominant theories of social justice. In later chapters, the health care policy implications of the differing perspectives on social justice will be considered.

DEFINING THE PROBLEM OF SOCIAL JUSTICE

The term *social justice* has many uses and interpretations, but in its most basic and universal sense, social justice is a philosophical construct—in essence a political theory or system of thought used to determine what mutual obligations flow between the individual and society. As such, social justice is distinct from the concept of individual justice, the latter pertaining only to obligations that exist between individuals (Rhodes, Battin, & Silvers, 2002). Also inherent in the concept of social justice, as it is generally construed within democratic societies, is the idea that civil society is predicated on the basis of a social contract that spells out the benefits, rights, and obligations of societal membership.[1] For example, at a very

---

[1] The idea of the social contract, as it evolved through the essays of Hobbes, Locke and ultimately Rousseau, holds that the only basis for the legitimate authority of governments and related social institutions is voluntary agreements between free and equal individuals.

basic level collective security as a benefit of membership in civil society is reciprocated through individual obligations pertaining to taxation and availability for military service.

Beyond these points pertaining to general definition, there is no absolute generally agreed-upon notion of what defines or constitutes "social justice," either as process or as an outcome. Were that the case, the problem of social justice would be limited to one of social engineering—ways of organizing social institutions to assure that the individuals, groups, and organizations composing society act in "just" ways in accordance with the rules of "absolute, true, and universal" social justice. However, unlike a theocracy comprised of culturally homogenous and like-minded individuals ascribing to a shared moral and political philosophy, a pluralist democracy must accommodate diverse points of view on what mutual obligations exist, what rules for the governance of mutual obligations should be codified, and how limited resources should be distributed. Thus, in a pluralist democracy, the problem of social justice is two-fold. First, there is the problem of achieving a conception of social justice that is mutually recognized and acknowledged by diverse individuals and groups as a legitimate basis for adjudicating claims on obligations and resources. Second, there is the problem of how to organize social institutions in accordance with the prevailing conception of social justice (Rawls, 2001).[2] This chapter is principally concerned with the first problem, namely, finding a perspective on social justice that accommodates fundamentally different world views, experiences and interests.

ALTERNATIVE THEORIES OF SOCIAL JUSTICE

As implied by the general definition of social justice as a philosophical construct, there are very different theoretical perspectives pertaining to the principles used to determine what we as individuals are owed as members of society, and what we in turn owe society at large. A second point of theoretical diversity concerns the just distribution of limited resources, an aspect of social justice that is obviously central to health care policy. The social justice perspective that frames the analysis of health care policy in this text, that advanced by John Rawls, will be contrasted with three very different but highly influential theoretical approaches to social

---

[2] The problem of social justice as it is defined here is based upon two critical concepts that John Rawls builds upon in his theory of social justice. The first is the idea of a *public conception of justice* and the second is the idea of a *well-ordered society*. According to Rawls, one requisite of a well-ordered society is that it is regulated by the prevailing public conception of social justice (see Rawls, 2001, p. 9).

justice: libertarianism, utilitarianism, and Marxism.[3] In the review of alternative theories of social justice that follows, the primary bases of comparison will be each theory's fundamental claims pertaining to the nature and overall purpose of civil society, what obligations flow upward from individuals to society, what obligations flow downward from society to the individual, and the theory's essential basis for the just distribution of limited resources.[4]

It should be noted in the review that follows the term "obligations" is used in a very broad sense to apply to all of those acts and actions that either individuals or social institutions have a responsibility to perform under the principles of a given theory of social justice. As we use the term obligations here, it is meant to apply to acts that might more narrowly be defined as "duties" rather than just obligations. A more detailed analysis of alternative theories would devote more attention to this distinction within each theory. However, for the limited purposes here the more general application of the term "obligations" is acceptable.[5]

I. The Libertarian Theoretical Perspective on Social Justice

The Nature and Overall Purpose of Civil Society

In the classical libertarian perspective, civil society is comprised of a network of natural and voluntary associations among autonomous and equal individuals that in various ways serve human needs (Boaz, 1997). In accordance with this perspective, societies must be governed, but only to the extent necessary to assure the protection of an explicit set of individual rights. As such, government's legitimate functions pertain only to basic protections against foreign or domestic threats to life, property, or the

---

[3] Obviously, these do not comprise an exhaustive list of alternative social justice frameworks. Those chosen reflect the author's judgment of the most historically influential in terms of health care policy. Regrettably this leaves out of the analysis some very compelling perspectives on social justice that are very relevant to health care.

[4] Broadly speaking, principles of social justice are of three general types: procedural, retributive/compensatory, and distributive. Principles pertaining to *procedural justice* concern the fairness of the process for determining what is just, independent of the outcome. Principles pertaining to *retributive/compensatory justice* are concerned with the determination of punishment and compensation for wrongs, injuries and losses. Principles that are concerned with the just allocation of limited benefits and resources pertain to *distributive justice*. In this text we are chiefly concerned with the latter.

[5] In the literatures of political philosophy and moral philosophy the definitional distinction between obligations and duties is contested ground. As Rawls would have it, obligations are incurred as the result of some voluntary action, whereas duties are acts that are "moral requirements" that apply to all persons irrespective of explicit consent or the moral status of the person (Steinberger, 2002).

exercise of personal autonomy (Nozick, 1974). For example, governments can legitimately do such things as levy taxes to provide military and police protection, legislate and enforce laws against theft, fraud, and breach of contract, and restrain actions by individuals or groups that in other ways deprive or interfere with the essential civil and property rights of others.

In the dominant libertarian vision of civil society, collective well-being is best achieved through the exercise of individual free will and self-responsibility in the context of a laissez-faire market economy. A market economy, unrestrained by burdensome taxes and regulation, alleviates poverty and promotes commonwealth through technological innovation, job creation, and the efficient production and distribution of goods and services yielded by the free flow of labor and capital. To the extent there are individual misfortunes[6] that result in poverty (and family resources are absent), mutual aid societies and other charitable organizations exist as an outgrowth of voluntary cooperation and such factors as individual religious conviction. However, because illness, unemployment, and even old age are risks that are intrinsic to human social existence, it is the role and responsibility of individuals in a free and civil society to self-protect through (1) such market mechanisms as insurance and savings, (2) sharing of family resources, and (3) participation in voluntary networks of mutual aid and protection (e.g. churches, fraternal organizations).[7]

What Obligations Flow Upward From Individuals to Society

Core to libertarian philosophy is the premise that individuals have "full self-ownership," meaning that individuals have a *moral right* to grant or deny use of any aspect of their person on whatever basis they determine aligns with their preference, individual moral philosophy, or self-interest. It also means that *individuals have full immunity or protection against the "nonconsensual" loss of their rights to self-ownership*—except where the individual violates the rights of others (Vallentyne, 2004). A second core premise of libertarian social philosophy is that individuals also have the moral right to acquire *property rights* in external things (objects outside the person) that if acquired legitimately *are also immune from nonconsensual loss.*[8] A third and related core premise of libertarianism

---

[6] Libertarians are loath to concede market failures, see Boaz, 1997, pp. 256–260.

[7] Libertarians decry the emergence of the welfare state and its displacement of social welfare functions that were formally assumed by other social institutions, most notably the family but also various types of mutual aid societies that have flourished throughout U.S. history. This point of view is hardly unique to libertarians, but this perspective is far more central to the libertarian views of the pernicious nature of government.

[8] This generally means acquired in ways that do not violate the rights of others.

concerns the use of coercion by governments, institutions, or individuals. In accordance with this third core premise, it is not permissible to employ coercion or the use of force to either: (1) benefit the person, (2) benefit others, or (3) prevent third parties from violating the rights of others (Vallentyne, 2004, p. 1). A fourth core premise, mentioned previously, concerns the minimalist role of governments, in essence, the position that governmental functions should be limited to the protection of life, property, and the exercise of personal autonomy (Nozick, 1974). Collectively these premises imply that the obligations that flow from individuals to society are limited to those that involve overt or explicit consent, and in the case of individual obligations to the government, are limited to those essential for the preservation of collective security and individual liberty, such as taxation for national defense and law enforcement. Indeed, other than those obligations assumed under explicit and free consent, the only other obligations owed by individuals to society at large are those that involve a duty not to violate the essential rights of others (Vallentyne, 2004).[9]

Notably, libertarians do not dismiss the idea that individuals have moral responsiblities, or that various obligations do not arise from their status as moral actors. In the libertarian thought, it is entirely compatible for a libertarian to *voluntarily* hold herself to a stringent moral philisophy that requires that in every action she places the well-being of others before her own narrow self-interest. It is also the case that libertarians place great emphasis on the notion that the free agency carries with it the full burden of accountability for whatever good or evil might result from one's actions (Clarke, 2003).

> The dignity that one has in virtue of being a free agent, then, consists in one's making a difference, by one's exercise of active control, to how things go in the world. It consists of one's actions' (and some of their consequences') being attributable to one as source and author, and, providing that one has an ordinary capacity to appreciate and act for moral reasons, in one's being responsible for one's action (and some of their consequences).[10]

---

[9] The strain of libertarianism presented here is the traditional form of libertarianism, sometimes called "right-wing libertarianism," which tends to be much more absolutist about unfettered individual appropriation of natural resources—and by extension the negation of equality of opportunity. There are "left-wing" versions of libertarianism that recognize and accommodate issues of compensation and equality of opportunity, even to the extent of equality of access to personal welfare (see M. Otsuka, 1998).

[10] Randolph Clarke (2003). *Libertarian Accounts of Free Will.* New York: Oxford University Press. p. 7.

Although one can clearly read the foregoing account of libertarian free will as a heavy imperative that individuals should strive to do good in the world and should pursue existence as atomistic and egocentric beings, the distinct thread of libertarianism is retained through the exercise of free will in selecting one's individual moral philisophy. The central point of libertarianism concerning the obligations that flow from the individual to the society at large is that obligations toward others in society are a matter of free choice, other than the nonconsensual obligation or duty to not violate the libertarian rights of others (Vallentyne, 2004).

What Obligations Flow Downward From Society to the Individual

As implied by the preceding summary of the libertarian perspective on the flow of obligations from the individual to society as a whole, as well as the libertarian perspective on the nature of society, the obligations that flow downward from the society to the individuals would seem to be quite limited. If, as libertarians argue, civil societies are spontaneous entities comprised of a network of natural and voluntary associations (Boaz, 1997), then it is difficult to find any basis for assuming what (if any) obligations toward individuals actually encumber society at large. However, in the classic libertarian framework there are two kinds of obligations that flow from society to the individuals: those that pertain to the preservation of a limited set of natural rights and those that arise from voluntary social contracts between individuals and the organizations, institutions, and communities they choose to join.

In the utopian society described by classic libertarian theorist Robert Nozick (1974), individuals are free to form, enter, and exit any of a multitude of diverse communities, each expressing a different vision of what values should govern individual lives and what values should govern communal relationships. As stated by Nozick (p. 312) there is no utopian society writ large with a single encompassing vision of ideal social existence, but rather a utopian society that is a collection of many different kinds of utopias that serve different individual preferences. In this vision of society, individuals are at liberty to choose which community to join or leave; membership in any one community can entail a large set of restrictions on individual freedom and extensive mutual obligations between the individual and the community at large. Accordingly, an individual may choose to join a highly socialistic community, or at the other extreme, may choose to join a highly laissez-faire community having minimal constraints on individual behavior and very few mutual obligations.[11] Thus,

---

[11] On this point see Nozick (1974), pp. 320–321.

libertarian theory really does not oppose the idea that an extensive set of entitlements and obligations can flow downward from society to the individual (or vice versa) per se, just as long as those more extensive entitlements and obligations are a function of a social contract enacted by voluntary membership in a community comprised of other like-minded individuals.[12]

In contrast to this benign view of the entitlements and obligations that might arise in voluntary communities, libertarians consider entitlements and obligations that flow through any kind of central government to be inherently suspect, if not pernicious. The philosophical basis for this libertarian aversion to central government is typically attributed to John Locke's (1690) *Second Treatise of Government*, wherein Locke argues that (1) individuals possess an essential set of natural rights that precede the formation of governments, (2) governments are formed to protect natural rights, and (3) governments that exceed their protectionist role and impinge on individual rights lose their basis of legitimacy (Boaz, 1997; Nozick, 1974). Although there are strains of libertarianism that are willing to extend the protectionist role to equality of opportunity (Otsuka, 1998; Vallentyne, 2004), advocates of classic libertarianism emphasize the idea of the "minimal state" described previously—one that is limited to "the functions of protecting its citizens against violence, theft, and fraud, and to the enforcement of contracts." (Nozick, 1974, p. 26).

Libertarian theory is popular among individuals who, for various reasons (and often good ones), believe governments do things badly. However, in the classic libertarian framework the reasons why governments are inefficient (and even pernicious) are tied to issues of human diversity and political pluralism. According to this line of reasoning, if it is presumed that individuals have a natural right to live life as they choose (as long as their actions are not harmful to the natural rights of others), and that society is comprised of individuals having diverse preferences and beliefs about what constitutes personal security and the requisites of happiness, then how is it possible to sustain a form of government that serves all individual ideologies and preferences? The answer is that central governments in fact cannot, and that by some method (be it democratic or authoritarian), central governments are bound to select and impose duties, mutual obligations, and limits to freedom that force some individuals to conform to the social ideologies of others. The objection to the central government being the purveyor of mutual social obligations, as

---

[12] "Like-minded individuals" is used here in a very limited sense, meaning persons with a similar social philosophy and set of preferences for human community. Nozick envisions his utopian communities as being comprised of highly diverse individuals in other dimensions, for example, in talents and occupational preferences.

opposed to communities and other voluntary forms of human association, is that individuals cannot "opt out" and seek other alternatives short of renouncing citizenship and fleeing—which itself defeats the very purpose of having a central government.

II. The Utilitarian Theoretical Perspective on Social Justice

The Nature and Overall Purpose of Civil Society

Classic utilitarians, like libertarians, assume that society is founded upon, and to a large extent justified by, voluntary relationships formed for purposes of mutual advantage (Barry, 1989; Roemer, 1996). It can be said the origins of the utilitarian perspective on social justice begins with Aristotle's notion of distributive justice, which in essence views the just distribution of the goods and benefits of society as a legitimate function of the state (Miller, 2002). That being said, Aristotle himself was not in any sense a utilitarian, because his criteria for the just distribution of goods and benefits rest on the merits of the individual rather than upon the *principle of utility*—the latter being the hallmark of classic utilitarianism introduced in its full form by John Stewart Mill in his (1863) essay entitled *Utilitarianism*.[13] In simple form, this principle states that utility (whatever is valued as a good thing) should be distributed in accordance with whichever scheme yields *the maximum good to the maximum number of people* (Rescher, 1966). The principle of utility, taken at face value, suggests that civil society should be organized in highly rationalistic terms (some would say even in calculated terms) to achieve the maximum social good for the most number of persons. Accordingly, the primary problem of distributive justice becomes one of economics, or in the words of eminent economist John Roemer, that system of resource allocation "which maximizes the sum total of utility over persons" (Roemer, 1996, p. 5).

Taken to this extreme, the doctrinaire utilitarian society would be relatively unconcerned with problems of either extremes of deprivation or extremes of abundance, as long as *the maximum good to the maximum number* outcome is served. While one might question the political viability or moral basis of such a system of social organization and governance, in effect this utilitarian doctrine has been underscored and emphasized as a rationale for a number of economic and social policies that clearly benefit

---

[13] It should be noted that John Stewart Mill did not himself introduce the basic utilitarian principle of "the greatest good to the greatest number of people," that is credited to the writings of English jurist and social philosopher Jeremy Bentham in 1776 (Fox, 1907). However, John Stewart Mill is credited with extending the utilitarian principle to a unified theory and popularizing utilitarian ideas among English intellectuals.

some groups over others, such as tax policies that by many accounts contribute to rising concentrations of wealth via such arguments as "a rising tide lifts all boats" (Pizzigati, 2005). The remarkable level of acceptance among Americans for this line of argument suggests that utilitarianism in fact has broad intuitive appeal as a significant foundation for social policy on a variety of fronts, including health care.

What Obligations Flow Upward From Individuals to Society

To get to an idea of what obligations flow upward from individuals to society (and vice-versa), three concepts are key. First is *consequentionalist theory*, in essence theories that hold that individual obligations are a function of their outcomes. The second key concept is the ethical principle of *rule utilitarianism*, meaning in essence that the rightness or wrongness of acts are evaluated in accordance with a set of rules that themselves have (over time) managed to achieve the maximization of the common good. Third is the now familiar idea of the *social contract*, described earlier as the idea that civil society is predicated on the basis of a social contract that spells out the benefits, rights, and obligations of societal membership. Thus, in accordance with the utilitarian premise that the ultimate function of society is the promotion of the maximum level of common good, the primary basis for determining the social rules (e.g. laws, social policies, civic duties) is whether or not they are genuinely intended for the common good—even if one's own happiness and well-being (or utility) are compromised. Conversely, this also implies that utilitarian ethics do not obligate one to act in accordance with rules that do not serve the maximization of the common good.

As an example, consider a tax that is levied for road construction, under the premise that there is a consensus among voters that building a particular arterial is essential to commerce and public safety. Even though a utilitarian citizen may not drive or even personally agree that the proposed arterial is needed, she is obligated to pay her share of the taxes because the decision to build the road was determined (1) by the rules of democratic process (presumably adopted because they maximize the common good) and (2) the utilitarian justification that the proposed road itself serves to maximize the common good. However, suppose that it is shown that the proposed road is actually an overly priced boondoggle, put before the voters to benefit a select contractor with a lot of political influence. Would our citizen-utilitarian still have the ethical obligation to pay the taxes levied for the boondoggle arterial? If the voting process itself were not corrupt the answer would seem to be yes—the premise being that accountability to the outcome of the democratic process remains justified under the ethical principle of *rule utilitarianism*. If on the other hand, both the democratic process was not adhered to and the road project was not in service of the common good, then our utilitarian citizen will not in any sense violate her ethical principles by refusing to pay taxes for the road because there is no aspect of social contract that was not violated (she still might be thrown in jail however).

The only other general obligations that flow upward from individuals to society are those that concern restraint from doing evil or harm, or *negative utilitarianism*. Simply stated, there is a utilitarian principle that also states that the rightness of actions should be also evaluated by producing the least harm to the least number of people, or performing actions that prevent the most harm to the most number of people. Accordingly, a social contract that is consistent with utilitarianism can also include obligations that are aimed at either constraining harmful behavior or even obligating the individual to perform duties that are aimed at preventing harm. As an example, it is legitimate from a utilitarian perspective that a village obligates every person who is physically capable to help pile sandbags along a river that is on the verge of flooding. From a health care policy perspective, negative utilitarianism underscores the justification of rules governing personal health behavior—including sexual conduct.

What Obligations Flow Downward From Society to the Individual

Utilitarianism does not prescribe a specific set of societal obligations toward individuals, but rather provides general ethical criteria for the evaluation of the laws and other social policies that distribute the benefits and resources of society. In this sense, though, utilitarian theory is an extremely potent determinant of societal obligations. Consistent with the ethical obligations of individuals, utilitarian principles hold that social arrangements and actions should (1) maximize the sum of happiness and well-being over the most number of persons or (2) do the least harm to the least number of persons or (3) prevent the most harm to the most number of persons. By strict utilitarian standards, this suggests that governments are not ethically obligated to respect any aspect of individual autonomy, happiness, or well-being that runs counter to the maximization of the general good of all—per the ruthless utopia depicted in Aldous Huxley's (1932) *Brave New World*.

However, most utilitarian thinkers promote a strain of utilitarianism that recognizes that there are some limits to the utilitarian principle where the so-called natural rights of individuals are at stake, such as life and liberty. For example, few utilitarian ethicists condone violent actions of governments or individuals that take the lives of innocents in order to prevent the deaths of many others, or suggest a rigid application of a strict cost–benefit analysis to the provision of all forms of health care.

Rather, most utilitarian thinkers temper their utilitarianism with other fundamental considerations of justice that are not themselves derived from utilitarian theory, such as recognition of a minimum subsistence threshold for the distribution of essential goods. Along this line, distributive justice philosopher Nicolas Rescher (1966) proposed a "qualified utilitarianism" that adds *all other things being equal* to the basic "greatest good to the greatest number" principle of utility—these other things referring to other relevant principles of justice (Rescher, 1966, pp. 115–117).

III. A Marxist Theoretical Perspective on Social Justice

There is no single Marxist theory of social justice per se, but rather a variety of interpretations of how the extensive political and historical works of Karl Marx and Friedrich Engels (spanning the nineteenth century from 1841 to 1895) lead to an implicit theory of social justice. The Marxist theory of social justice that is selected for this text is explicated in Rodney Peffer's (1990) *Marxism, Morality, and Social Justice*, which many would agree is a rigorous and exhaustive treatment of this subject.[14] However, it should be noted and emphasized that any scholarly interpretations of Marxist thought are generally (and often hotly) contested among Marxists and non-Marxists alike. As such, Peffer's Marxist theory of social justice stands as an exemplar of a Marxist social justice framework rather than the definitive Marxist theory of social justice.

The Nature and Overall Purpose of Civil Society

The central tenet of Marxist theory is *historical materialism*, which stated in the simplest terms claims that the particular social arrangements that compose different forms of society (social systems) are determined by the modes of production that are dominant in any given historical epoch. Over time, less efficient social systems (those that fail to maximize the dominant mode of production) give way to social systems that are more efficient with respect to the maximization of production (Peffer, 1990). The image of society that became the basis for Marxist theory was 19th-century England; a social system with a rigid class structure and ruthless class oppression that was greatly transformed by the Industrial Revolution that had taken place over the preceding 100 years. Thus, class exploitation and conflict lie at the heart of the Marxist perspective of the nature of society and compose a central theme of contemporary Marxist writings pertaining to issues of social justice.

[14] Published by Princeton University Press, Princeton NJ in 1990.

Although it can be said that the Marxist[15] perspective on the nature of society rests upon an explicit theory of economic determinism and class conflict, the classic Marxist perspective on the overall purpose of civil society can be gleaned only indirectly—since neither Marx or Engels can be said to have produced a unified moral theory.[16] However, one can gain a foothold on the Marxist conception of the purpose of society by examining (1) the central themes of Marx's critiques of 19th-century social systems, (2) the fundamental merits of the communist social system Marx viewed as morally superior to capitalism, and (3) the Marxist criteria for a morally justified revolution—as argued by Peffer (1990). Concerning the first point, insomuch as Marx viewed the capitalist social systems as pernicious and exploitive because a large segment of society suffers poverty and fails to find personal fulfillment or freedom and self-determination, it can be assumed that Marx regarded such things as legitimate claims or expectations of everyday citizens. Regarding the second point (the relative virtue of the communist social system over others), Marx's famous dictum that such a system would assure that "each contributes according to their ability and receives according to their need" strongly suggests themes of equity and commonwealth as core purposes of society (Wolff, 2003). Finally, as Peffer's interpretation of Marxist theory of social justice would have it, people have a legitimate basis for rebellion where governments: (1) fail to secure basic rights of well-being, or (2) fail to secure "maximum equal liberty" among citizens, or (3) fail to provide equality of opportunity, or (4) fail to eliminate unjust social and economic inequalities.[17]

Marxist thinkers differ greatly on the extent to which the social systems they endorse or believe will incorporate all aspects of doctrinaire Marxism. Peffer's approach to a Marxist theory of social justice rests

---

[15] For the limited purposes of this text, I will not discriminate between the particular contributions of either Marx or Engels to Marxist theory, but will refer to Marxism as incorporating the ideas of both.

[16] In fact, Marx deliberately avoided moral arguments because he believed that moral systems of thought were themselves products of economically determined social systems rather than the foundations of social systems. Moreover, he regarded his work as empirical theory and not moral philosophy. However, it seems that he was unable to escape moral arguments altogether (on this observation see Wolff's (2003) essay in chapter references).

[17] See chapter reference on Peffer, pages 416–418 and 452. Peffer constructs his Marxist theory of social justice largely from Marx's idea of maximum equal freedom (explicated on page 417 of Peffer) and the main tenets of John Rawls' theory of justice. As such, Peffer incorporates a modified version of Rawls' "difference principle," which in its original form holds that only those social and economic inequalities that provide the greatest benefit to the least-advantaged members of society are just (see reference for Rawls, 2001, *Justice as Fairness*, p. 42).

upon the model of a "democratic, self-managing socialist" society, which he argues is the social system that is most able (in the current historical epoch) to fulfill the Marxist principles of social justice he puts forth. In such a society the core tenets of socialism (that productive property is socially owned rather than privately owned and the formally working class is elevated to the ruling class), are joined with the political authority of the democratic state (Peffer, 1990, pp. 11–12). Notably, Peffer suggests that democratic, self-managing socialist society can either function as a socialist command economy or a socialist market economy as a matter of simple pragmatism rather than ideology—the choice should be whichever form is most efficient and compatible with the principles of social justice derived from Marxist theory. Briefly stated and somewhat paraphrased, Peffer's Marxist theory of social justice has four core principles:

1. Each person's rights to security and subsistence shall be respected.
2. There is to be a maximum system of equal basic liberties, which at minimum must include:
   • freedom of speech and assembly.
   • freedom of conscience and thought.
   • freedom of the person.
   • personal (as opposed to productive) property rights.
   • freedom from arbitrary arrest and seizure.
3. Equal rights to opportunity of position attainment and participation in decision-making within all social institutions of which one is a part.
4. Social and economic inequalities are justified if and only if they:
   • serve to benefit the least advantaged member of society.
   • fall below a level that undermines equal worth of liberty or the good of self-respect. (Peffer, 1990, p. 418)

What Obligations Flow Upward From Individuals to Society

In contrast to the libertarian and utilitarian frameworks reviewed previously, included and explicit in the Marxist social justice perspective, is the positive right of subsistence (see the first principle). Broadly defined, subsistence refers to being provided the material essentials necessary to sustain life (food, shelter, clothing). However, as explicated by Peffer, the positive right of subsistence is meant to *guarantee* each member of society "a minimum level of material well-being including basic needs, i.e., those needs that must be met in order to remain a normal functioning human being" (Peffer, 1990, p. 14). Positive rights that involve material resources are inherently reciprocal—meaning that as individuals not only

access to basic health care is a basic need

R= Pharmacy prescriptions
Hospitals

Tx = treatment

do we benefit from the guarantee of some minimum level of our own welfare, but we also assume specific obligations and duties toward the basic welfare of others. The second of the Marxist principles is basically consistent with the obligations individuals assume toward the natural rights of others as advocated by libertarians, except for the limited definition of property rights that excludes ownership of property that has a productive function. The third and fourth principles imply that individuals are also obligated to surrender their individual interests where their personal interests significantly clash with collective equity in the material, social, and political spheres of opportunity, and where their individual interests conflict with social and economic equalities more generally. In sum, these principles imply that individuals assume not only a moral burden for the basic well-being of others, but also the significant individual obligations that are necessary to promote the ethic of egalitarianism in all spheres of public and productive life.[18] As stated by Peffer, these principles convey a "natural duty" that extends to the support and promotion of just social institutions (p. 15).

What Obligations Flow Downward From Society to the Individual

Akin to libertarian theory, under Peffer's interpretation of Marxist social justice principles, society is obligated to respect and protect the so-called natural rights of individuals, those that pertain to fundamental liberties such as freedom of speech, thought, association, and dominion of one's person and personal property (see the second principle). However, in contrast to the libertarian perspective and as pointed out previously, the Marxist social justice principles do not suggest that society is obligated to respect or protect property rights that are in any way linked to the productive capacities of society—the latter being subject to collective ownership. Like other theories of social justice that assume an implicit social contract as the basis for legitimacy of political authority (the corollary of which provides the basis for legitimate revolution), the Marxist perspective obligates society to sustain and protect rights to personal security, that is, the provision of protections against coercive actions of others (individuals, institutions, or states) that would unjustly deprive the individual of life, liberty, or personal property. A distinctly Marxist societal obligation pertains to the provision of subsistence at a level necessary to sustain normal

---

[18] It should be noted that Peffer extends his Marxist principles of social justice to the international sphere, which he argues holds each individual to a "natural duty" to promote a "worldwide federation of democratic, self-managing socialist societies (see Peffer, pp. 14, 15).

human functioning, which in the classic context of Marxist theory would suggest a subsistence level that is sufficient to preserve individual human dignity (e.g., no poor farms, no slums, or other accoutrements of abject poverty).

As specified in the third principle, the Marxist social justice framework places significant emphases on society's obligation to promote and protect equity of opportunity for both status attainment and participation in political decision-making, consistent with the liberal social justice framework to be described shortly. However, the thread that is distinctly Marxist in Peffer's social justice framework is the emphasis (in the third principle) on equal rights of participation in all social decision-making processes within *all* social and economic institutions of which one is a part. As Peffer states it (1990, pp. 401 and 404), the Marxist approach to social justice extends the principle of collective self-determination beyond the political realm to all other realms of social and economic structure—most particularly the workplace. In practical application, the third principle argues that society has the obligation to restrain such social organizations as schools, workplaces, and social service agencies from engaging in nondemocratic forms of governance, and conversely, to positively promote democratic governance in such organizations.

The final set of societal obligations (embedded in the fourth principle) pertains to the eradication of *unjust* social and economic inequalities. Since this principle holds that there are very restricted circumstances under which social and economic inequalities can be considered just, it would seem that society is obligated to eliminate as much as possible all the social and economic inequalities that fall outside of the narrow circumstances specified. The exceptional circumstances are specified in the *Difference Principle*, a cornerstone of Rawls' theory of social justice. In essence, the difference principle holds that *only those social and economic inequalities that provide the greatest benefit to the least-advantaged members of society are just* (Rawls, 2001, p. 2). The Marxist modification of the Difference Principle (as postulated by Peffer) narrows the criteria for "just" social and economic inequalities by limiting the application of the Difference Principle to *only* those social and economic inequalities that do not undermine the social bases of self-respect. To illustrate, the original *Difference Principle* would suggest it is "just" to reward a manager with a higher salary for the same number of hours of work if this arrangement provided the most material benefits to the least advantaged of workers. The Marxist modification of the *Difference Principle* would suggest that the higher salary must not only produce the most benefits to the least advantaged, but also must not be so much higher as to undermine the social bases of respect for the other workers.

IV. The Rawlsian "Justice as Fairness" Theoretical Perspective on Social Justice

As acknowledged and explained earlier in the preface, Rawls' theory of social justice has been selected as the central social justice perspective of this text. The social justice theory of John Rawls, referred to by Rawls as a "Justice as Fairness" approach to a theory of social justice (Rawls, 1985), is also commonly regarded as the classic liberal theory of social justice. As explained by Rawls (p. 224), his theory of social justice is intended to be a *political* theory of social justice; that is, a moral conception of justice that applies to the political, social, and economic institutions of society as distinct from a moral system that applies to the actions of individuals. Notably, Rawls considers his theory of social justice to be limited to and specifically for the special case of a modern constitutional democracy (Rawls, 2001, p. 14). According to Rawls (1985, pp. 226–227), the central challenge of a political theory of social justice in the context of constitutional democracy is to reconcile the inherent pluralism that a free and democratic society promotes with the imperative to create *a public conception of justice*—the latter described as a "mutually recognized point of view from which citizens can adjudicate their claims of political right on their political institutions or against one another" (Rawls 2001, p. 9).[19]

The Nature and Overall Purpose of Civil Society

Consistent with the social contract doctrine of Locke and his predecessors, Rawlsian social justice theory views the purpose of society as a cooperative social and political arrangement conceived and enacted for mutual advantage. As described by Rawls, his essential concept of society is that of *a unified and fair system of cooperation for reciprocal advantage between free and equal individuals* (Rawls, 2001, p. 22). Notably, Rawls speaks of society only in political terms and as a political conception, which in essence is a closed system of coercive authority (and hopefully optimal mutual benefit) that one involuntary enters at birth and exits at the point of death (p. 40).[20] Because Rawls limits his theory to the case of modern constitutional democracies, his theoretical conception of society places a strong emphasis on society's inherently and irreversibly pluralistic

[19] The version of Rawls' theory of social justice that is presented here is the most recent formulation, published in 2001 before his death the following year.
[20] Obviously, individuals can generally choose to exit a given society through migration. However, even in democratic societies exit through migration comes at a psychological and/or material cost that for many individuals is prohibitive. Thus it is reasonable for theoretical purposes to treat even democratic societies as closed systems.

nature (Rawls, 1996). As an extension of this idea, Rawls rejects the notion that "cooperation for mutual advantage" implies society can be or should be communal in nature—because pluralism, optimal individual liberty, and a genuine general communalism cannot all three jointly coexist.[21]

Although Rawls' ideal society is founded upon the moral principles of individual liberty and equality, his theory acknowledges that democratic societies do not (and in fact cannot) assure an equal distribution of advantage and resources (both social and material) across all members of society. That is to say, even among democratic societies conceived on principles of equality and fair reciprocity, there exists an inherent hierarchy of advantage and various forms of social and economic inequalities that arise from arbitrary forces of history and individual endowments. However, pluralism, hierarchies of advantage, and social and economic inequalities do not preclude the evolvement of a society that is both "well ordered" and fundamentally just, a point that brings us to central concepts and principles of Rawls' theory of social justice.

As described by Rawls a *well-ordered society* is one governed and regulated by *a public conception of justice*, described previously as a "mutually recognized point of view from which citizens can adjudicate their claims of political right on their political institutions or against one another" (Rawls, 2001, p. 9). The paradox involves the achievement of "a mutually recognized point of view" or set of universally sanctioned justice principles in a society that is (1) inherently pluralist in culture and ideology and (2) already weighted with differences in relative advantage and political interest. To do so, Rawls builds his theory of social justice on a framework of six core concepts (described by Rawls as his "fundamental ideas") and two principles. In keeping with Rawls' presentation of his ideas (Rawls, 2001), we begin with a review of his six fundamental ideas.[22]

The first fundamental idea, *society as a fair system of cooperation*, was described previously as Rawls' essential concept of society, that is, "a unified and fair system of cooperation for reciprocal advantage between free and equal individuals" (Rawls, 2001, p. 22).

The idea of *free and equal individuals* (identified by Rawls as the fifth of his six fundamental ideas) is more complex than it appears. As

---

[21] While society can be hospitable to an array of communal associations, society itself is too pluralistic to be communal absent the arbitrary imposition of a universal set of values and beliefs (see Rawls, 2001, pp. 198–199). On this point Rawls shares some common ground with classic libertarian theory.

[22] For ease of presentation, this text departs from the exact order of presentation of Rawls.

explained by Rawls, it actually incorporates core conceptions of citizenship that originate with the writings of Aristotle in ancient Greece (see Rawls, 2001, p. 24 and pp. 142–143). Central to the Aristotelian idea of citizenship in a democratic society is full access to social and political participation and engagement in all the rights and duties that accompany citizenship. In the just society of Rawls, being "free and equal" requires that one has the capacity to fulfill the role requirements of active social and political citizenship as conceptualized by Aristotelian philosophy. The radical element of the Rawlsian notion of "free and equal" is the idea that freedom and equality cannot exist independently of the right and capacity to engage in all aspects of citizenship. For example, under this more restricted notion of free and equal citizenship, persons who are unable to exercise the right to vote (whether through physiological incapacity or electoral process manipulation) cannot be called free and equal.

A third fundamental idea of Rawls theory of social justice is the concept of *a well-ordered society*, which in its essence is a society governed by a generally recognized and broadly accepted "public conception of justice"—a concept mentioned in the introductory paragraph on Rawls' theory of justice as "a mutually recognized point of view from which all citizens can adjudicate their claims of political right on their political institutions or against one another" (Rawls, 2001, p. 9). In essence, "a public conception of justice" requires that there is some core set of principles of justice that are known, recognized, and accepted by all members of society. It further means that all members of society have an individual sense of justice that enables them to understand and apply the broadly shared principles of justice as they function in the social and political roles of citizenship.

Also as pointed out earlier, there is a central paradox in this conception having to do with pluralism—how can a society comprised of culturally and politically diverse individuals with distinct individual moral identities be expected to universally know, recognize, and accept *any* principle of social justice, let alone a fully explicated public conception of justice involving multiple principles? Rawls deals with this paradox by suggesting that citizens have two kinds of commitments and attachments that "specify their moral identity"—those that pertain to their conceptions of political and social justice and those that pertain to more personal aims (Rawls, 2001, p. 24). In contrast to moral attachments that are tied to more personal aims, the moral commitments and attachments that are tied to individual conceptions of political and social justice are more amendable to the achievement of some " overlapping consensus" among otherwise highly diverse individuals.

Although Rawls does not list his concept of an "overlapping consensus" as one of his six fundamental ideas, it is in fact core to his theory of social justice. In essence, an "overlapping consensus" refers to a political conception of justice that does not derive from any particular comprehensive religious or political doctrine—but derives sufficient support from diverse and often opposing religious, political, and moral doctrines to attract a critical mass of adherents and to endure over time (Rawls, 2001, p. 32). Simply stated, an overlapping consensus involves the rules of justice that diverse peoples can agree to agree upon.[23]

A fourth fundamental idea of Rawls' theory of social justice refers to *the basic structure of a just society*. First and foremost it should be emphasized that "the basic structure of society" is the end object and central subject of Rawls' theory of social justice. As described theoretically, the basic structure of society is the " background social framework" that provides the structural context for political and social cooperation between the various individual elements and associations that compose society. As such, the basic structure involves such institutions and processes as a political constitution, specification of property rights, the economic system, and the social and political constructions of the family system (Rawls, 2001, p. 10). Critical to Rawls' theory of social justice is the idea that the principles of social justice *do not necessarily* determine the actions of the particular associations and institutions that compose society. For example, families may choose to adopt a set of duties and obligations for children that, outside the family context, would be generally interpreted as unfair and pejorative elsewhere—just as churches, employers and social clubs might. The principles of social justice can indeed determine or trump the policies and actions of families and social organizations, but only where the general principles of social justice are clearly at stake. For example, a parent may choose to ground a child as punishment for some minor transgression without violating political principles of social justice. However, denial of the child's needed medical care as punishment does—because the latter involves fundamental concerns pertaining to the particular social obligations assumed by parents under any reasonable scheme of social cooperation as well as the basic rights the child holds as a prospective citizen.[24]

A fifth fundamental idea of Rawls' theory introduces *the idea of the original position*, which, like the other fundamental ideas thus far

---

[23] For example, although Americans have diverse religious views on the personal circumstances that justify divorce, there is clearly "an overlapping consensus" that the state's interests in promoting and preserving marriage does not supersede the exercise of individual rights pertaining to the dissolution of marriage.

[24] Rawls uses the denial of medical care of a child as an example of a situation where parental actions are constrained by political principles of social justice. See Rawls (2001, p. 10) on this point.

discussed, has layers of complexity that are left unaddressed in this limited rendition of Rawls' theory of justice. Briefly stated however, the "original position" involves the necessary and sufficient conditions for arriving at a "just" agreement that determines the structure of "a fair system of cooperation between free and equal citizens." That is to say, the original position refers to the point of view from which the social contract is negotiated and agreed upon. An original position that promotes fairness has formidable requisites that go beyond ordinary considerations of coercion and overtly unfair bargaining advantage. In essence, the ideal original position for the creation of a just social contract must be completely objectified—uninfluenced by immediate social contingencies, historical advantages, or any social factor that contributes to the bargaining advantage of any particular individual or group. This condition of unfettered objectivity is referred to by Rawls as the "veil of ignorance," emphasizing the point that the truly objective pursuit of fairness can be achieved only with complete absence of information about the effect of the agreement on any particular individual or group.[25]

The sixth and final fundamental idea that rounds out the foundation of Rawls' theory is *the idea of public justification.* "Public justification" is described by Rawls as a central feature of a well-ordered society that "establishes a shared basis for citizens to justify to one another their political judgments: each cooperates, politically and socially, with the rest on terms that all can endorse as just" (Rawls, 2001, p. 27). Rawls very deliberately makes a distinction between public justification and either (1) assent to the merits of valid argument or (2) what he terms "mere agreement" to a political judgment. The latter two are outcomes, whereas public justification is more truly a process of political engagement between free and equal citizens that yields a consensus on more fundamental principles of justice and related crucial aspects of the basic structure of a just society (Rawls, 2001 p. 29 and p. 46). In Rawls' theory of justice, the process of public justification is central. By extension, basic structural arrangements may be considered adequate and just to the extent they optimize the capacity of all individuals to participate in this process. This particular point has significant implications for a number of social institutions—including basic education and health care.

The Rawlsian model of a just society is shaped by two essential principles of justice, which for convenient reference are referred to as (1) the

---

[25] Had the ideal conditions prevailed in the framing of the U.S. Constitution, its authors would have known nothing of colonial history, the social characteristics of various groups of colonial Americans, or the history and characteristics of the continent's indigenous inhabitants. It is interesting to consider how some aspects of the document might have been different had this level of objectivity been achieved.

Equal Basic Liberties Principle and (2) the *Difference Principle.* The *Equal Basic Liberties Principle* simply states that "Each person has the same indefeasible claim to a fully adequate scheme of equal basic liberties, which is compatible with the same scheme of liberties for all" (Rawls, 2001, p. 42). Although there is considerable explication devoted to the delineation of which individual liberties are considered basic, on its face this first principle is consistent with a number of other theories as well as popular ideas of social justice. On the other hand, the *Difference Principle* (briefly described earlier in Peffer's Marxist theory of social justice) is far more unique and nuanced.[26] It reads as follows:

> Social and economic inequalities are to satisfy two conditions: first, they are to be attached to offices and positions that are open to all under fair conditions of equality of opportunity; and second, they are to be the greatest benefit to the least-advantaged members of society (Rawls, 2001, p. 42).

The *Difference Principle*, while it acknowledges that inequalities are unavoidable and in some instances even functional, sets a very high bar for justification. First, that privilege in status and power cannot be just if inherited or otherwise conferred in a process that does not provide equity of opportunity for all persons. In pragmatic terms, this principle implies that social class standing and the resources that accompany social class are under most circumstances inherently unjust—whether or not the privileged status in question ultimately serves a greater benefit to the least advantaged. In this regard, Rawls is careful to make the point that "fair equality of opportunity" in its moral weight precedes "the greatest benefit to the least advantaged" that is the other essential justification embedded in the *Difference Principle* (see Rawls, 2001, p. 43). Second, as previously stated, even where privileged status arises through a fair and equitable process of selection, it is deemed just only if it continues to benefit most those that are most marginalized in society. Although a more complete discussion of the health policy implications of Rawls' two principles of social justice will take place in the chapters that follow, it is easy to see how the *Difference Principle* might be applied to the analysis of status, power, and income inequalities that are embedded in the hierarchy of the health professions.

---

[26] Although Peffer employed a modification of the Difference Principle in his version of a Marxist theory of social justice, the Difference Principle is original to Rawls. Peffer does not suggest Rawls derived his Difference Principle from Marx, but rather argues that there are aspects of the Difference Principle that are compatible with Marxist theory. On this point see Peffer (1990, pp. 368–369).

Although the preceding paragraphs have sketched the main framework of Rawls' theory of social justice and vision of a just society, it is also important to reference the four-part process through which principles of justice are formulated and adopted. In Rawls' model of an optimally just society, the essential principles of justice are identified and adopted during the first stage by the various parties to the agreement[27] behind the previously described veil of ignorance—in essence to assure as much as possible that the principles adopted are unbiased with respect to the interests of particular persons or groups. In the second stage, described as the "constitutional convention" stage, the specific political arrangements that optimally serve the essential principles of justice are adopted—with some knowledge of and attendance to the nature and interests of various groups composing the body politic. In the third "legislative stage" specific laws are enacted that are either required or permitted by the principles of justice adopted in the first stage, and in the fourth stage the laws that are enacted at stage three are interpreted, applied, and followed in the respective roles of elected officials, administrators, the judiciary, and ordinary citizens (Rawls, 2001, p. 48). In essential respects, Rawls' ideal process serves as a justification of the historical process that yielded the American constitutional democracy—with the notable exception of a "veil of ignorance" during the first stage.

What Obligations Flow Upward From Individuals to Society

Under the Rawls' theory of justice, the obligations that flow from individuals to society either derive from obligations accounted for by the principle of fairness or derive from what he terms "natural duties" (Rawls, 1971). According to the general principle of fairness explicated in his original theory, individuals are accountable to the obligations imposed by social and political institutions when two conditions are met: the institution is "just" in that it satisfies the two fundamental principles of justice; and the individual in question has either voluntarily accepted the benefits of or taken advantage of the personal opportunities afforded by the arrangement (Rawls, 1971, pp. 111–112). As Rawls would have it, under such restricted criteria only a limited number of individuals have obligations that derive from such voluntary arrangements—public office holders and ordinary citizens that have clearly advanced their interests by accepting particular institutional arrangements. A classic case of the latter might be the extraordinary obligations physicians assume to provide emergency aid to victims of injury irrespective of the opportunity for payment.

---

[27] The term "parties to the agreement" refers to the representatives of free and equal citizens.

On the other hand, the obligations that fall under the rubric of "natural duties" apply to all persons under the general circumstances of a legitimate social contract. While Rawls suggests there are many "natural duties," those he highlights in his original theory and later writings include the duties of justice, fair play, mutual aide, and nonmaleficence (Rawls, 1971, 1999). Briefly stated, the principle of justice requires individuals to both support and comply with the just institutions of society that apply to each individual's circumstances. The principle of justice also "constrains [the individual] to further just arrangements not yet established, at least when this can be done without too much cost to ourselves" (Rawls, 1971, p. 115). The closely related duty of fair play holds that individual participants in the various social institutions that exist for purposes of mutual benefit, if they accept the rules of the institution as just or fair, are obligated to act in accordance with the rules of the institution.[28] The duty of mutual aid, as described by Rawls, involves helping another person when that person is in need or jeopardy, "provided one can do so without excessive risk or loss to oneself" (Rawls, 1971, p. 114). Finally, the duty of nonmaleficence (or do no harm) requires that individuals not engage in actions that either do harm to another person or are the cause of unnecessary suffering.

Of the aforementioned natural duties, the most radical departure from other theories of social justice is the clause of the duty of justice that obligates individuals to be advocates of social change. A principle of justice that "constrains [the individual] to further just arrangements not yet established" implies very directly that any individual's passive acceptance of unjust aspects of social structure or unjust institutions is in essence a violation of their duty of justice—even if the individual had nothing to do with the creation of the structural injustice in question. This aspect of Rawls' theory imposes a very different lens on the analysis of health and health care policy than is typically afforded, as will be evident in later chapters.

What Obligations Flow Downward From Society to the Individual

The obligations that flow downward from society to the individual are not systematically delineated by Rawls so much as they are discussed in reference to three general domains of social justice: *equal basic liberties*, *fair equality of opportunity*, and *equal distribution of primary goods*.

---

[28] Rawls uses the example of the tax-dodger who violates the duty of fair play when he accepts the benefits of government while not paying his share of the tax burden (see Rawls, 1999, footnote on p. 99). It seems that this example is not only apt, but given Rawls' political philosophy, one very close to his heart.

Although equal basic liberties and fair equality of opportunity are sub-sumed under equal distribution of primary goods, a more complete sense of the societal obligations toward the individual is gained through some explication of all three general domains of social justice. Given its primacy, the first to be considered will be *equal distribution of primary goods.*

As the term "primary goods" implies, these are the political, social, and material benefits of society that are deemed to be the most core or essential. The most specific definition of primary goods provided by Rawls identifies primary goods as those "things needed and required by persons seen in the light of the political conception of persons as citizens who are fully cooperating members of society, and not merely human beings" (Rawls, 2001, p. 58). As originally described (1971), primary goods were said by Rawls to encompass rights and liberties, opportunities and powers, and income and wealth. In later writings primary goods were assigned to five more elaborately described categories that include basic rights and liberties that are the essential institutional conditions for the adequate development and the full and informed exercise of the two moral powers of free and equal persons,[29] the freedom to pursue opportunities that are consistent with individual ends; power and authority; income and wealth; and "the social bases of self-respect"—meaning those aspects of basic institutions that are essential to self-worth (Rawls, 2001, p. 58).

Rawls offers two approaches to the explication of "basic liberties." One approach delineates an explicit list of basic liberties that is either logi-cally derived from Rawls' first principle of justice (Martin, 1985) or based upon a historical survey of common basic rights among the most success-ful democratic regimes (Rawls, 2001). As noted by Martin (1985), the "explicit list" approach yields what is commonly regarded in the United States as the basic civil rights: the right to vote, freedom of speech and assembly, liberty of conscience, the right of property, and the protec-tions against arbitrary arrest, servitude, and seizure of property that are established by the rules of due process. The other approach is analytical rather than explicit. In essence, basic liberties are defined generally as those basic rights and liberties "that provide the political and social conditions that are essential for the adequate development and full exercise of the two moral powers of free and equal persons" (Rawls, 2001, p. 45). Al-though the latter approach may not yield a radically different set of basic rights and liberties from those delineated in the first, it does build in more possibility of contextual adaptation and dynamic evolvement.

[29] The two moral powers Rawls refers to are in essence the moral exercise of political power, that is (1) the ability to understand, apply and act from the principles of political justice and (2) the capacity for the conception of the good in accordance with individually selected belief systems or moral doctrines (see Rawls, 2001, pp. 18–19).

The final domain of societal obligations toward the individual considered here, "fair equality of opportunity," is conceded by Rawls to be difficult and fraught with ambiguity. However, the explicit inclusion of this idea in Rawls' second principle of social justice clearly establishes its central place in Rawls' theory of social justice. As suggested by Rawls (2001, p. 43) the idea of "fair equality of opportunity" can best be understood if contrasted with the idea of "equality of opportunity" in the formal or legalistic sense. In the formal or legalistic sense, equality of opportunity involves institutionalized rules and practices that leave offices, occupations, and social positions open to all persons who have the requisite abilities and credentials. Although this might be de jure equality of opportunity, de facto equality of opportunity involves a far more complex appraisal of a given individual's genuine prospects; given such factors as the impediments (or privileges) of social class background, stigmatized social characteristics, and access to the other material and social benefits that are determinate of the opportunity in question. In stating that a just society owes each person "fair equality of opportunity" to offices and social positions that is commensurate with his or her natural endowments and motivations (Rawls, 2001, pp. 42–44), Rawls very directly lays not only the groundwork for an array of individual claims on society, but a radical social and political agenda as well.[30]

Taken to its logical end, the idea or principle of "fair equality of opportunity" produces an expansive set of societal obligations that flow to individuals (and particular groups) that in large part are determined by the sources and extent of their accumulated disadvantage. For example, interpreted in this light "fair equality of opportunity of education" implies a special and particular set of obligations pertaining to the schools that serve the poor that is the complete opposite of the current patterns of social investment in education. As argued by Norman Daniels (Daniels, 2002), the principle of social justice that entails fair equality of opportunity also extends societal obligations to the provision of health care—an argument to be revisited in later chapters of this text as the specifics of a just system of health care are considered.[31]

---

[30] As Rawls notes (2001, p. 44), fair equality of opportunity means that the free market economic system, as one aspect of the basic structure of society, must be constrained to prevent excessive concentration of wealth and political power. In the contemporary context of the United States, this necessitates the redistribution of concentrated wealth—the equivalent of class warfare in the lexicon of conservative political philosophy.

[31] Rawls initially did not include health care among either his list of basic rights or primary goods. In fact, the hypothetical circumstances for his theory did not account for disparities in health among the free and equal individuals that compose his model society. Daniels nonetheless (and very effectively) argues that Rawls' "fair equality of opportunity" principle

CONCLUDING COMMENTS—ALTERNATIVE THEORETICAL PERSPECTIVES ON "THE RIGHT TO HEALTH CARE"

Political theorists and moral philosophers make a distinction between *negative rights* and *positive rights*. Negative rights involve constraints on others to not impede our actions and preferences, do something to us, or take something from us. Negative rights also mostly apply to the actions of the state or governments and thus are commonly known as "liberty rights." Positive rights pertain to what is owed to us or what we can legitimately claim we should be provided. The "right to health care" typically is construed as a positive right, something society owes the individual as either an implied or an overt provision of the social contract. As it is conventionally understood, the right to health care entails a societal obligation to furnish individuals and/or populations with some established array of health care services that may be preventative, curative, or even restorative (Hessler & Buchanan, 2002). Debates about the "right to health care" can be roughly divided between those that are focused on whether *any* right to health care exists, and those that concern the scheme of specific entitlements and limits that derive from the right to health care.[32] While only the former are considered in this brief discussion, alternative social justice perspectives on specific entitlements will be considered later in the text in the context of health care reform.

As the reader might have concluded by now, the four social justice perspectives considered in this chapter (Classic Libertarian, Utilitarian, Marxist, and Rawlsian) indeed differ on their appraisal of health care as a basic right. The libertarian perspective, primarily because it is concerned with constraining the authority of the state, conceptualizes a very minimal social contract that clearly excludes any semblance of a right to health care. Notably, it presumes that persons who prefer a more extensive array of reciprocal obligations than provided by the minimalist state will self-select into the kind of human communities and voluntary associations that best fit their preferences (Nozick, 1974). Core also to the classic libertarian perspective is the idea that as the risks to human existence are

---

entails obligations pertaining to health care that draw on the same rationale that Rawls uses to justify the societal obligations pertaining to education (Daniels, 2002).

[32] There are those that contend the right to health care should be extended to the "right to health," for example, equal opportunity, some basic state of health, equal distribution of health life-years. The position taken here and explicated in later chapters is that health is in large part a function of other rights and societal obligations that pertain to material, social, and political provisions and entitlements. That is, if there is a right to health, it is derivative of other aspects of the social contract.

generally known and individuals exist as autonomous and self-responsible beings, it is incumbent on individuals and not governments to seek ways to self-protect and mitigate risk. As applied to health care, this suggests that the prudent individual will assure the provision of adequate health care (in accordance with their personal tastes) through such voluntary mutual benefit associations as nonprofit health insurance funds or commercial health insurance. Although a variety of challenges to this perspective are put forth concerning the plight of the more vulnerable populations (children, elderly and disabled), the classic libertarian perspective denies at every turn that there exists any general positive right to health care.

The second social justice perspective considered, utilitarianism, also does not establish health care as a basic right—but utilitarian theory does leave open the possibility that health care might be defined as a universal entitlement that is established by social policy. It was stated earlier in this chapter that utilitarianism does not prescribe any specific set of societal obligations so much as it provides the general ethical criteria for the evaluation of social policies that distribute the benefits and resources of society. Under the utilitarian ideal, if some scheme of universal basic health care were indeed proposed as an obligatory function of government, its ethical justification would turn on two criteria: (1) whether or not the agreed upon processes of deliberation and public consent had been followed and (if so) (2) whether or not the principle of utility had been satisfied in the proposed scheme, meaning that the proposed universal health care scheme distributes health care in a manner that yields *the maximum good to the maximum number of people* (Rescher, 1966) Notably, utilitarianism is the ethical perspective that is most consistent with public health analysis of the more advanced and desirable health care systems—in essence, those systems of health care that yield the highest levels of average population health. If the health care systems that yield the highest levels of population health also happen to provide universal access to health care,[33] this provides a utilitarian argument in favor of a universal positive right to health care. However, if the evidence were to suggest that the utility principle is best served by a more selective entitlement to health care, then the utilitarian perspective would argue against a universal positive right to health care.

Marxism is far less equivocal, although like most other political theorists and social philosophers of his day Karl Marx did not speak directly

---

[33] In fact, according to World Health Organization data (in particular see *The World Health Report 2000*), there is a strong correlation between universal access to health care and average population health outcomes. However, universal access to health care correlates with other aspects of social structure that appear to be determinants of more favorable population health. This point will be explored in great depth in later chapters.

of a right to health care. However, the ideal, if not a general positive right to health care, has been the centerpiece of every regime in history predicated on Marxism. This is so for a variety of reasons, the most fundamental of which are that Marxist principles call for both the collective ownership of the system of health care and the elimination of any disparities in the rewards of labor. That is, the health care system exists as a "mode of production" that involves labor and ergo collective ownership, and health care (if not provided outright by the state) is generally construed as a reward of labor. Although Marx theorized different principles of distribution at different stages in the evolvement of the communist state (Peffer 1990, p.78), perhaps his most infamous quote, "From each according to his ability, to each according to his needs" (Marx, 1938, p. 10), refers to the state of affairs he envisions in the final evolution of the communist society. As a statement of the Marxist ideal, this if nothing else establishes a positive right to health care as a clear tenet of any reasonably Marxist theory of social justice. Thus, the Marxist theory of social justice explicated earlier in the chapter (Peffer, 1990) specifies (under its principle pertaining to universal security and subsistence rights) a universal positive right to basic medical care (see Peffer, 1990, pp. 418 and 420).

As a final point on framing the Marxist perspective on health care, it must be said that Marxism goes much further than the other theories of social justice considered in establishing theoretical linkages between economic injustices, class structure, and injustices in the distribution of health. In classic Marxist theory, poor health is seen as consequent to the capitalist social system, because the capitalistic system directly spawns detrimental and demoralizing living and working conditions, and further, undermines the physical and mental health of workers through processes of disempowerment and alienation (Peffer, 1990, p. 52). Moreover, Marxist critiques of the organization of health care in market economies generally see their health care systems as inherently exploitive and reinforcing of class structure. In general, Marxist theorists directly and often quite coherently link the basic social and economic structure of a given society, the distribution of health and disease, and the organization of the health care system.

The final theory of social justice considered, that formulated in a series of treatises over the most recent 3 decades by John Rawls, in various ways argues for a positive right to health care. Embedded in Rawls' theory are two core arguments for a positive right to health care. One draws upon the *difference principle*, the idea that a necessary precondition for a "just" state of inequality is that the inequality in question "must be of greatest benefit to the least advantaged members of society" (Rawls, 2001, p. 43). Clearly, one is hard put to explain how significant disparities in access to health care for any one group of citizens would be of benefit to those that in all other respects are themselves the least advantaged members of society. However, suppose that there were competing claims between two groups upon a limited quantity of publicly funded health care services, such as elderly adults and poor children. Suppose further that it had been effectively demonstrated that in fact the poor children qualified as the "least advantaged" of all social groups considered, even including the elderly. If push came to shove, would not the difference principle be satisfied if it were shown that health care services for poor children would be best served by constraining the "right to health care" for the elderly? This in fact is precisely the situation with respect to the allocation of tax dollars to the Medicaid and Medicare programs, and as it happens children are the clear losers (unlike the elderly, they don't vote). In sum then, while Rawls' *difference principle* establishes a very high threshold for the justification of selective access to health care, it falls short of providing sufficient grounds for a general positive right to health care.

The second core argument for the general positive right to health care embedded in Rawls's theory of justice involves the core idea or principle of *fair equality of opportunity*, that is, society's obligation for providing for "the general means necessary to underwrite fair equality of opportunity and our capacity to take advantage of our basic rights and liberties, and thus be normal and fully cooperating members of society over a complete life" (Rawls, 2001, p. 174). Although in his earlier writings it might be said that Rawls was more equivocal in the emphasis he placed on health care as a primary good (meaning those things needed and required for persons to achieve their status and function as fully cooperating members of society), it is clear that in this final treatise Rawls considered a positive right to health care as an essential foundation of free and equal citizenship. To quote Rawls directly on this key point (Rawls, 2001, p. 174):

> ... provision for medical care, as with primary goods generally, is to meet the needs and requirements of citizens as free and equal. Such care falls under the general means necessary to underwrite fair equality of opportunity and our capacity to take advantage of our basic rights and liberties, and thus to be normal and fully cooperating members of society over a complete life.

As Rawls would have it, inequalities that arise under the *difference principle* (including those that pertain to disequities in access to health care) are always subject to the contingencies of competing ethical priorities over limited resources. In contrast, the means (or entitlements) necessary to "underwrite fair equality of opportunity," are morally primary over other considerations and as such are a societal imperative. It is very clear that Rawls' theory of social justice in its final iteration makes health care just such an imperative entitlement.[34] However, nothing in Rawls' theory of justice establishes prima facie any particular scheme of specific entitlements or for that matter limits that derive from the right to health care. Linking the application of Rawls' principles and arguments to specific aspects of health care policy will be a task taken up in later chapters.

REFERENCES

Barry, B. (1989). *Theories of justice*. Berkely, CA: University of California Press.

Boaz, D. (1997). *Libertarianism: A Primer*. New York: The Free Press.

Clarke, R. (2003). *Libertarian accounts of free will*. New York: Oxford University Press.

Daniels, N. (1981). Health-care needs and distributive justice. *Philosophy and Public Affairs, 10*, 146–179.

Daniels, N. (1985). *Just health care*. New York: Cambridge University Press.

Daniels, N. (2002). Justice, health and health care. In Rhodes, R.Battin, M. & Silvers A. (Eds.), *Medicine and Social Justice*. New York: Oxford University Press.

Fox, J. J. (1907). Benthamism. In John Cardinal Farley (Ed.), *Catholic Encyclopedia On-line* (2003 ed., Vol.II). New York: K. Knight.

Hessler, K., & Buchanan, A. (2002). Specifying the Content of the Human Right to Health Care. In R. Rhodes, M. Battin, & A. Silvers (Eds.), *Medicine and Social Justice*. New York: Oxford University Press.

Marx, K. (1938). *Critique of the Gotha Programme, by Karl Marx; with appendices by Marx, Engels and Lenin; a revised translation*. New York: International Publishers.

Martin, R. (1985). *Rawls and rights*. Lawrence, KA: University Press of Kansas.

Miller, F. (2002). Aristotle's political theory. In E. N. Zalta (Ed.), *The Stanford Encyclopedia of Philosophy*. Palo Alto, CA.

Nozick, R. (1974). *Anarchy, state, and utopia*. New York: Basic Books.

Otsuka, M. (1998). Self-ownership and equality, a Lockean reconciliation. *Philosophy and Public Affairs, 27*, 65–92.

Peffer, R. G. (1990). *Marxism, morality, and social justice*. Princeton, NJ: Princeton University Press.

Pizzigati, S. (2005). The rich and the rest: The growing concentration of wealth: A labor economist sees peril as a tiny minority of the population accumulates more and more wealth. *The Futurist, 39*(4), 38–43.

Rawls, J. (1971). *A theory of justice*. Cambridge, MA: Harvard University Press.

---

[34] It may be that Rawls' more explicit identification of health care as the equivalent of a primary good in his later writings may have been influenced by Norman Daniels' emphasis on the role of health care as a critical foundation of equal opportunity (Daniels, 1981, 1985).

Rawls, J. (1985). Justice as fairness: Political not metaphysical. *Philosophy and Public Affairs, 14*(3), 223–251.

Rawls, J. (1996). *Political liberalism.* New York: Columbia University Press.

Rawls, J. (1999). *Collected papers.* Cambridge, MA: Harvard University Press.

Rawls, J. (2001). *Justice as fairness.* Cambridge, MA: Harvard University Press.

Rescher, N. (1966). *Distributive justice: A constructive critique of the utilitarian theory of distribution.* New York: Bobbs-Merrill.

Rhodes, R., Battin, M., & Silvers, A. (2002). Preface. In R. Rhodes, M. Battin & A. Silvers (Eds.), *Medicine and Social Justice* (pp. vi). New York: Oxford University Press.

Roemer, J. (1996). *Theories of distributive justice.* Cambridge, MA: Harvard University Press.

Steinberger, P. (2002). Political obligations and derivitive duties. *Journal of Politics, 64*(2), 449–465.

Vallentyne, P. (2004). Libertarianism. In E. N. Zalta (Ed.), *The Stanford Encyclopedia of Philosophy.* Palo Alto, CA

Wolff, J. (2003). Karl Marx: Life and works. In E. N. Zalta (Ed.), *The Stanford Encyclopedia of Philosophy.* Palo Alto, Calif.

CHAPTER TWO

The Historical Evolvement of the U.S. Health Care System

A remarkable feature of the U.S. health care system is that in many respects, it largely evolved in the absence of any strong role of government. Until the middle of the 20th century, American hospitals received very little investment or attention from either the state or the federal government; the medical profession was, for all practical purposes, unregulated and unlicensed until the last decades of the 19th century; the government was not involved in the financing of health care for ordinary citizens (i.e., those not wards of the state, not covered by Indian treaties, nor veterans with war-related injuries) until private health care insurance plans had emerged as the dominant form of personal health care finance in the 1930s. Although federal financing and regulation of the U.S. health care system has now ascended to dominance, this is a relatively recent development spanning just the last 60 years. Thus, this chapter is divided into two segments. The first is devoted to the emergence of the fundamental parts of the U.S. health care system: its hospitals, its professional labor force, and its system of employment-based health care insurance financing. The second segment of this chapter concerns itself with the historical evolvement of the federal government in health care, and ultimately the effects of federal legislation on the contemporary structure of the health care system.

THE HISTORICAL EVOLVEMENT OF THE BASIC COMPONENTS OF THE HEALTH CARE SYSTEM: HOSPITALS, DOCTORS, NURSES, AND HEALTH INSURANCE

A Brief History of the American Hospital System

The centerpiece of the American health care system is its roughly 5,800 hospitals, of which just over three-quarters are either public or private not-for-profit (AHA, 2005). The majority of hospitals (60%) exist as voluntary organizations and operate on a nonprofit basis, reflecting the philanthropic, ethnic, and religious origins of the American hospital.[1] Although there are many historical narratives of the evolvement of the American hospital system, the definitive history offered by Rosenberg's (1987) *The Care of Strangers,*[2] suggests that the evolvement of the American hospital in its most essential features occurred over three distinct periods: the pre-Civil War period from 1800 to 1850, the midcentury period from roughly 1850 to 1870, and the critical 50-year-long era of hospital care expansion between 1870 and 1920 (Rosenberg, 1987). The history offered here will extend the American hospital's chronology to a fourth period, the second major expansion of the hospital care that occurred during the post–World War II era between 1946 and 1970.

The American Hospital in the Pre-Civil War Era

During the first century of the nation's existence, there was a very small number of hospitals, largely because hospitals existed to provide shelter and care for the destitute—those without the resources of either kin or community. In fact, the first census of hospitals in 1873 found only 178 hospitals with a collective capacity of less than 50,000 hospital beds, including those classified as mental hospitals (Rosenberg, 1987). The character of the early American hospital reflected the fact that medicine had very little to offer in the way of cure, and that most of what medicine did have to offer, either to heal an injury or help cure a disease, could more readily and more safely be provided in the home. The developmental progression of the American hospital, though more rapid in America than in Europe, essentially followed a similar path from a specialized form of an

---

[1] The term voluntary organization derives from the notion of a voluntary association or gathering of citizens for some shared purpose, generally civic, political, charitable, or religious in nature. Thus the term voluntary hospital, which throughout this book will be used interchangeably with the term private not-for-profit.

[2] Rosenberg, C. (1987). *The Care of Strangers: The Rise of America's Hospital System.* New York: Basic Books.

almshouse to eventually a place of care and cure that served all segments of society (Starr, 1982, p. 151).

The immediate precursor of the early American hospital, the almshouse, existed as a shelter of last resort for the poor that (as the name implies) was created and supported as an extension of Christian charity. As such, almhouse residents were comprised of abandoned elderly, orphaned children, unwed mothers spurned by their families, the insane, and those too ill or disabled to work. Although some colonial almshouses developed what amounted to charity care wards for the sick and injured, the civic and religious leaders of colonial America's large cities did not consider the almshouse the appropriate place to care for those who, through no fault of character or moral defect, found themselves ill and unable to support themselves. Thus the earliest American hospitals had a common purpose: a place of refuge and care for the worthy poor. The early American hospitals that fit this description include Charity Hospital in New Orleans (1736), Pennsylvania Hospital in Philadelphia (1752), New York Hospital (1771), and Massachusetts Hospital in Boston (1821) (Rosenberg, 1987; Starr, 1982).

Religiously motivated charity was not the only stimulus for the founding of hospitals in early America; the need for public order was also a significant concern. The well-ordered city could not have sick and destitute immigrants collapsing in the doorways, the insane babbling in the market places, or the abandoned women delivering their newborns in the street. A third impetus to the founding of hospitals was tied to the various waves of new immigrants, who emigrated with both an ethos of "taking care of our own" and the reality of being in an alien city without the presence and care of kin in the event of illness or injury. Thus, the origins and affiliations of many 19th-century hospitals can be traced to the efforts of different ethnic societies and associations, such as Philadelphia's German Hospital, founded in 1860 (Rosenberg, 1987). A fourth source for the founding of hospitals was various faiths and religious orders, usually as an expression of religious mission but also in response to Protestant bigotry encountered in established hospitals. This was the story behind the founding of many of the early Catholic and Jewish hospitals. Finally, as the industrial revolution progressed, hospitals were organized by different industries, particularly among those industries like mining, textiles, and railroads that had high accident rates (Rosenberg, 1987).

The 1850–1870 Period: The Era of Hospital Reform

The main social purposes of the hospitals of the pre-Civil War period included the provision of shelter and care for the incapacitated poor, providing a social laboratory for the training of physicians, and as a means of discharging the obligations of religious piety. Medicine had very limited range of genuinely curative interventions, and death by contamination and infectious disease was common. Although Pennsylvania Hospital in Philadelphia was superior to most by the standards of the time, death rates from such routine surgeries as limb amputations was exceeded 25% (Rosenberg, 1987). In 1869, the term " hospitalism" was coined by British physician James Simpson to refer the septicemias, gangrenes, and other forms of infections that were endemic to hospitals of the pre-1870 era (Brieger, 1972). The sources of death from contamination and infectious diseases could be largely attributed to the absence of sterile surgical techniques, crowded ward conditions with an abundance of effluvia in open buckets, reuse of soiled linen, and poor ventilation.

Ironically enough, the transformation of the 19th-century hospital from an institution of last resort to an edifice of healing can largely be attributed to the lessons learned over two bloody wars, the Crimean War (1854–1856) and the American Civil War (1861–1865). Although the discoveries of pathogenic microbes and antiseptic techniques in the 1860s by Pasteur and Lister ultimately propelled the medical profession to the acceptance of germ theory, this acceptance was slow in coming and preceded by the pioneering hospital reforms advanced by Florence Nightingale. Nightingale, known more generally as the founder of the nursing profession, made at least equal contributions as a hospital reformer. Formally trained as a nurse, Nightingale volunteered her services to the British army as nursing supervisor during the Crimean War. Although Nightingale's reforms were not informed by germ theory, she believed disease and death were caused by overcrowding, poor food, the presence of filth, and poor ventilation. Under Nightingale's ruthless tutelage the British military hospitals became the models of hygiene and order and the death rates of British soldiers plummeted. Nightingale's *Notes on Hospitals,* published in 1859, contained the essential lessons on the organization of nursing and hospital reform that were adopted by the Union Army over the course of the Civil War (Brieger, 1972). As a result, during the final year of the Civil War over 1 million soldiers were treated in the military hospitals of the Union Army with a mortality rate of only 8% (Starr, 1982). The convincing successes of the Civil War military hospital, coupled with the tireless advocacy of Nightingale and her followers, by the early 1870s had fundamentally transformed the organization of the 19th-century American hospital and had also provided the basic foundations for the later professionalization of nursing.

The First Era of Hospital Expansion: 1870–1920

In the first survey of U.S. hospitals, conducted in 1873, there were 178 hospitals in existence. By 1920 the number of hospitals exceeded 4,000

(Rosenberg, 1987). Although some of the growth in the number of hospitals can be attributed to population growth in the wake of massive immigration, the primary factors have to do with the ascendance of the medical profession, the effects of hospital reform on survival and recovery, and the marriage of the interests of the medical profession and private philanthropy.

By the 1870s, the gradual acceptance by the medical profession of germ theory and related developments in aseptic and antiseptic techniques were coupled with the development of surgical anesthesia—first used in 1846 to aid the surgical excision of a tumor (Brieger, 1972). The use of sterile techniques permitted patients to survive more complex and invasive surgeries, and anesthesia permitted both patients and surgeons to endure it. As a result, heretofore fatal conditions like appendicitis and abdominal tumors often became curable and successful surgery for a variety of conditions became more common (Cassedy, 1991). Parallel developments in clinical pathology and disease-specific diagnosis and treatment, coupled with innovations in surgery, gradually made the hospital the prime locus of curative medical practice for the most serious illnesses. With the invention of the X-ray machine in 1896, by turn of the century hospitals had finally become embraced by the middle and upper classes rather than shunned by them. This in turn fueled a huge popular demand for hospital expansion and new hospital construction.

Despite the growth in demand for hospital care, neither states nor the federal governments had traditionally assumed more than a peripheral role in the construction of hospitals. Other than asylums for those deemed mentally ill and hospitals for the quarantining of those with diseases like tuberculosis, states and the broad public saw hospitals as the business of municipal governments and private charities—largely because hospitals had functioned as a specialized form of the almshouse. Had the turn of the century medical profession no alternative for the funding of hospital expansion and construction but the government, it is likely that the hospital system in the United States would have evolved to a far more equal mix of voluntary and public hospitals—which in turn in later decades could have tipped the balance in favor of a federalized system of health care insurance. History instead took another turn, one that involved the marriage of private philanthropy and medical free enterprise.

As noted by Starr (1982), philanthropy is the means by which personal wealth can be parlayed for social status and social influence. Throughout the nation's first century, hospitals had historically been a preferred destination for philanthropy, both because more than other charities they appeared to serve the "worthy poor" and because their boards of trustees brought together the elites of science and politics. Coincidentally, as the demands for hospital expansion escalated toward the close of the 19th century, the era of economic expansion known as the

Gilded Age (1866–1901) had created a new class of wealthy elites (many of them immigrants) eager to transform their wealth to status and influence. Physicians, who by this same period became economically aligned with the growth of hospitals, were only too eager to turn to a source of hospital financing that would as much as possible keep government out of the business of health care. Where possible, physicians would often organize investor-owned hospitals that would rely on profits from private pay patients. However, the driving source of expansion were the voluntary hospitals that, while representing different kinds of ethnic and religious loyalties, nonetheless had the common thread of extensive reliance on private philanthropy.

The most significant exception to the general pattern of the nongovernmental funding of hospitals pertained to mental hospitals. Prior to the Civil War, the mentally ill that were not tolerated in almshouses were relegated to jails, and the almshouses that did tolerate the mentally ill were often themselves deplorable establishments. Through the revolutionary and tireless state-by-state campaign of social reformer Dorthea Dix (1802–1887), over the latter half of the 19th century the state mental hospital became the national pattern for the care of the mentally ill. Although state asylums are rightfully regarded as having a very dark history, during the latter half of the 19th century they were conceptualized as curative institutions that were a humanitarian alternative to the jails and poorhouses that heretofore had warehoused the mentally ill.

The Second Era of Hospital Expansion: 1946–1970

The economic consequences of the Great Depression and World War II had basically stagnated civilian hospital growth for nearly 2 decades, despite the continued increase of the national population. Despite the Truman administration's strong preference for amendments to the Social Security Act that would extend health insurance coverage to all Americans, there was a stronger political consensus in Congress to fund the expansion and modernization of the nation's hospitals. Moreover, federal investments in the expansion of hospitals in ways that would not invite federal control over the delivery of health care were more acceptable to the interests of the powerful AMA lobby. The result was the Hill–Burton Act of 1946 (formally titled the Hospital Survey and Construction Act of 1946), which involved a multibillion dollar infusion of federal dollars into the modernization and expansion of the nation's hospitals. Discussed in more detail later in this chapter, this legislation basically provided federal matching funds for the expansion of hospital capacity in accordance with plans administered by the individual states. Between 1947 and 1971, this legislation generated an estimated $9.1 billion in local and state matching funds in addition to the $3.7 billion federal investment, three quarters of these monies going for hospitals (Starr, 1982).

Other social forces that contributed to the expansion of hospital capacity during this era include suburbanization, the expansion of hospital insurance benefits, the post-WW II birthrate increase, technological innovations in hospital care technology that further fueled demands for hospital care, and parallel federal investments in the expansion of the health care labor force. As a result, by 1970, the number of acute care hospitals had peaked to more than 5,800, of which just over 60% were not-for-profit (U.S. Census Bureau, 1972). Notably, by 1970 most hospitals had been upgraded to many of the basic architectural standards that are still in place today. That is, large wards had been replaced by semiprivate rooms, specialty care units (e.g., intensive care, telemetry, psychiatry) had become the industry standard, as had the physical structures to accommodate very sophisticated diagnostic and surgical technologies.

The Brief Overlapping Histories of Medicine, Nursing, and Health Insurance

The primary labor force components and the financing component of the health care system each have their own very complex histories, but in critical analysis their narratives must intersect and overlap. This is because the political economy of the American medical profession to a large extent fashioned the institutional characteristics of nursing and health insurance to serve the material interests of physicians. While recent decades have witnessed a sea change in the level of professional autonomy and social status achieved by the nursing profession and in many respects the practice of medicine is now subordinate to the bureaucracy of health insurance, the fundamental truth remains—both the nursing profession and the essential structure of health insurance exist (even in their current forms) in large part as derivatives of the political economy of the American medical profession. Given its dominant role, the early history of the medical profession is the logical place to start.

The Medical Profession: The Colonial Period Through Abraham Flexner (1760–1910)

The 150-year period between roughly 1760 and 1910 spans the time from colonial medicine to the historical point at which it can be said that the American medical community had clearly emerged as a powerful profession with a coherent social and political agenda. The narrative that follows is very different from the countless other published histories of medical care that place emphasis on the ascendance of modern medical practice as a triumph of human achievement over ignorance and disease. Since this is about the policy-relevant aspects of medical history, the narrative offered here must tilt toward the role that the ascendance of the *medical profession* played in the unique structures of American health care policy—largely as portrayed in Paul Starr's eloquently documented 1982 classic, *The Social Transformation of American Medicine.*[3]

In the colonial America of the mid-18th century, there were at least a few thousand persons described as physicians, but only a small proportion them actually possessed medical degrees. In fact, the title of "doctor" was not generally used in the American colonies until a few years before the American Revolution (Twiss, 1960). By the year of the nation's founding in 1776, there were estimated to be 3,500 physicians, of which 400 possessed medical degrees (Twiss, 1960). Persons who practiced colonial medicine typically learned their profession (such as it was) as an apprenticeship, a practice that continued well into the century that followed. The selection of persons for medical apprenticeships was at the individual discretion of practicing physicians, within broad normative criteria—i.e. that the candidates be white, male, of good character, intelligent, industrious, and literate. It was also preferred that the prospective physician's family background be reputable and prosperous, though not necessarily wealthy. The following passage, quoted from a prominent early 19th-century physician's essays on medical education, is illustrative (Brieger, 1972, p. 10):[4]

> But it is not sufficient that boys selected for the study of medicine should have a good constitution, they ought, equally, to be endowed with vigorous and inquiring minds. Without these, whatever may be the appearance of success, they must at last make incompetent physicians... A student of medicine should not only be of sound understanding but imbued with ambition. A mere love of knowledge is not to be relied upon, for the greatest lovers of knowledge are not infrequently deficient in executive talents and go on acquiring without learning how to appropriate.

---

[3] This chapter provides what amounts to a synopsis of key observations and arguments of Starr's history, even then painted in very broad strokes. Interested readers are urged to read the original work, along with a set of retrospective critical essays published in the 29th volume (August–October, 2004) of *The Journal of Health Politics, Policy and Law.*

[4] This passage in quoted from an essay of Daniel Drake (1785–1852) titled *The Selection and Preparatory Education of Pupils,* published in a book that was a collected set of Drake's essays in 1832. Drake was a prolific author of publications devoted to medicine and medical education, and a legendary figure in early American medicine. The source for Drake's essay is a reprint of the original version, published by medical historian Gert Brieger in *Medical America in the Nineteenth Century* (1972: Johns Hopkins University Press).

Although race is not alluded to in this passage, that the candidate be White and generally Northern European was a given. In all other respects this passage captures the essence of the ideal early American physician; a male of vigorous constitution, an inquiring mind, and a clear talent and disposition toward medical free enterprise.

The problem that plagued the early American medical profession, also alluded to in this passage, was that the ranks of those claiming to be physicians were polluted with incompetents and outright quacks. Broadly speaking, an incompetent physician is one who was practicing medicine in an honest state of perpetual ignorance, whereas quackery involves the willful pretense of knowledge and/or use of false credentials (Cassedy, 1991). Both involve issues of control over the professional credentialing process, and they undercut both the public confidence in professional medicine and the capacity of competent physicians (by the standards of the time) to earn a living. A related problem that retarded the legitimization of the early American medical profession was of course the limited state of medical knowledge and limited range of curative therapeutics. This in turn perpetuated the continued prevalence of folk medicine as the preferred alternative to the services of a physician, as well as reliance on other kinds of healers—ranging from mystics to women who, despite being spurned by the nascent medical profession, were gifted practitioners of the medical arts.

As the nation developed, the situation that characterized American medicine during the pre-1865 antebellum period can be described as a polyglot of competitive schools of therapeutic thought, some clearly outside the mainstream medicine of French and British origin and some embraced within. As noted by Cassedy (1991), these different "sects" of therapeutic belief tended to be aligned with social class. For example, homeopathic medicine (which emphasized personal attention and conservative use of pharmaceutical remedies) was preferred by the middle and upper classes. In contrast, rural and lower class patients preferred therapies which were more aligned with their trust of folk remedies, eclectic medicine, and a botanically oriented system of medicine called Thomsonianism (Cassedy, 1991, pp. 36–39). Notably, neither the government nor university-sanctioned medical education in the form of medical schools played more than a peripheral role in the organization of the medical profession until after the Civil War.

With the ending of the Civil War, the medical profession entered what might be called its Enlightenment period, which like the Enlightenment era of 17th-century Europe was exemplified by the ascendance of intellectual and scientific achievement. As previously discussed in the section devoted to the development of hospitals, the significant advancements in surgery made possible by the application of antisepsis and anesthesia greatly contributed to the rising status of formally trained physicians—as well as contributed to a rising demand for their services. Although surgical anesthesia was an American innovation, most of the critical 19th-century advancements medical science originated in Europe. Thus, the period immediately following the Civil War witnessed a vast increase in the numbers of Americans traveling to Europe to acquire education in the medical sciences, most of whom returned to ultimately populate the faculties of American universities and revolutionize the scientific foundations of American medicine (Cassedy, 1991).

The ground-breaking advancements in medical science of the post–Civil War period were complemented by demographic and economic developments that set the stage for the private practice of medicine to flourish. Rural or so-called horseback medicine had always existed as an economically marginal enterprise, both because of the range of travel involved in maintaining a medical practice and because barter rather than currency was often the medium of exchange. For medical practice to become lucrative, increased levels of population concentration, improvements in transportation, and the replacement of barter systems with currency all needed to evolve. These changes epitomized the 1865–1900 era of industrial expansion, Western migration, and immigration that transformed the nation to a modern industrial state. Thus, as the latter half of the 19th century commenced, the medical profession had science, demography, and industrial expansion on its side—what it lacked was organization and direct control of the credentialing process.

Although the market for the private practice of medicine was beginning to flourish, the period between 1865 and 1900 was rife with medical sectarianism. In the battles between different sects of medicine over claims to legitimacy and control over the credentialing process, the principal protagonists were homeopathic physicians, eclectics,[5] and the so-called allopathic physicians representing the orthodox medical traditions of Western Europe (Rothstein, 1972). Although numbers favored the adherents of allopathic medicine (they controlled 80% of the roughly 130 medical schools that existed in the late 19th century), no group was able to gain a particular advantage over the mechanisms of state licensure, which in any case were often devoid of adequate enforcement provisions (Rothstein, 1972; Starr, 1982). The American Medical Association, which represented orthodox medicine, was itself too weak and divided during

---

[5] Eclectics, like homeopaths, were a sect of physicians that had managed to develop to the point where eclectic medicine had its own medical schools. Eclectic medicine, which had its roots in botanical medicine, had no coherent theory of physiology and disease so much as it had a range of medical ideas on illness and therapeutics drawn from multiple traditions (Rothstein, 1972).

this period to enforce its sanctions against the local medical societies that failed to expel their eclectics and homeopaths. Clearly, unless medicine could ultimately speak with a unified voice, it could not gain firm control of its credentialing.

Ultimately, the AMA yielded to pragmatism, and in 1903 it adopted a revised version of its constitution that eliminated provisions that had heretofore excluded nonallopathic physicians. As a result, the AMA ranks swelled to the point where the organization could soon claim without serious challenge that it represented the national voice of the medical profession. This in turn gave the AMA the unity and political clout it needed to achieve uniform standards of medical licensure in each state, including dominion over what acts by the various groups of other healers constituted the illegal practice of medicine. Even more significantly, the AMA's new constitution (approved in 1901) created a structure whereby the membership and representation at the state and national levels re-quired membership in the county medical society (Rothstein, 1972). In effect this provision permitted the AMA to purge from its ranks any mem-bers who could not either gain or retain membership in its local medical society. Although this had the very desirable effect of ridding the profes-sion of its quacks and incompetents, it also permitted the local medical societies to enforce nonscientific norms of membership having to do with gender, race, ethnicity, and political views that conflicted with the interests of unfettered medical free enterprise. Taken in tandem, these two devel-opments assured that for the critical decades to come, the medical profes-sion remained largely the exclusive dominion of white males—collectively committed to extending the profession's political influence and economic advantage.

As described by Paul Starr, the achievement of *professional sovereignty* refers to the capacity of a profession to extend and trans-form its authority into social privilege, economic power, and political influence (Starr, 1982, p. 5). In the case of the medical profession of the 20th century, it fully exploited its authority in the shaping of a health care system that yielded medicine its disproportionate share of economic rewards and social privileges. Although the achievement of the medical profession's unique level of authority is best left to the original teller of the tale, at minimum it required the acquisition of legitimate authority. In the case of medicine and many other professions it entails the posses-sion of a universally recognized credential that represents mastery over a definitive body of knowledge. After it had achieved professional consoli-dation in the first years of the new century, the most significant problem confronting the AMA remained the weak claim to legitimate authority car-ried by the medical school diploma. Of the roughly 160 medical schools that were in existence at the turn of the century, at least half or more were either proprietary diploma mills devoid of anything akin to even a minimal medical education or at the very least schools that were grossly deficient in faculty credentials, laboratories, and integration of clinical training.

The AMA dealt with the issue by turning to the Carnegie Foundation for the Advancement of Teaching, which in turn commissioned educational specialist Abraham Flexner to conduct an investigation of the nation's medical schools and make recommendations (Rothstein, 1972; Starr, 1982). Flexner visited 152 medical schools in the United States and 8 in Canada, the result of which was the infamous Flexner 1910 report on medical education (Cassedy, 1991). The report was a devastating critique of the state of American medical education and recommended that the training and credentialing of physicians be consolidated into a small number of top-quality schools. Although the AMA did not go as far as Flexner recommended, within a few short years the number of medical schools was cut in half, and those that remained were generally affiliated with universities, prestigious colleges, and teaching hospitals. Within 2 years of the publication of Flexner's report, about 80% of medical school graduates completed their training in hospital internships, thus cementing together the prestigious triad of universities, hospitals, and medical schools (Starr, 1982).

Gender, Medicine, and the Early Professionalization of Nursing

History abounds with ironies, among them the stark contrast between the historically subordinate status of the nursing profession and the invaluable contributions of nursing knowledge to the survival chances of hospitalized patients—all to the ultimate benefit of the medical profession's further achievements in occupational prestige and economic reward. As discussed previously in this chapter's section on the development of hospitals, Florence Nightingale was at once a pioneer of nursing and a pioneer of hospital reform. This makes sense, in that the boundaries between defining the body of knowledge and essential skills of nursing and the reform of hospital care were even more permeable in the 19th century than they are today. As Nightingale rationalized and organized the labor and training of nurses, she attacked with equal vigor and certainty the sources of disease and death endemic in the physical arrangements, food, supplies, and customary hygienic behaviors of the various ranks of hospital workers. Because the effects of Nightingale's efforts (in combination with later developments in anesthesia and antiseptic surgical practice), the mid-19th hospital was transformed from a death house to an institution of healing and hope.[6] In particular, surgery was transformed from a procedure of desperate resort to a curative miracle that only medical doctors trained in science and surgery could perform. Thus, the medical profession could at last differentiate itself from other kinds of healers in a way that was convincing to the general public.

These developments, which fostered both the ascendance of hospital care and the ascendance of the medical profession during the last quarter of the 19th century, also made hospitals the institutional locus of nursing training and credentialing. Paralleling the expansion of hospitals during the same era, between 1873 and 1900 the number of nurses' training schools had grown from 3 to 432 (Cassedy, 1991; Starr, 1982). Although many of Nightingale's principles of nursing education were largely incorporated into the structure and curriculum of hospital based schools of nursing, Nightingale's philosophy of nursing education favored independent schools of nursing where only nurses trained nurses (Cope, 1958; Hobbs, 1997). Nightingale saw very clearly that in institutions dominated by male physicians, the knowledge and skills of women would be discounted and subordinated to the interests of both the medical profession and the extension male of privilege.[7] In fact this became a dominant theme that burdened the evolvement of the nursing profession throughout most of the century that followed, and likely will continue to haunt the nursing profession until gender balance in all domains of medicine is realized.[8] The precepts of Nightingale's philosophy of nursing education were no match for the medical profession's financial interests in having a ready source of essentially free hospital labor, thus the hospital school model of nursing training prevailed for decades to come. Although the exploitation of cheap labor was in many respects the primary reward of the hospital training school model, the real damage to both the nursing profession and

---

[6] Also ironically, Nightingale herself wholly rejected germ theory's central premise that disease was attributable to microscopic contagions. To Nightingale, the sources of disease were seen and smelled in the filth and disorder that characterized European and American hospital wards through most of the 19th century (Cope, 1958).

[7] Nightingale was not at all a feminist in the contemporary use of the term. In fact, she believed that medicine and surgery were best left to men, whereas the hospital ward and the sickroom were clearly the dominion of women (Hobbs, 1997).

[8] The enormous gains made in the status of nursing as a profession made over the past half-century have not been dependent upon the transformation of medicine, but have come from within through formidable nurse-driven advancements in nursing research, clinical practice, and education. However, it seems reasonable to conclude that as long as men dominate the ranks of the medical profession, either in numbers or in prestigious specializations, the interaction between gender privilege and occupational status will remain a burdening factor in the ascendance of the nursing profession.

the evolvement of the health care system was in the long-term effect of this institutional arrangement—the subordination of autonomous nursing knowledge and practice to the interests of the medical profession.[9]

Medicine and the Early Evolvement of Health Insurance

Until nearly the end of the 19th century, the concept of health insurance was not generally known and certainly not an issue of any significant political concern. As late as the last quarter century of the 1800s, most hospitals that existed were already charitable institutions of last resort, and the primary locus of medical practice was the patient's home. Those unable to afford the services of a private physician either did without (which was often the safest road to recovery), bartered what they could for a physician's services, or they sought medical care at a "dispensary."[10] Medical dispensaries, like almshouses, originated in England as a charitable provision for the poor. Their primary function was to provide medical care for the poor as an alternative to hospital care, and to provide the medical profession with human grist for medical education.[11] In this way the 19th-century medical dispensary was the forerunner of the emergency department of a public teaching hospital. Although as of 1900 there were about 100 dispensaries in the United States, by 1918 their numbers had expanded by hundreds more—ultimately accounting for the care of 4 million patients annually (Davis & Warner, 1918).

The increased demand for dispensary care in the first decades of the 20th century signaled that the nation's reliance on a wholly private fee-based model medicine, augmented by the arbitrary judgments of private medical charity, must come to an end. The forces that led to this dilemma included immigration-driven population growth, industrialization, rising literacy, and a greatly increased level of public confidence in the medical

---

[9] In this brief history the origins of the gender balance in the medical profession are not explored. Suffice it to say that as late as 1940 only 6% of the students in U.S. medical schools were women and that the AMA did not extend membership to women until 1915 (Cassedy, 1991). In part, this could be readily attributed to general subordinate status of women that was quite literally written into the U.S. Constitution until the triumph of the Women's Suffrage Movement in 1920. However, it can also be argued that exclusion of women from the medical profession served an instrumental purpose. That is, the large presence of women (as a subordinated gender) in the medical profession would have undermined the profession's struggles to attain professional sovereignty.

[10] Although individual acts of charity in the form of free medical care by physicians has always been an important source of health care for those unable to afford it, it has also been perennially arbitrary and inadequate to the need.

[11] The term dispensary is derived from the initial function of the first dispensary as it was founded in London in 1696, the dispensing of medicines to the poor.

profession. Responding to a growing consensus that some alternative to the wholly private fee-based model of medical care must be found, in 1912 the Progressive Party of Theodore Roosevelt included a call for national health insurance as a part of its platform. After some initial waffling, the AMA ultimately (in 1920) declared its definitive opposition to a plan of compulsory health insurance (Litman, 1991). In fact, opposition to any plan that would involve government health insurance ultimately became the dominant rallying cry for the AMA membership for decades to come.

The AMA's progressive era opposition to health insurance had many reasons, two of them dominant. The first involved the genuine belief (and enduring public relations refrain) that the government financing of health care would relentlessly undermine the authority of the physician to practice medicine in a manner consistent with the patient's best interest. The second, less visible to the broad public, was the AMA's conviction that government financing of health care would bring an end to the lucrative rewards of private fee-based medicine. The political strategy of the AMA, then as today, was three pronged: Label publicly sponsored forms of health insurance as radical socialism, emphasize the predatory tendencies of government bureaucrats, and remind the public that the doctor–patient relationship was sacrosanct and never the business of government. In a nutshell, this strategy entailed convincing the voting public that a vote for a plan of national health insurance was a vote against the beneficent wisdom of their family doctors. A curious ally of the AMA during this initial run at a national plan of health insurance was labor patriarch Samuel Gompers, founder and first president of the American Federation of Labor. Although Gompers did not speak for or agree with many other leaders in organized labor on the issue of compulsory health insurance, at the time his was labor's most powerful voice. Gomper's opposition national health insurance was at once philosophical and strategic; health insurance coverage was emerging as an important bargaining issue and government sponsorship of health insurance represented an infringement upon labor's right to engage in collective bargaining (Litman, 1991).

The temporary Progressive Era alliance between organized labor and the AMA on the issue of health insurance was short-lived,[12] but it came at a critical juncture. As suggested by Starr (1982), with America's entry into World War I, the Progressive Party's capacity to focus the public's attention on domestic economic issues dwindled, as did its political power. By the early 1920s, the most vociferous supporters of national health insurance had become a political fringe movement, and the AMA had

---

[12] This was not so much of a formal alliance as it was a temporary convergence of interests.

by then consolidated its membership around the national health insurance issue and refined its strategy to defeat it. This strategy, which in its various permutations defeated the national health insurance agendas of subsequent presidential administrations (including F.D.R., Truman, and Clinton), continued to play upon the public's distrust of government, notions of creeping socialism, and most of all the idea that doctors (unlike the government) would always act in the best interests of patients.

What was more acceptable to the AMA, though not without some level of internal controversy as to the specifics, was the voluntary model of health insurance. From the standpoint of the AMA, the most ideal financing model for health care would involve private insurance for catastrophic illnesses that required hospital care, private payment of physician's services, and care for the poor as a matter of private charity. To the AMA, the appeal of this model was that hospital care would be affordable and the solvency of hospitals assured, while at the same time physicians would be permitted to engage in medical free enterprise—unencumbered by government regulation or oversight. This model was also supported by the American Hospital Association (AHA), which had been founded in 1899 as a professional association for hospital superintendents. By the 1930s, when the nation had arrived at a crossroads between an AMA model of health care financing and a social insurance model favored by the Franklin D. Roosevelt administration, the AHA had evolved toward a business model of hospital administration that favored the more conservative hospital insurance solution to health care (Litman, 1991; Shi & Singh, 2001). Although the nascent AHA of the 1930s did not have the political clout of the AMA, the convergence of perspectives between the AHA and the AMA on the issue of a voluntary health insurance model versus the social insurance model advocated by the Roosevelt administration ultimately helped the AMA retain the upper hand. Roosevelt's plans to extend the Social Security Act to a universal health insurance entitlement were thus obstructed until the nation's impending entry into World War II dominated the national agenda—a war that Roosevelt did not live to see to the end.

The dominant structures of voluntary health insurance that ultimately evolved were the nonprofit Blue Cross and Blue Shield plans, the former providing hospital insurance coverage and the latter providing insurance coverage for physician services. Notably, both Blue Cross and Blue Shield plans originated as artifacts of a process of innovation and diffusion rather than the outcomes of a comprehensive national health care planning process. In the case of Blue Cross hospital coverage plans, they began as an innovative strategy to create a fund for the hospital care of school teachers at Baylor University Hospital in Dallas, Texas, in 1929 (Litman, 1991; Shi & Singh, 2001). Over time, and ultimately through the coordinative efforts of the AHA, Blue Cross hospital insurance evolved from a single-hospital plan sponsored by independent hospitals to a Blue Cross network of plans, and ultimately to a Blue Cross Association that operated independently of hospitals (Shi & Singh, 2001; Starr, 1982). The first Blue Shield plan appeared in California in 1939, a decade after the original model for Blue Cross hospital insurance was established in Texas (Shi & Singh, 2001). In significant part, the delay reflects the medical profession's reluctance to endorse even voluntary health insurance for physician's services, until it became obvious that it was needed as a strategy to forestall the emergence of publicly sponsored health care insurance. Following the California model, the nonprofit Blue Shield plans were sponsored by state and county level local medical associations, leaving physicians largely in control of the range of benefits offered and the fees paid (Shi & Singh, 2001; Starr, 1982). In fact, these plans were generally structured in ways that allowed individual doctors to maximize their fees in accordance with the income level of their patients (Starr, 1982). Finally, aside from protecting the autonomy of physicians, physician control of the dominant form of health insurance for outpatient care ensured that physicians could continue to exclude competitive providers from the outpatient care market for decades to come.[13]

Ultimately, both the complementary protections of Blue Cross and Blue Shield plans and the rising importance of health insurance benefits as a bargaining tool for labor established the dominant role of employment-based voluntary health insurance in the financing of health care. Notably, both general forms of insurance emerged from the provider side rather than the consumer side of health care—thus also establishing the dominance of provider interests over the public interest in the financing and delivery of health care. Eventually, the health insurance industry itself emerged as an autonomous player in the political economy of health care with its own interests—sometimes aligning on side of the provider interests in health care (e.g., the AHA, the AMA, and in more recent decades PhRMA)[14] and other times not. However, the tie that binds them all is the perennial claim (of each) that they represent the public interest in affordable and high quality health care, juxtaposed with their common opposition to the fundamental reforms in health care financing that would be necessary to accomplish just such an end.

---

[13] Ultimately, as health insurance benefits assumed a larger share of the total compensation of workers, the labor movement began to assert more control over structure of Blue Cross plan benefits through collective bargaining. This offset the power of physicians until the labor movement itself began to decline in the 1970s, at which point health care inflation and consumerism emerged as another source of constraint on the power of physicians.

[14] The Pharmaceutical Research and Manufacturers of America.

THE HISTORICAL EVOLVEMENT OF THE FEDERAL GOVERNMENT IN HEALTH CARE

The exercise of federal authority in health care at various points in history can be thought of as arising from two kinds of agendas. The first is an overt agenda that is direct and specific with respect to its immediate health care policy goals. The second kind of agenda, which tends to be more latent, involves the framing or reframing of the political philosophy that defines the general purpose and boundaries of the federal role in health care. The earliest example of this dual agenda structure is seen in the first major piece of health legislation passed by the federal government: the act passed by the Fifth Congress in 1798 that taxed the wages of American seamen in order to establish the U.S. Marine Hospital Service. At the overt level, this legislation established the health care infrastructure needed to attend to the health care needs of the nation's maritime labor force. On the level of political philosophy, this act also established the legitimacy of a federal role in the provision of health care where there is compelling national interest—in this earliest case the protection and enhancement of the seagoing commerce that was the lifeblood of the new republic. In essence, since the viability of the maritime industry was wholly dependent upon the health of the ordinary seamen that manned the ships, the Fifth Congress created what amounted to the first prepaid medical care system in American history. Later examples of federal actions that also were based on what was perceived as a compelling national interest include the National Quarantine Act of 1878, the 1917 amendments to the War Risk Insurance Act that provided medical care benefits to veterans disabled as a result of military service, the Vocational Rehabilitation Act of 1920 that served to put disabled workers back into the industrial labor force, and the World War Veterans Act of 1924 that further extended hospital benefits to disabled veterans (Litman, 1991).

The overt policy agenda that has motivated the array of federal legislation in health care over the past 2 centuries has served one or more of six very general goals:

- expansion of the essential components of health care system infrastructure: facilities, technology and human resources.
- expansion of health care access.
- enhancing health care system cost control and cost effectiveness.
- promotion of public health, public safety, and consumer protection.
- promotion of research in health and health care.

- federal program retrenchment and reductions in health care access.

Each of these six general policy goals rose to prominence during different historical periods. For example the dominant policy goals during the 2 decades following World War II involved significant federal investments in the infrastructure of the health care system, while the decade between 1965 and 1975 reflected a more significant emphasis on the expansion of health care access for the poor, the disabled, and the elderly. Since 1975 the policy goals driving federal health care legislation placed a significant emphasis on cost containment as a counter to rampant health care inflation—albeit with only limited success. As a result of the general failure of policies aimed at health care cost containment, as well the ascendance of political and social conservatism, the dominant federal health care policy goals are now swinging toward federal program retrenchment and significant reductions in health care access.

In order to provide a general historical overview of the role of federal legislation in the development of the health care system, a series of four tables is provided that show the critical federal health care legislation that was enacted over the different periods composing U.S. post-colonial history. Each of the tables covers a specific historical period, and shows which of the six policy goals are served by each article of federal health care legislation passed. While over ninety specific articles of legislation are shown on the table, they represent only the more significant articles of federal legislation pertaining health care enacted over the nation's history. In reviewing the tables, the reader should pay primary attention to differences in trends within each historical period and the broad categories of legislation that have over time defined the federal role in health care. Although it is beyond the scope of this text to discuss the specifics of each piece of federal legislation shown, there will be some comment on the most influential or illuminating articles of federal legislation.

Federal Health Care Legislation in Early Nationhood Through the New Deal and World War II

The first period considered, shown on Table 2.1, covers nearly 150 years of the nation's history and reveals a very minimal federal role in health care. Only 23 significant pieces of federal legislation pertaining to health care were enacted, mostly during the period following World War I. The most active arenas for federal activism in health care during this period pertained to policies that were tied to commerce, war, treaty obligations, or threats to public health. Up until the Sheppard–Towner

Table 2.1 Federal Health Care Legislation in Early Nationhood Through the New Deal and World War II

Federal Legislation	Expansion of Infrastructure	Expansion of Access	Cost Control Effectiveness	Public Health/ Safety/ Protection	Health/Health Care Research	Retrenchment/ Reductions in Access
1798 U.S. Marine Hospital Service	X	X				
1824 Bureau of Indian Affairs (BIA), which ultimately assumes federal responsibility for health care for Native Americans	X	X		X		
1878 National Quarantine Act	X			X		
1902 Public Health and Marine Hospital Service Merger	X			X		
1906 Federal Food and Drugs Act				X		
1912 Children's Bureau Est.				X	X	
1912 Public Health and Marine Hospital Service Renamed to U.S. Public Health Service	X			X	X	
1917 Medical Benefits Added to War Risk Insurance Act		X				
1920 Smith–Fess Vocational Rehabilitation Act		X				
1921 Sheppard–Towner Act	X	X		X		

Legislation / Event				
1921 Snyder Act expands federal appropriations and role in Native American Health Care	X	X	X	
1924 World War Veterans Act	X	X	X	
1929 Repeal of Sheppard–Towner Act[1]				X
1930 National Institute of Health est.		X	X	
1933 Federal Emergency Relief Act		X	X	
1935 Social Security Act		X	X	
1936 Walsh–Healy Act		X		
1937 National Cancer Institute esb.			X	
1938 LaFollette–Bulwinkle Act		X	X	
1938 Food, Drug and Cosmetic Act		X	X	
1941 Lantham Act[2]	X			
1941 Nurse Training Act	X			
1944 Public Health Service Act	X	X		

[1]Strictly speaking, the Sheppard-Towner Act was not repealed, but was not reauthorized despite its popularity among women of child bearing age. Opposition to the renewal was a victory for the American Medical Association, which considerd Sheppard-Towner a threat to medical free enterprise.
[2]The 1941 Lantham Act (Pub. L. No. 77-137) provided funds for a wide range of public works projects, including the construction of both public and private not-for-profit hospitals (Perlstadt, 1995).

Act's passage in 1921, the population groups that were entitled to even a minimal level of federal support for the direct provision of health care were limited to those serving in the military and some disabled veterans, federal prisoners, Native Americans living on tribal reservations, and American merchant seamen. Examples of federal legislation aimed at the provision of health care for these populations include the establishment of the U.S. Marine Hospital Service in 1798, the creation of the Bureau of Indian Affairs in 1824,[15] the 1917 revisions to the War Risk Insurance Act that extended medical benefits to disabled soldiers, and the Snyder Act of 1921 that expanded federal appropriations to Native American health care.

There were a variety of reasons for the very limited federal involvement in health care that characterized most of U.S. history. These reasons included the marginal role that the federal government occupied in most peoples lives until the Progressive Era, the very limited benefits that organized medicine could provide in the event of serious illness, and the prevailing belief that the provision of health care was a matter of either medical free enterprise or nongovernmental charity where dictated by individual misfortune (Rosenberg, 1987; Rothstein, 1972; Starr, 1982). Pertaining to the very limited benefits that 19th-century medicine had to offer in the event of serious illness, demographic historian Samuel Preston pointed out that had medicine more to offer, the survival chances of the children of physicians would have been significantly better than the children of those unable to afford medical care—which they were not (Preston & Haines, 1991).

The first major departure from the federal government's very limited and selective involvement in health care did not occur until the second decade of the 20th century, with the passage of the Smith–Voss Vocational Rehabilitation Act in 1920 and the Sheppard–Towner Act of 1921. While the Smith–Voss Act's provision of vocational rehabilitation services to injured workers was certainly a new federal foray into an area that heretofore had been distinctly absent of government involvement at any level, the underlying interest of the federal government in Smith–Voss was tied far more to the promotion of commerce and productivity than to the health and welfare of workers (Litman, 1991). In that sense the Smith–Voss Vocational Rehabilitation Act was consistent with the rationale that had led to the creation of the U.S. Merchant Hospital Service in 1798. The Sheppard–Towner Act, however, was an altogether radical expansion of

---

[15] In creating the Bureau of Indian Affairs (BIA), Congress established the bureaucracy through which the federal government was supposed to have channeled its treaty obligations to Native Americans—including obligations pertaining to the health and welfare of tribal members. However, most of what the BIA did over its history was to the (often deliberate) detriment of Native Americans.

the federal role in health care—at least in symbolic terms if not in dollars allocated.

Early Federal Funding of Maternal Child Health: The Sheppard–Towner Act of 1921

In 1921 the U.S. Congress passed legislation that provided federal funds to states that would enable states to sponsor an array of maternal child health programs. "The Congressional Act for the Promotion of the Welfare and Hygiene of Maternity and Infancy of November 23, 1921," or the Sheppard–Towner Act as it was it became generally known, provided a modest $1.2 million dollars per year for states to fund an array of community maternal and child health-promotion programs with the broad aim of reducing infant and child mortality (Almgren, Kemp, & Eisinger, 2000).

The reasons behind the radical departure of the U.S. Congress from its historical reluctance to play a larger role in either the organization or financing of health care are a complex mixture of naïve assumptions about the voting behavior of the nation's women, worries about the high levels of infant mortality among the native born White American population (fears that were rooted in racism and xenophobia), highly effective political activism of the progressive reformers affiliated with the settlement house movement, and the judicious interjection of empirical science to the process of political deliberation. Concerning the first factor, naïve assumptions about the voting behavior of women, Sheppard–Towner was passed at the apex of the women's suffrage movement—and it was assumed by the males of Congress that once women won the vote they would continue to vote largely as a block on whatever seemed to be defined as a female political issue. In fact, the primary advocates of the Sheppard–Towner legislation, the Hull House–trained leadership of the federal Children's Bureau, worked closely with their allies in the suffrage movement to make sure that the passage of Sheppard–Towner was of highest priority among the newly enfranchised female voters (Almgren et al., 2000). The leadership of the Children's Bureau also had science on their side. Through what was then a highly innovative series of community studies, the Children's Bureau established a compelling case for the preventative strategies embedded in the Shepard-Towner Act. For a brief moment in history, just long enough to marshal sufficient support to overcome the vigorous objections of the American Medical Association, an act was funded by Congress that federalized the provision of health care to women and children.

Although states were permitted enormous discretion in the mix of prevention programs funded under Sheppard–Towner, in general they followed a series of health education strategies developed by the federal Children's Bureau on the basis of the evidence garnered from community studies undertaken by that agency in the decade preceding the enactment of Sheppard–Towner. The health education strategies funded under Sheppard–Towner included maternal and child health conferences for physicians and other public health workers, publicly funded maternal and child health clinics, health education classes for women of child-bearing ages and their daughters (who would often act as the prime infant care provider), classes for midwives, and the distribution of maternal and child health promotion literature (Almgren et al., 2000).

In the end though, the Sheppard–Towner Act was repealed in what became a continuous string of political victories for the medical profession over the interests of public health (Starr, 1982). At the behest of the American Medical Association, the Sheppard–Towner Act was repealed in 1927 with a sunset clause that permitted it to continue through 1929—despite the widespread popularity of its programs among women in rural communities nationwide. The demise of Sheppard–Towner at the hands of social conservatives and the AMA was in large part due to their joint opposition to the establishment of any precedent for publicly funded health care—even one as laudable as basic maternal child health (Lindenmeyer, 1997). In particular, the AMA was eager to preserve the relatively new domain of "well-baby care" as the exclusive province of medical free enterprise. Another reason for Sheppard–Towner's demise was likely the belated discovery by the men of Congress that the women's suffrage movement, as powerful as it was, did not endure the other political and economic divisions among women. Although Sheppard–Towner was initially successful politically because the men of Congress were persuaded by social welfare activists that this legislation was potentially critical to winning and retaining the votes of newly enfranchised women, as the first decade of women's voting rights transpired this strategy gradually unraveled.

In historical appraisal, the rise and fall of Sheppard–Towner had little to do with either its rationale or its effectiveness as a public health program. Although the infant mortality rate plummeted during the years of Sheppard–Towner's existence, recently available historical evidence suggests that the beginning of the decline in infant mortality actually preceded implementation of the Sheppard–Towner Act. However, the historical evidence is consistent with the conclusion that the public health initiatives undertaken by the Children's Bureau and its public health allies, as well as other contextual factors (like the rising literacy rates among women), likely played a significant role in initiating the decline in infant mortality during the decade that immediately preceded the implementation of Sheppard–Towner (Almgren et al., 2000; Lindenmeyer, 1997; Meckel,

1990). Though the public health interventions sponsored by Sheppard–Towner were indeed on target and likely were effective on a small scale, they were never funded on a scale that would reach more than a small fraction of women of child-bearing age (Lindenmeyer, 1997). A final significant critique of the Sheppard–Towner Act was that its programs were largely targeted on the maternal and child health issues of white women living in agrarian communities, rather than either the new urban poor or African American families.

Despite these shortcomings, there remains a greater historical relevance to the Sheppard–Towner Act. First, the structure of Sheppard–Towner and its early political success were outcomes of empirical investigations undertaken by female social scientists and social welfare activists that ultimately emerged as intellectual leaders of the emerging profession of social work.[16] Secondly, the Sheppard–Towner was an early policy application of multilevel theories and methods of prevention that in later decades became known as "prevention science" (Kemp, Almgren, Gilchrist, & Eisinger, 2001). Third and lastly, Sheppard–Towner served as an early pioneer of what ultimately emerged as an expanded federal role in national public health and federalized health care for the poor, elderly, and disabled during the post-WW II era. In this sense the advocates of the Sheppard–Towner had the last word over the AMA.

The Emergence of the Federal Role in Health and Health Care Research

The medical profession's longstanding opposition to the federal government's involvement in the provision of health care does not extend to federal funding of health and health care research. In fact, with the passage of legislation that funded the National Institute of Health in 1930, the Congress established the foundations of an enduring partnership between the hospital and clinics affiliated with American universities, a massive federal research bureaucracy, and medical free enterprise. In benign appraisal, the establishment of the National Institutes of Health (NIH) in 1930 and later legislative acts that expanded the NIH bureaucracy to include such sub-institutes as the National Cancer Institute (1937), the National Heart Institute (1948), and the National Institute of Mental Health (1949) propelled the United States to prominence in the domain of the health sciences research. In more critical perspective, it can be argued that the federal government's investment in health research has also fueled the establishment of an exploitive "medical–industrial

---

[16] Julia Lathrop, a pioneer of empirical methodology in social policy, and Grace Abbott, who later wrote the *Child and the State* and became the longtime editor of *Social Service Review*.

complex" that historically has privileged the health care industry, the investor class, and the medical profession over the public interest (Abraham, & Abraham, 1995; Starr, 1982; Wohl, 1984). No matter what lens is employed in historical appraisal of the federal government's leading role in funding health and health care research, with the establishment of the National Institutes of Health in 1930 the Congress elevated the funding of health and health care research to one of the federal government's critical functions.

The New Deal and the Emergence of Federalized Health Care

The fears on the part of the American Medical Association that the provision of health care would one day become federalized nearly materialized in the wake of the Great Depression and the New Deal legislation of the 1930s. Throughout his administration, President Franklin D. Roosevelt had intended that the social and economic guarantees of the federal government would extend to the provision of health care—and had he had his way the Social Security Act of 1935 would have included the provision of universal health insurance. Although the AMA's strategy of threatening to scuttle the Social Security legislation package as a whole if it included health care insurance was successful at dissuading the Roosevelt administration from this course, the Social Security Act's (SSA) passage in August of 1935 still managed to established the precedent whereby economic security became the role of the federal government where market systems failed. This in fact was an essential precedent for the later establishment of the Medicare and Medicaid programs were enacted in 1965, and the various smaller federal acts in the years between that gradually expanded federal funding of health care for the poor, old, and disabled.

These later acts included amendments to the Social Security Act permitting state payments to health care providers to the welfare recipients in 1950, and the Kerr–Mills legislation of 1960 that permitted federal grants to states for care of "medically indigent" elderly.[17] Notably, the SSA also managed to include some funds for local and state public health efforts like those that in prior years had been vigorously opposed by the AMA.[18]

[17] The term "medically indigent" applies to persons who are unable to afford payment for essential health care.

[18] Title V (Part 1) of the Social Security Act of 1935 included provisions for the federal funding of maternal and child health programs that were administered by states and subject to the approval of the federal Children's Bureau—very much like the provisions of the Sheppard–Towner Act that the AMA had ultimately defeated a decade previously.

Federal Health Care Legislation in the Post-World War II Era of Prosperity

Much of the health care legislation in the period following World War II reflects the interplay between two general policy agendas. One policy agenda involved a fallback strategy undertaken by the proponents of national health care insurance and their congressional allies to incrementally expand federal funding of health care to eventual universal coverage. The second policy agenda involved expansions of the health care system infrastructure that were broadly supported by the public, the medical profession, and the hospital industry.

With respect to the first agenda, although both the Truman and the Roosevelt administrations favored amendments to the Social Security Act that would have created a program of national health insurance, the fact that neither administration was able to overcome the opposition of the AMA and its allies ultimately left incremental universal coverage as the only strategy to pursue. The ultimate goal of this incremental strategy was not just to eliminate the coverage gaps left by the employer-based health insurance, but to eventually transform health insurance to a federal entitlement. The federal health care legislation that was passed toward this end included the 1950 amendment to Social Security, the act that established the Indian Health Service in 1955, the (Military) Dependents Act of 1956, the Federal Employees Health Benefits Act of 1958, the previously mentioned 1960 Kerr–Mills amendments to the Social Security Act, and finally in 1965 the amendments to the Social Security Act that established the Medicaid and Medicare programs. While the incremental coverage was successful in terms of eliminating significant gaps in health insurance coverage for persons poor enough to qualify for public assistance and persons over age 65, as history has shown the incremental strategy never did achieve universal health insurance coverage or transform to a universal federal entitlement to health care. In fact, in retrospective appraisal it can be argued that the health care insurance programs associated with the incremental coverage strategy in a variety of ways undercut the evolvement of a national health care insurance program—despite their huge beneficial impacts on the poor and elderly that were eligible for these programs.[19]

As Table 2.2 shows, the immediate post-World War II decades were characterized by enormous federal investments in health care system

---

[19] The most compelling arguments concerning the ways in which programs associated with the incremental strategy undercut the evolvement of universal health care coverage involve the inflationary structure of the Medicare program, and helping to sustain the political viability of the employer-based system of health care insurance coverage.

Table 2.2 Federal Health Care Legislation in the Post-World War II Era of Prosperity

Federal Legislation	Expansion of Infrastructure	Expansion of Access	Cost Control Effectiveness	Public Health/ Safety/ Protection	Health/Health Care Research	Retrenchment/ Reductions in Access
1946 National Mental Health Act	X	X		X	X	
1946 Hill-Burton Act	X	X		X		
1946 National Health Act					X	
1949 Hospital Construction Act	X					
1950 SSA Amendments		X				
1950 National Science Foundation Est.					X	
1954 Hill-Burton Act Expansion	X	X				
1955 Polio Vaccination Assistance Act				X		
1955 Indian Health Service Esb.	X	X		X		
1956 SSA Amendments		X				
1956 (Military) Dependents Medical Care Act		X				
1956 Health Amendments Act	X					
1956 National Health Survey Act					X	
1958 SBA Loan Program Expansion	X					

Legislation				
1958 Grants in Aid to Schools of Public Health	X			
1958 Federal Employees Health Benefits Act		X	X	X
1960 Kerr-Mills Amendments to SSA		X		
1961 Community Health Services and Facilities Act	X			
1962 Health Services for Agricultural Migratory Workers Act	X	X		
1963 Health Professions Educational Assistance Act	X			
1963 Maternal and Child Health and Mental Retardation Planning Amendments	X	X	X	
1963 Mental Retardation Facilities Construction Act/Community Mental Health Centers Act	X	X	X	
1964 Nurse Training Act	X			
1964 Hill-Burton Act Expansion	X			

infrastructure—both in human resources and in hospital facilities. The earliest investments, most notably the Hill–Burton Act of 1946 and its later amendments, poured millions of dollars annually into the construction of public and voluntary hospitals in communities nationwide. Later investments, including the 1963 Health Professions Educational Assistance Act and the 1964 Nurse Training Act, helped train a generation of health care professionals. Because of its enormous influence on shaping the institutional structure of the U.S. health care system, the Hill–Burton Act merits particular attention.

The Hospital Survey and Construction Act of 1946 (The Hill–Burton Act)

In very basic terms, this act allocated funds to states for the construction and modernization of hospitals, with the broad goals of improving the hospital capacity of the nation and eliminating disparities between states in hospital resources. Hill–Burton funds were allocated to states according to a formula that considered existent hospital resources and per capita income, and required states to submit a comprehensive hospital facilities development plan. Within states, eligibility for Hill–Burton funds was predicated on a community's ability to raise a significant (as originally written a two-thirds) proportion of construction funds. During the first 25 years of the Hill–Burton Act's existence, $3.7 billion in federal funds was allocated to hospital construction accounting for 30% of all hospital construction projects (Starr, 1982).

> The origins of the Hill–Burton, named for Senators Lister Hill of Alabama and Harold Burton of Ohio, can in large part can be traced to the prewar New Deal legislative agenda to establish a general plan of economic and social security that included a national program of health care for all Americans (Perlstadt, 1995, p. 80).

While the Roosevelt administration was able to incorporate limited provisions for health care into the Social Security Act of 1935 pertaining to maternal child health, as already mentioned the national health care program component failed to gain the political traction needed to overcome AMA opposition. The AMA was far friendlier to the idea of federal funding for hospital construction, just as long as the federal funds did not open the door to a strong federal role in the planning of health services. Another New Deal component to the origins of the Hill–Burton Act had to do with a significant concern on the part of the Roosevelt administration (and subsequently the Truman administration) that to avert a postwar depression, there needed to be significant amount of preemptive federal investment in public works programs to counter the effects of massive demobilization. No politician, conservative or progressive, wanted a repeat of the 1932 Bonus Army occupation of Washington, DC, or the violence and political retribution that followed.[20]

Although historical narratives of the Hill–Burton Act differ on what players and forces occupied the most significant roles in the crafting and passage of this landmark legislation, in Perlstadt's (1995) rigorous analysis of the history of this legislation the main partners were the then fledgling American Hospital Association (AHA), the U.S. Public Health Service and its allies in the American Public Health Association, and the Senate Subcommittee on Wartime Health and Education chaired by Senator Claude Pepper—a member of the progressive wing of the Democratic party. In its final form the Hill–Burton Act attended to the central agendas of all three partners. For its part, the AHA got what it wanted in a federal plan that would fund the construction of both voluntary (private not-for-profit) hospitals as well as public hospitals without a commitment to either publicly sponsored health insurance or federal involvement in local hospital management. The Public Health Service, which had advocated the allocation of hospital construction funds on a regional need basis, won provisions in Hill–Burton that would target funding to states with fewer hospital beds relative to the population. The progressives for their part were able to win a victory for health services for the poor in the Hill–Burton Act provisions that (1) obligated hospitals to admit patients without discriminating on the basis of race, creed, or color and (2) required that hospitals furnish a reasonable volume of services for persons unable to pay (Perlstadt, 1995, p. 92).

Despite the fact that the AMA was not a major partner in the negotiations that ultimately yielded the Hill–Burton Act, its political agenda to promote the sovereignty of medicine and protect medical free enterprise from the specter of socialized medicine was very well served by the Hill–Burton Act. First, the Hill–Burton Act further reinforced the incrementalist alternative to the provision of health care for the poor and those without health insurance—as opposed to the progressive approach that would have included universal health insurance as a further extension of the Social Security Act. Second, as Hill–Burton funds were poured into

---

[20] The "Bonus Army," as it was called, was comprised of roughly 20,000 unemployed World War I veterans and their dependents who marched on Washington in the spring of 1932. Their central demand involved early dispersal of war service bonuses that had been voted on by a (then) grateful Congress in 1924. The marchers were dispersed after General Douglas MacArthur, in defiance of orders from President Hoover, commanded his troops to burn their encampments. Hoover and the Republican party, and not MacArthur, paid the political price as public outrage over the incident helped fuel the election of Roosevelt and the congressional Democrats the following November (Zinn, 1999).

hospital construction, physicians derived enormous direct economic benefits from the opportunities to expand their practices to include hospital care—without significant federal involvement in either hospital service planning or hospital utilization management. Thus, under the provisions of Hill–Burton physicians were largely free to promote and ultimately effect the kinds of investments in hospital facilities that were most favorable to their economic interests. Often this involved the channeling of Hill–Burton funds into more affluent and less medically needy communities, and toward the kinds of hospital facilities that served the economic interests of medical free enterprise over the interests of public health.

In his historical appraisal of the hospital construction provisions of the Hill–Burton Act, Paul Starr[21] notes that while in principle the provisions of the act were "redistributive" in that formula for allocating funds among states placed a higher priority on those states with lower per capita income, in reality the allocation of hospital construction funds within states favored more affluent communities (Starr, 1982, p. 350). In large part this outcome was a consequence of provisions in the law that required that communities pay a large share of hospital construction expenses—in more affluent communities as much as two-thirds (Starr, 1982). A second major deficit of the Hill–Burton Act pertains to the weakness of its antidiscrimination provision which, until the Supreme Court intervened 1963, allowed hospitals that had received Hill–Burton funds to refuse admission to African Americans if "separate but equal facilities were available in the area" (Starr, 1982, p. 350). The most significant historical criticism of the Hill–Burton Act, again offered by Starr but echoed by many others since, is that the Hill–Burton program "retarded the integration of the hospital industry," in that the regional planning provisions included the act did not extend to the continued coordination of hospital facilities and service planning once the funds were allocated (Starr, 1982, p. 351). In effect, this permitted uneconomical and marginally competitive hospitals to keep operating and, even more significantly, helped lay the groundwork for the costly "capital-based competition" between hospitals that later ensued in the wake of the Medicare program.[22]

---

[21] Throughout this chapter and others, multiple references are made to Paul Starr's observations and arguments concerning the history and organization of the U.S. health care system, as published in his landmark *The Social Transformation of American Medicine* (Basic Books, 1982). This is arguably the most authoritative and controversial history and critique of the U.S. health care system and the medical profession written to date.

[22] Capital-based competition, as described elsewhere in this book, involves investments in medical technology and facilities that are aimed at gaining or preserving a hospital's market share of patient referrals. Frequently (and more often), these investments are made to attract referring physicians. Capital-based competition is distinct from price- or outcome-based competition, both of which have greater potential to reduce health care costs. Capital-based

Later Hill-Burton Amendments and the Evolvement of the Nursing Home Industry

In 1954, the Hill–Burton Act was extended to the construction and modernization of nonprofit and public nursing homes and ambulatory care facilities, with a dramatic impact on the structure of the long-term care component of the health care system. By the mid-1950s the combination of such factors as postwar advancements in antibiotic therapies, the effect of Social Security pensions on the capacity of retired elderly to live independently in such places as boarding homes, and the geographic mobility of the adult children of elderly translated to an increased level of demand for residential nursing care of frail elderly (Almgren, 1990; Vladeck, 1980). In the face of an inadequate supply of voluntary and public sector nursing homes, the lack of community-based long-term care services, and the inadequate and often dangerously constructed former boarding homes that composed the for-profit sector of the nursing home industry, Congress passed a new version of the Hill–Burton legislation that poured millions into the nonprofit institutional long-term care industry. Because the 1954 Hill–Burton provisions demanded hospital-level facility standards to qualify for funding, it in essence created a highly institutionalized model of care for the frail aged that was later extended to the for-profit sector of the industry.

Although the for-profit owners of boarding homes and investors planning to build nursing homes were not eligible for Hill–Burton funds, federal construction subsidies were extended to the proprietary sector of the nursing home industry in the late 1950s in the form of legislation that provided Small Business Administration loans. This legislation, in concert with amendments to the Social Security Act in 1950 and in 1956 that provided federal matching funds for provision of custodial care in proprietary nursing homes, fueled the growth of the for-profit nursing home industry—an industry that over time became dominated by corporate nursing home chains. In contrast to the hospital industry, which historically has had a very small for-profit ownership sector, the nursing home industry evolved to a high proportion of for-profit ownership—today comprising 66% of the industry (Kaiser Family Foundation, 2006).

In retrospect, it must be said that while the Hill–Burton Act and its later revisions were enacted with the best of intentions, the structure of the legislation that provided massive federal subsidies for institutional

competition may or may not be tied to better health care outcomes depending upon a large array of contextual factors. However, it is inherently inflationary and in historical perspective has proved exceedingly detrimental to equitable access to essential health care.

expansion in absence of federal control yielded a variety of unintended consequences. In the hospital component of the health care system, the Hill–Burton Act contributed significantly to geographic disparities in hospital resources and also sowed the seeds of the capital-based competition between hospitals that flourished with the later introduction of Medicare. In the long-term care segment of the health care system, the investments of Hill–Burton funds that favored the development of a quasi-hospital institutional model of care for frail elderly ultimately created the template for the modern and dominantly for-profit nursing home industry. The road not taken in long-term care until decades later—investments in community based long term care—now struggles to compete for public dollars against a deeply entrenched and politically influential investor driven nursing home industry (Almgren, 1990; Kane, Kane and Ladd, 1998; Vladeck, 1980). While the Hill–Burton Act provided critical momentum for construction and remodeling of badly needed hospitals nation wide and in many ways expanded access to health care for generations of Americans, the Hill–Burton Act is also saddled with an unfortunate legacy of incrementalism, missed opportunities, and latent inflationary effects on the national cost of health care.

Federal Health Care Legislation Through the Rise and Fall of the Great Society

As Table 2.3 shows, the period between 1965 and the late 1970s is characterized by Congressional actions that favored significant investments in health care system infrastructure, health care access, and health care research. Legislation aimed at curbing the growth of health care inflation did not emerge until the early 1970s, and even then without much political will or measurable effect.

By the mid-1960s, the U.S. health care system had been relentlessly expanding its capacities in facilities, technology, and resources year after year for nearly 2 decades. As a result, the average life expectancy of Americans was accelerating and the principal barriers to health care access had largely shifted from the availability of hospitals and trained staff to the availability of health care insurance. For the majority of Americans, those of working age and their dependents, access to health care was enhanced through the postwar rise in real wages and the increasingly common availability of health insurance coverage as a fringe benefit of employment (Starr, 1982, p. 372). Congressional actions during the prior decade had also yielded expansions in the health care access for veterans, Native Americans, federal employees, and the poor. The most significant segment of the population left out were the nonpoor aged, who nonetheless were threatened by poverty as their individual health care needs escalated year by year. This set the stage for the historically greatest expansions of federal funding of health care, the 1965 amendments to the Social Security Act that established the Medicare and Medicaid entitlements.

The Emergence of the Medicare and Medicaid Compromise

At the point that the Kennedy administration assumed power in 1961, there remained a significant level of public support for amendments to the Social Security Act that would expand its entitlements in universal health insurance. Moreover such a plan remained on the radar screen of the remnants of New Deal era politicians that remained in Congress. Faced with the very real possibility of a formidable pro-universal health insurance coalition comprised of labor, the elderly, the remnants of New Deal era politicians in Congress, and a progressive White House, the AMA and its allies ultimately had to acquiesce to a compromise that would yield *some* ground to further federalization of health insurance. For their part, the liberals also needed to compromise. The AMA's past tactics that played on the public's fears of a creeping socialist agenda and governmental interference in the doctor–patient relationship had been very effective in sidelining attempts to create a universal entitlement to health insurance in the Roosevelt and Truman administrations, and until 1964 the Democratic party lacked the clout in Congress to even approach enacting such an agenda (Starr, 1982). The final compromise contained elements of both liberal and conservative ideology; universal entitlement to health insurance for the elderly recipients of Social Security and for the poor, a means tested medical care assistance program that left a large share of the cost and much of the eligibility discretion to the states. It might be said that the AMA and liberal camps both held their respective noses and signed on to this legislation, each claiming a partial victory and plotting for the further battles to come. With AMA opposition to the further expansion of federal financing of health care held in abeyance, in 1965 Congress passed the amendments to the Social Security Act that provided medical care for the elderly (Title 18) and grants to states for the funding of medical care for the poor (Title 19) by a final vote of 307 to 116 in the House of Representatives and by a vote of 70 to 24 in the Senate (Litman, 1991).

While there are many distinctions between the Medicare and Medicaid programs, the fundamental one involves the difference between a social insurance model and one dependent on year-to-year appropriations and means-tested eligibility. The former, like the Social Security old-age pension entitlements, enjoys the status of a return on paid investments and brings with it the sense of "entitlement" in the truest sense of the

Table 2.3 Federal Health Care Legislation Through the Rise and Fall of the Great Society

Federal Legislation	Expansion of Infrastructure	Expansion of Access	Cost Control/ Effectiveness	Public Health/ Safety/ Protection	Health/Health Care Research	Retrenchment/ Reductions in Access
1965 SSA Medicare and Medicaid Amendments	X	X				
1965 Community Mental Health Services and Facilities Act	X	X				
1965 Mental Health Centers Act Amendments	X					
1965 Health Professions Educational Assistance Act Amendments	X					
1965 Heart Disease, Cancer and Stroke Amendments	X					
1965 Older Americans Act	X	X		X		
1966 OEO Neighborhood Health Centers Amendments	X	X		X		
1966 Comprehensive Health Planning and Service Act	X	X				
1966 Allied Health Professions Act	X					
1967 & 1968 SSA Nursing Home Amendments	X					
1968 Health Manpower Act	X					
1968 National Science Foundation Expansion					X	
1969 Medicaid 75th Percentile Fee Schedule			X			

Act					
1970 Community Mental Health Service Act	X	X			
1970 Occupational Safety & Health Act (OSHA)				X	
1970 National Institute of Alcohol Abuse & Alcoholism Esb.	X	X		X	X
1970 National Health Core Esb.	X	X			
1971 Economic Stabilization Act	X		X		
1971 Comprehensive Health Manpower Act	X				
1972 SSA Amended to Establish Peer Review Organizations	X		X		
1972 Emergency Medical Services Systems Act	X	X	X		
1972 SSA Amended to offer Medicare HMO Option			X		
1973 Health Maintenance Organization Act	X		X		
1974 National Health Planning and Resources Development Act	X		X		
1974 National Institute on Aging Esb.					X
1976 Indian Health Care Improvement Act[1]	X	X		X	X
1976 Health Professions Educational Assistance Act	X		X		
1977 Rural Health Clinics Act	X	X			

[1]The 1976 Indian Health Care Improvement Act (IHCIA) was preceded in 1975 by the Indian Self-determination and Education Assistance Act, which established the intent to expand local tribal governance of health care services to Native Americans (Kuschell-Haworth, 1998).

term. Medicare was constructed as just such a program, combining pay-roll contributions to a hospital insurance trust fund (Medicare Part A) with a second benefit that involved voluntary premium deductions from Social Security pension checks (Medicare Part B).[23] Moreover, eligibility for Medicare is essentially universal for all Americans that reach a minimum age, with rich and poor alike reaping the benefits. Medicaid on the other hand is burdened with extreme state-to-state variations in eligibility criteria and coverage, a financial structure that is completely based on tax revenues, and the stigma of demonstrable poverty as the essential precondition for eligibility. Despite these shortcomings, there is no question that with the implementation of Medicaid those in deepest poverty at last had a level of access to health care that in many respects was comparable to the level of health care access achieved for the middle class—at least in most parts of the country.

Community Mental Health Legislation

The early 1960s was also a watershed period for the expansion of community mental health services, in large part as a legacy of the Kennedy administration's particular commitment to the reformation of the mental health system and serendipitous advancements in psychopharmacology that made deinstitutionalization feasible. President Kennedy's particular commitment to the radical reformation of the mental health care is generally believed to have arisen from his family's tragic experience with the then conventional treatment of mental illness. In the early 1940s Kennedy's younger sister had undergone a lobotomy when she and Kennedy were young adults. Since the mid-1950s there had been a series of breakthroughs in the development and use of psychotropic medications that diminished the prevalence of the most debilitating symptoms of severe and persistent mental illness—thus undercutting the necessity and rationale for the institutional confinement of the severely mentally ill and the abuses that followed. Due to Kennedy's unprecedented direct advocacy of radical reformation of the mental health system to a community mental health service model, in 1963 Congress passed the Community Mental Health Centers Construction Act/ Mental Retardation Facilities Construction Act (PL 88-164). This legislation shifted the federal role in mental health from primarily the funding of research to the financing mental health care infrastructure. In 1965 and then again in 1970, further amendments to the Mental Health Centers Act increased the level of

---

[23] While the costs of Medicare Part B are federally subsidized, the fact that enrollment in Part B is voluntary and involves premium cost sharing on the part of program participants seems to remove the stigma that is usually associated with other forms of government subsidy.

federal funds for facilities construction and created seed grants for mental health centers to increase their staffing levels (The Brookings Institution, 2006). With the availability of SSA Title 19 (Medicaid) matching funds for payment of community mental health services for the many mentally ill that were poor, continued revolutionary advances in psychopharmacology, and a series of judicial decisions that greatly restricted use of involuntary institutionalization, by the early 1970s the dominance of a community based approach to the care of the mentally ill was firmly entrenched.[24]

Expansions in Health Services for Native Americans

During the 1970s Congress passed two acts that improved upon what heretofore had been a grossly inadequate response to the federal government's treaty obligations pertaining to the health and welfare of Native Americans. The first act, the 1975 Indian Self-Determination and Educational Assistance Act, affirmed that it was the federal government's obligation to promote the maximum level of Native American participation in the governance of federal health, welfare, and education programs serving Native American communities. In essence this act made Indian Health Service programs accountable to tribal governance. The Indian Health Care Improvement Act (IHCIA), passed in 1976, was largely motivated by public health research findings that highlighted the gross disparities between the health status of Native Americans and the general population (Northwest Portland Area Indian Health Board, 2006). Although the IHCIA provided an array of appropriations pertaining to health programs and services on behalf of Native Americans, the most significant aspect of the IHCIA was its declaration that it was a policy of the United States to achieve of health status parity for Native Americans (Northwest Portland Area Indian Health Board, 2006).

The Emergence of Cost Control in Health Care

By the early 1970s, it was becoming increasingly apparent that some of the critics of Medicare program had been correct in their prediction that there were aspects of the program that were inherently inflationary. As

---

[24] Although the community mental health approach was generally attractive to state politicians on humanitarian grounds and ultimately mandated by the judicial branch of government, the main incentives were always financial. By the accounts of its many critics, over time the community mental health movement devolved to an abrogation of public responsibility for the mentally ill and a principal factor in the growth of the homeless population.

initially designed there were two aspects of the Medicare program that were particularly inflationary.

The first inherently inflationary feature of Medicare involved a "cost-plus" form of reimbursement, similar to the federal government's often infamous payments to defense contractors. In essence, hospitals providing care to Medicare beneficiaries were reimbursed for the services they provided based upon the costs they were able to justify under the most generous of guidelines. Under cost-plus reimbursement, hospitals had no particular incentive to avoid providing unnecessary care and in fact had strong incentives to provide as much care as was conceivably defensible. Indeed, it became a widespread practice in the hospital industry to reward ancillary department heads for their ability to get physicians to order ever higher levels of supplies, tests, and treatments. This feature of Medicare fueled a hospital care culture that "more care was better" and also led hospitals to be less resistant to rising staffing levels and rising wages. Although it was left to physicians to determine the necessity of hospital admissions, the procedures performed, and the length of hospital stay, the structure of Medicare Part B reimbursement ensured that physicians would have strong financial incentives to use hospital services for patients and an absence of financial incentives for early discharge.

The second inherently inflationary aspect of Medicare reimbursement involved the "capital pass-through" provision of Medicare, which in essence allowed (and indeed encouraged) hospitals to invest in new technology and facility upgrades by recovering these expenses through quite generous Medicare allowances. In simple terms, Medicare provider payment rules permitted hospitals to include in their allowable costs whatever dollar investments in new technology, equipment, and facilities the hospital deemed necessary for providing care for Medicare beneficiaries. Thus, hospitals had the equivalent of a blank check from Medicare to invest in whatever facility improvements and purchases of technology could be defended as essential to improved patient care. During the 1970s in particular, it appears that hospital administrators and their physician constituents pushed the blank check nature of capital pass-through to its limits, thus fueling health care inflation to *its* limits (Garrison & Wilensky, 1986).

In the interest of fairness, it should be acknowledged that the capital pass-through provisions of Medicare were very deliberately intended to serve as a mechanism through which federal dollars could be infused into the health care system to fund modernization, improvements in capacity, and advancements in health care technology. In fact, it is indeed the case that the enhanced purchasing and investment capacity of hospitals available under the Medicare capital pass-through mechanism played a crucial role in providing incentives for the development of new innovations in health care technology, such as computerized tomography (CT) scanners. Although these policy goals were well served by the capital pass-through provisions of Medicare, an unintended consequence was the fueling of rampant capital-based competition between hospitals.

Capital-based competition between hospitals, described here and elsewhere in this volume as the use of advantages in physical facilities and/or health care technologies to either preserve or expand a hospital's share of the health care market, is a major driver of health care inflation. As a simple example, suppose Hospital A chooses to acquire a linear accelerator[25] for the treatment of a variety of cancers at the cost of roughly $2 million for the base equipment and related facility improvements. Hospital B, concerned that it will lose some of its market share of cancer patients to Hospital A, chooses to invest in a similar upgrade that involves a like purchase of a linear accelerator. There are now two virtually identical multimillion dollar linear accelerators within 10 miles of each other, each being paid for in substantial part by Medicare capital pass-through funds—with no demonstrable net benefit to the survival of cancer patients as a result of having two identical linear accelerators available rather than one. There is however, a substantial local contribution to Medicare cost inflation. Although this might seem like a ludicrous example, it is exactly the kind of capital-based competition that has led to the oversupply of expensive health care technologies in many communities across the United States, in many respects to the ultimate detriment of health care quality and access (Bryce & Cline, 1998).[26]

By the early 1970s health care inflation was finally recognized as a significant public policy issue, complicating a more general problem of rampant inflation that characterized all sectors of the national economy. While Congress did deal with the inflationary aspects of the Medicare program directly at that point, it did pass the Economic Stabilization Act in 1970, which permitted the Nixon administration to implement various forms of price control across key sectors of the economy, including health care. Recognizing that direct price controls were at best a short-term solution to health care inflation (as well as antithetical to the

---

[25] A linear accelerator is a device that precisely focuses a stream of fast-moving subatomic particles. As applied to cancer therapy, it can be employed to destroy or at least retard the growth of some types of cancerous tumors.

[26] The capital pass-through mechanism was not unique to Medicare, but also was embedded in the hospital pricing practices for the health insurance industry as a whole during this period. During the 1970s this was a nonissue, because insurance companies were able to pass these costs onto the purchasers of health insurances by increasing the health insurance premium prices.

laissez-faire sentiments of the Republicans that elected him), in 1971 Nixon urged Congress to promote the provision of health care through Health Maintenance Organizations (HMOs). In a stinging defeat to the AMA, in 1972 Congress both extended Medicare benefits to newly established HMOs and established Professional Standards Review Organizations (PSROs) to monitor the quality and the necessity of care provided to beneficiaries of Medicare, Medicaid, and other government health programs (Litman, 1991; Starr, 1982). In an even larger defeat for the AMA, in 1973 Congress passed the Health Maintenance Organization Act, which provided direct federal subsidies for the establishment and expansion of HMOs (Litman, 1991). Finally, as a restraint to the capital-based competition between hospitals that had fueled problems of oversupply in health care facilities and technology in some geographic areas and undersupply in others, in 1974 Congress passed the National Health Planning and Resource Development Act . This act established a national network of "Health Systems Agencies" (HSAs), which were responsible for the development of annual plans for the improvement of local health resources and oversight of the local "certificate of need" review process (The Brookings Institution, 2006).[27] As a result of these various legislative acts, by the mid-1970s hospitals and other institutional providers were (1) made financially accountable to Medicare and Medicaid for patient care that was either unnecessary or of substandard quality and (2) were largely precluded making large new investments in technology and facilities without the formal sanction of local health care planning authorities. Although the effects of these restraints on health care inflation ultimately proved negligible in the short run, the actions of Congress during much of the 1970s at least signaled the end of any assumptions by either political party that health care providers could be relied upon to self-regulate or spontaneously act in the public interest.

Federal Health Care Legislation Through the Era of Managed Care

By the close of the 1970s, the health care sector of the domestic economy had nearly doubled since 1960, and was fast approaching the 10%

---

[27] A "certificate of need" process involves a public review and approval process for the purchase of highly expensive health care technologies or health care facility construction projects in excess of a given amount. Prior to the 1974 National Health Planning and Resource Development Act, this process was carried out individually by a minority of states. Without the issuance of a "certificate of need" that sanctioned specific investments in new technologies or facility upgrades, hospitals would not be able to bill Medicare and Medicaid for their use.

proportion of the GDP. As a result, a 30-year national policy that had been characterized by an emphasis on the expansion of health care infrastructure and access gave way to a policy agenda aimed at cost control (see Table 2.4). Although the federal legislation that established mandatory peer review of hospital care proved successful in curbing the more severe abuses of the Medicare and Medicaid programs and also provided important impetus to the adoption of more cost-effective approaches to patient care, the general trend in health care inflation continued unabated. Similarly, the imposition of a national "certificate of need" process over major new investments in health care facilities and technology proved insufficient to the task. In many parts of the country, politically powerful hospitals and other health care investment groups intent on expansion and the acquisition of new technology found ways to subvert the process. As a result, the certificate of need process to a significant extent fueled rather than restrained the growth of disparities between affluent communities and poor ones in the quality of facilities and the level of technology available.

The Emergence of the Prospective Payment and the New Era of Managed Care

The primary problem faced by the just-elected Reagan administration and the Congress was that the cost accounting and reimbursement structure of the Medicare program, like that of health care insurance industry as a whole (with the exception of HMOs), financially rewarded both physicians and hospitals for providing more care rather than less. Although by the early 1980s it was generally apparent that mandatory peer review and other forms of federal regulatory oversight would not be enough to cure health care inflation as long as financial incentives of health care tilted toward expanding its use remained, neither the health care insurance industry nor the Congress was eager to reverse the financial incentives too far toward withholding the provision of health care. In the end though, Congress elected to act boldly and directly in a series of legislative acts that culminated with the restructuring of the Medicare hospital benefit to a *prospective payment system* (PPS) in 1983.[28]

---

[28] The 1983 amendments to the Social Security Act that established the prospective payment system were preceded by the 1982 Tax Equity and Fiscal Responsibility Act (TEFRA), which implemented a hospital reimbursement system that was based on a cost per discharge that was weighted by each hospital's case mix (distribution of cases by severity and related costs). This gave hospitals several months to adapt their utilization review systems to identify ways to eliminate sources of unnecessary patient care expenditures and realign their array of hospital services toward those that were economically viable.

Table 2.4 Federal Health Care Legislation Through the Era of Managed Care

Federal Legislation	Expansion of Infrastructure	Expansion of Access	Cost Control/ Effectiveness	Public Health/ Safety/ Protection	Health/Health Care Research	Retrenchment/ Reductions in Access
1980 Omnibus Reconciliation Act		X	X			
1981 Elimination of Public Service Hospitals & Free Medical Care to Seamen			X			X
1982 Tax Equity and Fiscal Responsibility Act (TEFRA) Funds Hospice Care & Imposes Hospital Cost Controls	X	X	X			
1982 Health Resources and Services Administration (HRSA) Esb.	X					
1983 DRG Based Prospective Payment System for Medicare Esb.			X		X	
1985 Consolidated Omnibus Budget Reconciliation Act (COBRA)[1]		X		X		
1986 Medicare reimbursement provisions added for disproportionate share of poor and graduate medical education	X	X				
1986 Medicaid eligibility coverage extended to poor pregnant women, infants and young children		X				
1987 Omnibus Budget Reconciliation Act (OBRA)[2]	X	X	X	X		
1988 Medicare Catastrophic Coverage Act[3]		X				

1988 Health and Human Services (HSS) Issues Restrictive Rules to Family Planning barring abortion related services.						X
1989 OBRA Esb. Agency for Health Care Policy and Research (AHPR)					X	
1989 Repeal of Catastrophic Coverage Act						X
1990 Americans With Disabilities Act		X				
1992 Reauthorization of the Indian Indian Health Care Improvement Act[4]	X	X		X		
1996 Personal Responsibility and Work Opportunity Reconciliation Act (TANF)		X		X		X
1996 Health Insurance Portability and Accountability Act		X	X			
1996 The Veterans' Health Care Eligibility Reform Act[5]		X				
1997 SSA Amendments Establishing State Children's Health Insurance Program (SCHIP)		X				
1997 Balanced Budget Act creates Medicare Part "C" Benefit Options & Expands Mandatory Enrollment in Medicaid Managed Care			X			
2003 SSA Amendments establishing Medicare Part D –Prescription Drug Benefit[6]		X				X

(continued)

Table 2.4 (*Continued*)

Federal Legislation	Expansion of Infrastructure	Expansion of Access	Cost Control/ Effectiveness	Public Health/ Safety/ Protection	Health/Health Care Research	Retrenchment/ Reductions in Access
2005 Deficit Reduction Act Introduces Unprecedented Cuts in Medicaid[7]						X

[1]COBRA 1985 was a sweeping piece of legislation that contained several significant health care system provisions, including makes hospice a permanent part of Medicare, allowing states the option to provide a Medicaid hospice benefit, allowing employees and their dependents to continue employer based health insurance despite disruptions in employment, and regulations that sanctioned hospitals for "patient dumping", i.e. transferring patients to other hospitals for the specific purpose of avoiding uncompensated care costs.

[2]OBRA 1987 was also included several key health care provisions: further expansion of Medicaid that required states to extend eligibility to poor women and young children, encouraged expansion of Medicaid clinics to the homeless, extensive regulatory upgrading of the nursing home industry including significant staffing upgrades, nursing home pre-admission s creening standards, and Medicaid funding for community based services for aged persons at high risk for nursing home care.

[3]Although the Catastrophic Coverage Act provided prescription drug coverage, expansion of nursing home care coverage and additional health care service coverage -this legislation also imposed increased premium charges that were means tested. Despite the significant benefits to the health care and financial security of seniors, the overwhelming majority of seniors viewed this legislation and an unfair financial burden on the elderly and a retreat from the federal commitment to affordable health care for older Americans.

[4]Since its initial authorization in 1976, the Indian Health Care Improvement Act (IHCIA) has been reauthorized numerous times. However, the 1992 reauthorization explicitly reinserted key language from the original (1976) authorization that identified the achievement of health status parity between Native Americans and the general U.S. population as a fundamental obligation to Native peoples and a central goal of federal policy (Kuschell-Haworth, 1998; Northwest Portland Area Indian Health Board, 2006).

[5]The Veterans' Health Care Eligibility Reform Act of 1996 restructured the Veterans Affairs health care system from a hospital based system to a population based system, and realigned eligibility standards to a system of eight priority groups that included eligibility criteria based on financial need and non-service connected disablement. This is seen as a critical acknowledgment of the VA health care system's commitment to all low income and disabled veterans, not just those disabled as a direct result of military service.

[6]Although the rationale and centerpiece of 2003 revisions to the Medicare was the addition of the prescription drug benefit that will add billions to the cost of the Medicare program, it also contained provisions that place a higher financial burden of the poorest and sickest of the elderly by raising their out-of-pocket costs. Thus this legislation can be said to have expanded access to health care for some elderly while reducing access for others.

[7]According to Congressional Budget Office estimates, this legislation will cut Medicaid by a total of 26.4 billion dollars over a ten year period, with significant reductions in access to health care for the poor (Congressional Budget Office, 2006).

The PPS method of hospital reimbursement pays hospitals for episodes of inpatient care of Medicare beneficiaries in accordance with each hospital episode's assignment to any one of 467 diagnosis-related groups (since expanded to roughly 500) (Shi & Singh, 2001). The DRG is determined at discharge and involves a select array of factors that include the patient's discharge diagnosis and other case characteristics that have proved to be predictive of hospital care costs (e.g. patient age, sex, type of surgery if any, presence of co-morbid conditions). Because this method of reimbursement is based on a standard fee per DRG rather than either the amount of hospital services provided or the length of hospital stay involved, neither hospitals nor physicians are financially rewarded for the ordering of unnecessary tests and procedures, providing unnecessary treatments, or keeping the patient in the hospital longer than is essential. Under PPS, hospitals may lose money on some episodes of care and make money on others, but in general the profits and losses offset each other if the hospital puts into place effective mechanisms of cost control and quality assurance. During the first year of its implementation, Medicare PPS reduced the average length of hospital stay for Medicare beneficiaries from 10.0 days to 9.1 days and proved quite effective at restraining the growth in Medicare program hospital utilization (Morrisey, Sloan, & Valvona, 1988; Sheingold, 1989).

The early success of the Medicare PPS system in placing constraints on hospital costs and forcing hospitals to put into place strong mechanisms of cost control ushered in the new era of managed care. Parallel developments in the health care insurance market such as the rapid shift from the community-rated insurance products to employer-based insurance pricing and the emergence of preferred provider hospital contracts ultimately saw hospitals bidding against one another to retain their market share of privately insured patients. Beginning with Medicare PPS and ultimately diffusing over the next decade throughout the private insurance market, the primary risk of health insurance abuse turned 180 degrees from the provision of unnecessary care to the withholding of it. It was this worry,[29] validated in some instances and overblown in others, that ultimately led to the retreat of managed care in the latter half of the 1990s.

Other Congressional Efforts at Cost Control

Even though the Omnibus Budget Reconciliation Act of 1987 sought in a variety of ways to improve the quality of care in the nursing home industry and further expansions of Medicaid program eligibility for children, it

---

[29] Combined with incredible bureaucratic excess.

also authorized funds for states to develop community-based long-term care services for persons who would otherwise be at risk for nursing home placement (Litman, 1991). Because the largest financial burden for nursing home care is assumed in roughly equal share by states and the federal government through the Medicaid program, both states and the Congress had a strong incentive to develop community-based long-term care programs as a cost effective alternative to nursing home care.[30]

In order to deal with the rising demands of the Veterans Affairs health care system and move away from the antiquated hospital-based structure of the VA system, in 1996 Congress passed the Veterans' Health Care Eligibility Reform Act. In effect, this legislation transformed the Veterans Affairs health care system from a hospital-based system to a population-based system that allocates care by an explicit set of eligibility priorities.

The most recent cost control legislation passed by Congress (that does not involve drastic reductions in eligibility), the Balanced Budget Act of 1997, expanded the criteria for mandatory enrollment in Medicaid managed care programs and also created Medicare "Part C" benefit options. Under Medicare Part C (also called Medicare+Choice), beneficiaries who participate in Medicare Part A and Part B were given the option of enrolling in a Medicare approved managed care plan (HMO or PPO) that would provide expanded benefits,[31] or for a limited number of people enrolling in a medical savings account (MSA) program (Shi & Singh, 2001). Although Congress had hoped to retard the growth in Medicare expenditures by providing incentives for beneficiaries to move to managed care alternatives, the first years of the program were replete with an array of setbacks in implementation.

Selective Expansions in Access/Infrastructure

The health care cost control theme that characterized the political agenda of Congress during the last 2 decades of the 1900s did not preclude some instances of expansion in either access or infrastructure—though by the standards of the 1950s and 1960s they were quite modest. First, the previously mentioned 1982 TEFRA legislation funded a Medicare hospice benefit, which has since been expanded in scope and also extended to Medicaid. In addition, Congressional actions in 1986 and 1997 witnessed important eligibility expansions in Medicaid, the most critical of which involved the Social Security Act amendments establishing the State

---

[30] There is an ongoing debate as to whether community-based long-term care systems yield net savings, but in passing these provisions Congress at least gave the benefit of the doubt to this argument.

[31] Medicare + Choice has since been renamed Medicare Advantage.

Children's Health Insurance Program (SCHIP).[32] Although the SCHIP program significantly expanded Medicaid eligibility for children of all ages in low-income families, it also came in the wake of another "near miss" in the establishment of a federalized universal health program—the so-called Clinton plan. In this sense, the SCHIP expansions of Medicaid eligibility were consistent with Congress's long record of preferring an incremental response to disparities in health care. In particular, the kinds of incremental solutions that would not run counter to the preferences of the health care establishment, that is, the nonpublic hospital industry, the conservative sectors of the medical profession, the health insurance industry, and the pharmaceutical industry.

Two other acts of Congress during this period addressed significant public health crises affecting particular segments of the U.S. population. The 1990 Ryan White Comprehensive AIDS Resources Emergency (CARE) Act provided funds for an array of community-based social and health care services to persons suffering from HIV disease and AIDS. The Ryan White CARE Act was amended and reauthorized in 1996 and 2000, and as of 2006 serves over 500,000 persons per year (HRSA HIV/AIDS Bureau, 2006). The 1992 Reauthorization of the Indian Health Care Improvement Act addressed the lingering health disparities suffered by Native Americans. In addition to authorizing funds for the expansion of access and infrastructure, the language of this legislation established the achievement of health status parity for Native Americans as an obligation of the federal government and as a central policy goal. Despite the continued gap between the level of federal funding and the magnitude of health and health care disparities between the general U.S. population and Native Americans, this legislation represented an important advancement in the cause of Native American health.

Although considered civil rights legislation rather than health care legislation, the 1990 Americans With Disabilities Act (PL 101-336) carried with it an array of provisions that in effect expanded access to health care for persons with disabilities. This is because the Americans With Disabilities Act (ADA) prohibits disability-based discrimination and upholds equal opportunity in an array of spheres that affect health care access, such as employment, government services, public accommodations, transportation, and commercial facilities. Because of the ADA, a disabled person is more likely to be eligible for employment-based health insurance, is more likely to have the transportation accommodations needed to access medical care, and is less likely to be discriminated against by health care providers who prefer not to treat persons with some stigmatizing

[32] See chapter 3 on health care finance for a more detailed description.

disabilities. Although employers and health care providers have success-fully used the courts to narrow the definition of disablement subject to ADA protections, in its 1998 Bragdon decision (Bragdon v Abbott, 118 S Ct 2196) the U.S. Supreme Court both extended ADA protections to persons with HIV seeking health care and left the door open to other health conditions (Gostin, Feldblum, & Webber, 1999).[33] Of equal importance, the courts have interpreted the definition of "public accommodations" to extend to hospitals, clinics and the offices of health professionals.

The largest and most controversial expansion in the federal role in health care during this period was the passage of amendments to the Social Security Act in 2003 that established Medicare Part D, generally referred to as the "Medicare Drug Benefit." This was not the first time that the Congress had passed legislation extending Medicare benefits to outpatient prescription drug coverage. The earlier attempt by Congress to expand Medicare benefits to drug coverage occurred with the passage of the Catastrophic Coverage Act of 1987. Although this legislation provided expanded nursing home coverage and home health care benefits in addition to prescription drug coverage, it also involved the imposition of increased Medicare premium charges that were means tested. In response to widespread outrage among Medicare program beneficiaries, Congress repealed the Catastrophic Coverage Act in 1989. In stark contrast to the rhetoric of the GOP-dominated Congress and the George W. Bush administration about the critical need to rein in entitlement spending, in the summer of 2003 Congress, by the narrowest of margins, passed the largest expansion of Medicare program's entitlements since 1965. In political terms, the Medicare Modernization Act of 2003 was crafted to serve two masters: the large voting block of Medicare beneficiaries seeking federal help with the ever-increasing costs of their prescription drugs and a pharmaceutical industry eager to see an expansion of the purchasing power of Medicare beneficiaries without the threat of federal price controls. The predictable result was a fiscally irresponsible and politically deceptive compromise that in the end is estimated to add $400 billion to federal Medicare program spending from 2004 through year 2013 (Congressional Budget Office, 2004). Despite the enormous burden that the expanded Medicare entitlements added to the federal budget deficit, the complexity of the program baffled consumers and retail pharmacists alike and still left many Medicare beneficiaries at risk for catastrophic personal

---

[33] Bragdon, a dentist, had refused to fill the tooth cavity of a woman who had disclosed she was HIV positive unless the services were performed in a hospital at significant extra expenses to the patient. In a 5–4 split decision, the Supreme Court held that a person with HIV fell under the impairment provisions of the ADA and that the refusal to provide services due to risk to the health care provider must be based on convincing scientific evidence.

expenditures. Those least served by this legislation, aside from federal tax payers, were the many Medicare beneficiaries living in poverty who were forced to assume an increased share of their pharmaceutical expenses as a result of this legislation (Steinberg, 2005).[34]

Reductions and Retrenchments Affecting Access to Health Care

Congress opened the 1980s with an act (in 1981) that eliminated the U.S. Public Hospital system, which its critics had long claimed was redundant, expensive, and inefficient. The systems facilities were in fact largely antiquated and operationally inefficient, but the closure of U.S. Public Hospitals also signaled a further devolvement of the national health care safety net—just at the point when the voluntary sector of the hospital was becoming less willing and able to absorb its share of the costs of uncompensated care.[35] A second major reduction in access to health care, specific to women seeking family planning services, occurred when the Department of Health and Human Services adopted rules that blocked federal funds to family planning clinics that engaged in any actions that facilitated women's access to abortions (Litman, 1991). Because the family planning clinics affected provided low-income women with an array of reproductive health care services that were unrelated to abortion, the failure of Congress to counter this action by the Reagan administration represented a significant retreat from the federal commitment to women's health.[36]

In limited but important ways, the 1996 amendment to the Social Security Act that eliminated traditional Aids to Families With Dependent Children (AFDC) in favor of the Temporary Assistance to Needy Families (TANF) also represented a retreat from access to health care for poor families, though its negative effects depended on the SCHIP and TANF

---

[34] Under the provisions of the Medicare Modernization Act of 2003, low-income elderly who qualify for Medicaid assistance for prescription drug coverage are transferred to a federally approved prescription drug plan in 2006. As a result, most will be required to pay a co-pay fee of up to $5 on every prescription. For the poorest and sickest of elderly, this may mean the choice between food and pharmaceuticals.

[35] The capacity of the voluntary (private not-for-profit) hospitals to absorb the costs of uncompensated care (bad debt and charity care) has always been dependent upon the ability of hospitals to "cost-shift," i.e. recover their losses through higher charges to insured patients. By the early 1980s, the health insurance market was shifting toward more competitive provider contracts with hospitals that reduced the ability of hospitals to cost shift—thus reducing their capacity to provide uncompensated care.

[36] The failure of Congress to counter these HHS rule changes is consistent with the Congressional record beginning with the Hyde Amendment of 1976, which in its various updates has restricted the federal part of Medicaid funding for abortions to pregnancies that result from rape or incest, or endanger the life of the mother (National Abortion Federation, 2006).

eligibility criteria specific to each state. In some states, involuntary termination from TANF also terminated Medicaid benefits to poor families (Center for Public Policy Priorities, 2003).

The most severe retreat from access to health care is the most recent, the 2005 Deficit Reduction Act. According to Congressional Budget Office estimates, the provisions of the Deficit Reduction Act (DRA) will trim more than 26 billion dollars from Medicaid over the next decade and result in large-scale reductions in Medicaid benefits and eligibility, thus affecting millions of the working poor and their health care providers. (Congressional Budget Office, 2006). The centerpiece of this act involves provisions that permit states to impose health care cost sharing requirements on Medicaid recipients, and other provisions that are clearly intended to discourage otherwise eligible persons from applying for Medicaid, such as increasing proof-of-citizenship requirements. While some aspects of the DRA may be more defensible,[37] on the whole the DRA represents an historically unprecedented blow to the federal health care safety net for the poorest of Americans.[38]

The DRA perfectly illustrates the dual agenda nature of federal health care legislation explained at the beginning of this section. The overt policy agenda, as identified in the title of the DRA, is "deficit reduction" at the federal level and the curbing of growth in the Medicaid program that imposes a particular burden in state budgets. The latent agenda of the DRA, which involves the framing of the political philosophy that defines the general purpose and boundaries of the federal role in health care, further reinforces the dominance of a political philosophy that seeks to diminish the role of the federal government as the ultimate guardian of access to health care for America's poor families.

CONCLUDING COMMENTS—PROSPECTS FOR A RENEWED CONSENSUS ON ACCESS TO HEALTH CARE

The last century of federal health care legislation was in large part characterized by a continuous struggle between incrementalism and progressive structural reform, framed by an overlapping political consensus that the assurance of health care access for all Americans should be the central goal

---

[37] The DRA imposes more restricted limits on the transfer of assets in order to qualify for Medicaid nursing home care funding. The pre-DRA generous allowances for nursing home care related asset transfers were of greatest benefit to the middle and upper class families.
[38] The DRA also introduced changes to the Medicare program aimed at reducing costs by $6 billion over the 5-year period beginning with 2006. However, the changes proposed do not represent a significant retreat from program benefits.

of federal health care policy. The new century seems to have ushered in a radically different perspective on the central goal of federal health care policy, one that subordinates the assurance of access to health care for all Americans to the goal of reducing government—both in the marketplace and in the provision of basic economic security. This third perspective on health care, falling under the policy rubric of ideological retrenchment, is embodied in the policies of the George W. Bush administration. Ideological retrenchment places a particular emphasis on private market solutions to issues of health care access and cost that is linked with an attack on the most politically vulnerable of federal health care entitlements—the financing of health care for the poor. As such, the Medicaid program cuts in the Deficit Reduction Act of 2005 represent a significant victory for this third perspective. Although the next logical step for this end of the political spectrum would extend entitlement reductions to Medicare, for a variety of reasons this appears politically unfeasible in the short term. The much touted Medicare Part D benefit is plagued by a legacy of political deception and huge costs, the Bush administration's popularity is at an all-time low in the wake of the Iraq war, and the political capital expended on the unsuccessful attempt to restructure Social Security has long been exhausted. Thus, as the first decade of the new century unfolds, none of these three perspectives (ideological retrenchment, incrementalism, and progressive reform) appears to be either dominant or in ascendance. The question is, which of these perspectives will finally arise to assume the major place in shaping health care policy?

In historical terms alone, the incrementalist approach to solving the nation's health care policy challenges seems like the horse to bet on. That is, at multiple points in history incremental solutions to the health care policy have accommodated the economic priorities of the entrenched health care interests as well as the competing priorities of liberals and conservatives. However, it should be acknowledged that the health care policy challenges facing the next presidency and Congress are in many respects unprecedented and are not particularly amenable to incremental solutions: Health care inflation continues unabated, the failures of the private employer-based insurance market have now undermined the economic security the middle class, and the basic structures of the health care system are ill equipped to accommodate the strain certain to be imposed by the new generation of aged.[39]

Given this reality, it may be that the framework that shapes the health care policy legislation of the new century will be decided by a contest

---

[39] U.S. Census interim population projections estimate a doubling of the population that is aged 65+ over the first 3 decades of the 21st century.

between the ideological extremes of retrenchment and progressive health care reform. While the explosive federal deficits created under the Bush administration have made the case for further reductions in health care entitlements appear compelling, meaningful reductions in federal health care costs cannot be achieved in absence of significant impacts on the middle class elderly. Moreover, the private market solutions to the health care that were touted as the preferred alternative to the Clinton plan have clearly failed to deliver. Middle class nonelderly families are no longer immune from disruptions in health care insurance coverage, they are absorbing an ever-larger share of health care costs, and tales of middle class families spiraling into bankruptcy due to medical expenditures are gaining increased media attention. Historically at least, to the extent that the economic security of the middle class becomes threatened and in that sense linked to the ordinary daily experience of the poor, a progressive consciousness emerges and structural policy reforms follow—thus suggesting that the prospects for a renewed political consensus on the need for radical health care reform are not all that dismal.

REFERENCES

Abraham, J. (1995). The production and reception of scientific papers in the academic–industrial complex: The clinical evaluation of a new medicine. *The British Journal of Sociology*, 46(2), 167–190.

Almgren, G. (1990). *Artificial nutrition and hydration practices and the American nursing home: Currents of social change and adaptation by an industry in transition*. Unpublished doctoral dissertation, University of Washington, Seattle.

Almgren, G., Kemp, S., & Eisinger, A. (2000). The legacy of Hull House and the Children's Bureau in the American mortality transition. *Social Service Review*, 74(1), 1–19.

American Hospital Association (AHA). (2005, November 14). *Fast facts on U.S. hospitals from AHA Hospital Statistics*. Retrieved January 23, 2006, from http://www.aha.org/aha/resource_center/fastfacts/fast_facts_US_hospitals.html.

Brieger, G. (Ed.). (1972). *Medical America in the nineteenth century*. Baltimore: The Johns Hopkins Press.

The Brookings Institution. (2006). *Government's 50 greatest endeavors: Enhance the nation's health care infrastructure*. Washington DC: The Brookings Institution Governance Studies Program.

Bryce, C. L., & Cline, K. E. (1998). The supply and use of selected medical technologies. *Health Affairs*, 17(1), 213–224.

Cassedy, J. (1991). *Medicine in America: A short history*. Baltimore: Johns Hopkins University Press.

Center for Public Policy Priorities. (2003). *Comments on proposed DHS rules regarding TANF and Medicaid.* Retrieved March 14, 2006, from http://www.cppp.org/research.php?aid=320.

Congressional Budget Office. (2004). *A detailed description of CBO's cost estimate for the Medicare prescription drug benefit.* Washington DC: Congress of the United States.

Congressional Budget Office. (2006). *Congressional Budget Office cost estimate: S. 1932 Deficit Reduction Act of 2005.* Washington, DC: United States Congress.

Cope, Z. (1958). *Florence Nightingale and the doctors.* London: Museum Press.

Davis, M., & Warner, A. (1918). *Dispensaries: Their management and development.* New York: Macmillan.

Garrison, L. P., Jr., & Wilensky, G. R. (1986). Cost containment and incentives for technology. *Health Affairs, 5*(2), 46–58.

Gostin, L., Feldblum, C., & Webber, D. (1999). Disability discrimination in America: HIV/AIDS and other health conditions. *Journal of the American Medical Association, 281,* 745–752.

Hobbs, C. (1997). *Florence Nightingale.* New York: Twayne.

HRSA HIV/AIDS Bureau. (2006). *Ryan White CARE Act: Purpose of the CARE Act.* Retrieved March 15, 2006, from http://hab.hrsa.gov/history/purpose.htm.

Kaiser Family Foundation. (2006). *Statehealthfacts: Distribution of nursing care facilites by ownership type, 2003.* Retrieved February 15, 2006, from http://statehealthfacts.org.

Kane, R., Kane, R., & Ladd, R. (1998). *The Heart of long term care.* New York: Oxford University Press.

Kemp, S., Almgren, G., Gilchrist, L., & Eisinger, A. (2001). Serving "the Whole Child": Prevention Practice and the U.S. Children's Bureau. *Smith College Studies in Social Work, 71*(3), 475–477, 499.

Lindenmeyer, K. (1997). *A right to childhood: The U.S. Children's Bureau and child welfare, 1912–1946.* Urbana: University of Illinois Press.

Litman, T. (1991). Appendix: Chronology and capsule highlights of the major historical and political milestones in the evolutionary involvement of government in health care in the United States. In Litman T. & Robins L. (Eds.), *Health Politics and policy* (2nd ed.). Albany, NY: Delmar.

Meckel, R. (1990). *Save the babies: American public health reform and the prevention of infant mortality, 1850–1929.* Baltimore: Johns Hopkins University Press.

Morrisey, M. A., Sloan, F. A., & Valvona, J. (1988). Shifting Medicare patients out of the hospital. *Health Affairs, 7*(5), 52–64.

National Abortion Federation. (2006). *Public funding for abortion: Medicaid and the Hyde Amendment.* Retrieved March 14, 2006, from http://www.prochoice.org/about_abortion/facts/public_funding.html.

Northwest Portland Area Indian Health Board. (2006). *Legislative history of the Indian Health Care Improvement Act.* Retrieved February 28, 2006, from http://www.npaihb.org.

Perlstadt, H. (1995). The development of the Hill-Burton legislation: Interests, issues and compromises. *Journal of Health and Social Policy*, 6(3), 77–96.

Preston, S., & Haines, M. (1991). *Fatal years: Child mortality in the late nineteenth century America*. Princeton, NJ: Princeton University Press.

Rosenberg, C. (1987). *The care of strangers: The rise of America's hospital system*. New York: Basic Books.

Rothstein, W. (1972). *American physicians in the nineteenth century: From sects to science*. Baltimore: Johns Hopkins University Press.

Sheingold, S. H. (1989). The first three years of PPS: Impact on Medicare costs. *Health Affairs*, 8(3), 191–204.

Shi, L., & Singh, D. (2001). *Delivering health care in America* (2nd ed.). Gaithersburg, MD: Aspen.

Starr, P. (1982). *The social transformation of American medicine*. New York: Basic Books.

Steinberg, M. (2005). *Trouble brewing? New Medicare drug law puts low-income people at risk*. Washington, DC: Families USA.

Twiss, J. (1960). Medical practice in colonial America. *Bulletin of the New York Academy of Medicine*, 36, 538–551.

U.S. Census Bureau. (1972). *Statistical abstract of the United States, 1972*. Washington, DC: Author.

Vladeck, B. (1980). *Unloving care: The nursing home tragedy*. New York: Basic Books.

Wohl, S. (1984). *The medical industrial complex*. New York: Harmony Books.

Zinn, H. (1999). *A people's history of the United States* (twentieth anniversary ed.). New York: HarperCollins.

CHAPTER THREE

The Contemporary Organization of Health Care: Health Care Finance

There is no paradox that equals the system of health care finance in the United States. According to estimates released in 2005, the United States spends about $1.7 trillion in health care annually, or an average of about $5,700 per year for every person residing in the United States (Smith, Cowan, Sensenig, & Catlin, 2005; U.S. Census, 2005). In relative expenditures per capita, the United States spends 11 times the most recent World Health Organization estimates of the global per capita average, and over two times the average of per capita expenses for Australia, Canada, Germany, Japan, Norway and the United Kingdom (World Health Organization, 2005a). Although the United States spends more dollars per capita than any other OECD member nation, the United States ranks lowest among OECD[1] countries in the proportion of its citizens having some form of public or private insurance for routine health care (Anderson & Poullier, 1999; OECD, 2004a). The purpose of this chapter is to provide the reader with a general understanding

---

[1] The OECD refers to the *Organisation for Economic Co-operation and Development*, an international organization of thirty democratic countries that espouse the common goal of promoting world economic progress, democratic forms of governance, and market economies. The origins of the OECD are in the post-WWII reconstruction of Europe sponsored by the U.S. and Canada through the Marshall Plan. The OECD is used extensively here as a comparative frame of reference for U.S. health care policies since OECD countries share the common characteristics of democratic government, mature industrial development, and a market economy. However, within the OECD there is significant variation with respect to the government's role in the provision of health care, the distribution of wealth and income, and structure of the social welfare system.

of the dynamics of this paradox, its origins, and the ways in which it is sustained.

In order to accomplish this, the chapter will review the system of health care finance in the United States, both in terms of its current organization and in the evolvement of its unique structure. The topics will include the magnitude and distribution of health care expenditures in the United States, the relative contributions of government and private sector forms of insurance, the fundamentals of risk and insurance, alternative models of health insurance finance and provider structures, and a detailed description of Medicare, Medicaid, and more recent policy initiatives in the public financing of health care (e.g. SCHIP, the Medicare Prescription Drug Improvement and Modernization Act, and Medical Savings Accounts). The central aim is to provide the foundation necessary for an informed assessment of the policy alternatives for health care system reform, the issue that is the principal focus of the book's final chapter. The logical place to begin is a basic review of how the United States spends its health care dollars.

HEALTH CARE EXPENDITURES

The United States spends about 15% of its GDP (gross domestic product) on health care. Relative to the other OECD countries, the United States spends about 1.8 times as much of its GDP on health care (OECD, 2004a). The brunt of the $1.7 in U.S. health care expenditures (73% of all health care dollars) are allocated (in this order) to hospital care, physician services, prescription drugs, and nursing home care. Of the remainder, by far the largest category of health care expenditures is for administrative costs (7.4% or $119.7 billion; Smith et al., 2005). A general grasp of the allocation of expenditures by payment source can be obtained from Table 3.1, which delineates the main sources of payment for health care services: private insurance, Medicaid and Medicare, other public programs, and then "out of pocket" expenses. Starting with the largest consumer of health care expenditures, hospital care, it can be seen that public programs actually account for more hospital expenditures than private insurance.[2] It is also apparent that private insurance plays a much larger role than public programs in the purchase of physician's services and outpatient prescription drugs.

Medicare, the federally funded program for older adults, clearly plays a marginal role in the payment of health care expenditures that fall outside

---

[2] Included in hospital service expenditures are pharmaceuticals related to inpatient care.

Table 3.1 Distribution of Health Expenditures by Type and Payment Source in 2003

	Other Private	Out of Pocket	Pvt. Health Insurance	Medicare	Medicaid	Other Public	$Billion
Hospital Care	4.2%	3.2%	34.4%	30.3%	17.0%	11.0%	515.9
Physician's Services	6.9%	10.2%	49.7%	20.0%	7.1%	6.2%	369.7
Dental Care	0.0%	44.3%	49.1%	0.1%	5.7%	0.8%	74.3
Nursing Home Care	3.1%	28.1%	7.7%	12.5%	46.4%	2.3%	110
Home Health Care	4.9%	16.2%	17.6%	31.6%	24.5%	5.1%	40.8
Retail Prescription Drugs	0.0%	29.7%	46.3%	1.6%	18.9%	3.6%	179.2
Administrative Costs	1.2%	0.0%	68.4%	6.9%	15.5%	8.0%	119.7

Data Source: Smith, C., C. Cowan, A. Sensenig, and A. Catlin. 2005. "Health spending growth slows in 2003." *Health Affairs* 24(1):185–194: EXHIBIT 5 Expenditures For Health Services And Supplies, By Type Of Service And Source Of Funds, Calendar Year 2003.

of hospital, physician, nursing home, and home health services—although this is likely to change as the Medicare program's new drug benefits are phased in. On the other hand, Medicaid, the joint state and federal program primarily for those with low incomes, is clearly an important source for the payment of health care services in a number of areas: hospital care, physician services, nursing home care, and outpatient prescription drugs. Out-of-pocket expenditures are clearly relevant as a source of payment in a number of areas of health care expenditure, most notably in physician services, dental services, prescription drugs, and nursing home care. Finally, it can be seen that the largest source of administrative expenditures for health services is not government programs, but rather the net costs of private health insurance products (i.e., premium costs that are not paid out in health care benefits).

In order to get a general sense of how the U.S. system of health care finance is organized relative to other industrialized democracies, some general comparisons between the United States and other OECD countries in health care resources, expenditures and finance are provided. The first to be considered will be health care system resources, specifically the relative numbers of physicians and hospital beds. As Figure 3.1 shows, the United States clearly lags behind other OECD countries in both the numbers of practicing physicians per 1000 persons and the number of acute hospital beds despite the primacy of the United States in health care spending. Also, although the United States leads other nations in the world in the development of new health care technologies and in total health care expenditure per capita, it does not necessarily lead the world in the diffusion of the technologies it invents (OECD, 2003).

Turning to comparisons of health care expenditures over time, Figure 3.2 shows that both for the United States and other OECD countries, health care inflation has been on the rise and increasing over the last 4 decades. Notably, the United States has consistently outpaced the other OECD countries in the percentage of its GDP that it allocates to health care and in the general pace of health care expenditure inflation (OECD, 2004b). Finally, it can be seen that the gap between U.S. health care expenditures and the OECD average began to widen in 1980 and has increased significantly thereafter. Two obvious questions are raised by the trends shown in Figure 3.2. First, have the additional health care expenditures for health care in the United States contributed to greater gains in national health? Secondly, why are the differences in health care expenditures so large between the United States and the other OECD member states?

The answer to the first question is clearly "no," if by defining the term "national health" we use broad measures of population health endorsed by the World Health Organization like life expectancy at birth, child

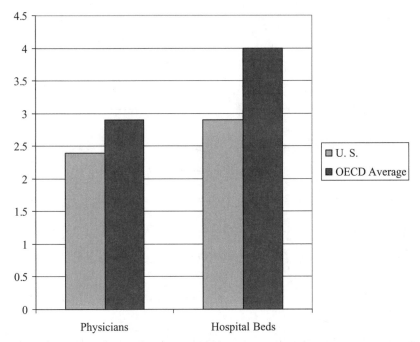

Figure 3.1 Practicing Physicians and Acute Care Hospital Beds per 1,000 Persons: U.S. vs. OECD Average.
Source: *OECD Health Data 2004*. Data from "Table 4: Practicing physicians, Density per 1000 population" and "Table 5: Acute care beds, Per 1000 population." Organization for Economic Co-Operation and Development, Paris, France. These estimates are based on OECD data available for the year 2001: 27 OECD countries for physicians and 23 OECD countries for hospital beds.

mortality, and "working age mortality"[3](World Health Organization, 2005b). Figure 3.3 shows how the U.S compares to the other OECD member states on all three of these national health indices. Although life expectancy for U.S. males is basically identical to that of the OECD member average, all other indicators of population health show the United States clearly lags behind the rest of the OECD countries. That is, death rates for male and female children under the age of 5 are higher in the United States relative to the OECD average, as are the death rates for

---

[3] The concept of "working age mortality" was introduced by Guest, Almgren and Hussey in their analysis of urban mortality patterns in the city of Chicago (Guest, Almgren, & Hussey, 1998). Working age mortality refers to adult mortality during the age range where labor force participation is highest, typically between the ages of 15 and 65.

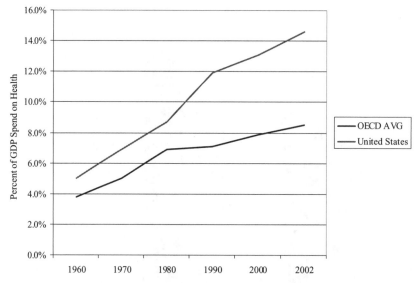

Figure 3.2   Trends in Health Care Expenditures as a Percent of the GDP: Comparison of U.S. with the OECD Average.
Source: *OECD Health Data 2004*. Data from "Table 10: Total expenditure on health, %GDP." Organization for Economic Co-Operation and Development, Paris, France.

working age adults. While it is true that differences between death rates among national populations reflect a variety of factors that are outside of health care quality and access (e.g. difference in the distribution of income among nations and the strength of the social welfare safety net), it seems reasonable to conclude that investments in health care in the United States clearly have far less of a payoff in national health benefits than other OECD countries that spend a far smaller proportion of their GDP on health care. This of course brings us back to the second question posed, why are health care expenditures in the United States so large relative to other industrialized democracies?

In simple terms, there are really only three general answers to this question: either Americans utilize more health care than citizens of other modern democracies, or Americans spend more for the health care that they use, or they do some combination of both. In order to determine which of these possibilities is true, a group of health care policy researchers from Johns Hopkins University School of Public Health and the Woodrow Wilson School of Public Policy at Princeton used recently released OECD data to compare health care expenditures and utilization of health care services between the U.S residents and those of other OECD countries (Anderson, Reinhardt, Hussey, & Petrosyan, 2003). The logic of the

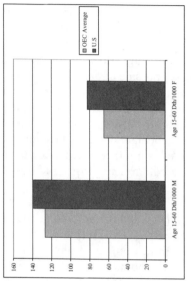

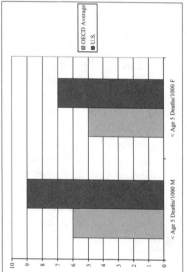

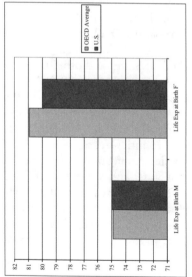

Figure 3.3 WHO Basic Indicators of National Health: Child Mortality, Working Age Mortality and Life Expectancy at Birth. (Source: World Health Organization. 2005. "World Health 2005, Annex Table 1 Basic Indicators for All Member States." Geneva, Switzerland: World Health Organization. All indicators are based on 2003 estimates. For child mortality, Turkey and Mexico are excluded from the average calculation because they are extreme outliers on this particular indicator.)

researchers' analysis was straightforward: essentially if the level of health care utilization relative to other OECD countries matched its higher levels of expenditures, then it would be safe to conclude that the explanation of expenditure difference between the United States and the lower OECD average lies on the demand side of the health care economy equation—in essence Americans spend more on health care because they use more health care. If on the other hand, the level of health care utilization among Americans is not higher than the OECD average, then the excess in U.S. expenditures is really embedded in the supply side of the equation, that is, the costs of the services delivered. Their analysis of health care service utilization was focused on three broad indicators of health care utilization: the median number of visits to physicians per person per year, the median number of hospital admissions, and the median length of hospital stays (in days) per hospital admission. Although a number of other health care utilization indicators might have been used, physician visits and hospital care are the two primary sources of per capital health care expenditures, with pharmaceutical expenditures still a distant third.[4]

The results of the investigators' analysis are both surprising and illuminating. As it in fact happens, relative to the OECD median, Americans were shown to have almost exactly the same number of physician visits per capita per year. Even more surprisingly, population rates of hospital admission and average lengths of hospital stays are *lower* than the OECD median. In terms of these key measures of health care utilization, the authors of this landmark study find that Americans appear to be paying more for less, or stated in another way differences in expenditures between the United States and other OECD member states really are about prices (G. F. Anderson et al., 2003). Although it can be argued that differences in price can and often do reflect differences in quality, any differences in the relative quality of health care between the United States and other OECD countries are not reflected in an array of population health indicators (World Health Organization, 2005b). The authors of this study speculate that a significant source of the price differential in health care between the United States and rest of the OECD community is embedded in the "highly fragmented and complex U.S. payment system" (Anderson et al., 2003, p. 98), something that is obvious to almost anyone seeking health care in the United States. This leads us to the primary task of this chapter— a general review of the system of health care finance in the United States.

---

[4] This might seem somewhat counterintuitive, because of the amount of public attention devoted to pharmaceutical expenditures. However, much of this attention is based on the fact that expenditures for prescription drugs are more likely to be "out of pocket."

AN OVERVIEW OF HEALTH CARE SYSTEM FINANCE
PART I: EMPLOYMENT-BASED HEALTH INSURANCE

Payment for health care in the United States comes from five general sources: out-of-pocket expenditures, employment-based private health insurance, Medicare, Medicaid, and public finance programs other than Medicare and Medicaid—most notably the Veterans Administration. As Figure 3.4 makes obvious, the dominant source of payment for health care is the private health insurance market. In fact, recent estimates show that the private insurance market covers 37% of all domestic health care expenditures, whereas the combined share of health care expenditures covered by the two largest public health care finance programs (Medicare and Medicaid) is 34% (Smith et al., 2005). Understanding how the private health care insurance market works is key to understanding the system of health care finance in the United States, not only because of the private health care insurance market's dominance as a payment source for health care—but also because the key principles that govern the private insurance market also extend to various aspects of public health care finance. Specifically, these principles pertain to the dynamics of "risk

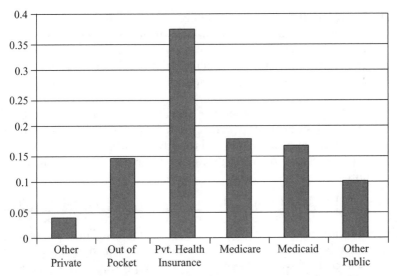

Figure 3.4 Distribution of Health Care Expenditures by Payment Source. (Data Source: Smith, C., C. Cowan, A. Sensenig, and A. Catlin. 2005. "Health spending growth slows in 2003." *Health Affairs* 24(1):185–194: EXHIBIT 5 Expenditures For Health Services And Supplies, By Type Of Service And Source Of Funds, Calendar Year 2003.)

and insurance"—in the most basic sense not unlike those governing the automobile, homeowner, and life insurance markets. Although there are critical differences between the incentives governing the health insurance market and the markets for other forms of insurance that have huge health care policy implications, the underlying principles of insurance apply to all.

Basic Principles of Risk and Insurance

Insurance markets exist because individuals are "averse" to large expenditures for events that *might* occur over some given period, but in the individual case have a low probability of occurrence—again over this given period. Thus, many of us carry renter's or homeowner's insurance against the possibility of a break-in and burglary, because we are strongly averse (e.g. feel we cannot afford) the loss of material things that are costly for us to replace. If the price of the break-in and burglary insurance seems more affordable to us than cost of the loss should a break-in occur, we are inclined to purchase insurance. In fact, if the risk of loss is less affordable to us than the cost of the insurance premium, then purchasing break-in insurance is a prudent and rational thing to do. This kind of scenario works for both the consumer and the insurance company because:

1. The risk of the insured event (a break-in and burglary) is low over the period of coverage (in the case of home owner's or renter's insurance generally either 6 months or 1 year).
2. The consumer views the actual cost of the event as prohibitive and therefore is strongly averse to assuming the risk of loss (i.e. self-insuring).
3. The " fair actuarial" insurance premium (or the main part of the price of insurance) that is determined from a calculation of the risk of the event occurring and the cost of the loss should it occur is low—in fact low enough not to create a disincentive against purchase.

It should be noted that while the risk of a break-in and burglary might be very high over the entire period one owns or rents a home, over each period of insurance coverage the risk is quite low. Thus, insurance products of this sort are purchased and sold over specified periods.

Embedded in this example are several key principles of insurance markets. The first concerns the actual price of the insurance, or as identified in point number three the "fair actuarial premium" or FAP. In simple algebraic terms, the FAP $= P_i {}^* C_i$, where P_i is the estimated probability of event i occurring and C_i is the estimated cost of event i should it occur—again as calculated over a specified period of insurance coverage.

Let's say the FAP for a break-in and burglary in a given low-crime middle class neighborhood is $4.00 per month or $48.00 over the one year period of coverage—not an unreasonable estimate in a low-crime middle class neighborhood. In our hypothetical neighborhood, while the average cost of a break-in and burglary is $4500.00, the probability of a break-in and burglary estimated from local crime rates and prior insurance claims is .0106. Note that the low FAP reflects both the low probability of a break-in and burglary occurring and the modest average level of loss when one occurs—few people in our hypothetical neighborhood keep large stashes of money or own expensive jewelry.

A second principle embedded in this example concerns the risk of *moral hazard*. In the parlance of insurance theory a problem of " moral hazard" arises when the state of being insured for a given event leads the insured to being less averse to the event occurring—thus altering their risk- related behavior. In the context of this example, a "moral hazard" problem would arise if, as a result of being insured against burglary, the homeowner or renter worried less about leaving the front door locked because the insurance company covers the cost of stolen property. In this simple example the moral hazard is minimal because for a variety of reasons besides theft, people generally don't like the idea of uninvited strangers walking into their homes and will still lock their doors. That is, people tend to remain equally "risk averse" to unauthorized home entry despite the fact that they are insured against theft. People also tend to be risk averse to car accidents, fires, and events involving personal injury or death despite being insured for these things—but what about health care? For reasons that will shortly be explained in more detail the moral hazard problem in health care insurance is far more complex than for most other forms of insurance. Suffice to say at this point that under a variety of circumstances individuals are not necessarily averse to an event that leads to an episode of health care and further, that many kinds of health behavior are influenced by having health care coverage.

A third principle of insurance that can be drawn from the example of household insurance concerns the problem of *adverse selection*. In very basic terms, when an insurance company markets a specific insurance product, in this example household insurance in the event of break-in and burglary, they assume that each person sold the insurance product has a level of insured risk and cost that is consistent with that used to calculate the fair actuarial premium or FAP. Of course insurance companies do not have perfect information on each purchaser, but the FAP is based on the average risk and cost as pooled across large number of insurance purchasers that share common predictive characteristics (e.g. being of a certain age, living in a low- crime location, and having no prior criminal history involving insurance fraud or property theft). Adverse selection occurs when individual purchasers actually have a level of insurance risk that is significantly in excess of the risk and cost assumed in the FAP calculation. Normally, individual instances of adverse selection are offset by comparable instances of favorable selection due to the mathematics of random chance. However, if there is some systematic and unfavorable selection bias in either the nature of the insurance product or the way that it is advertised, the insurance company is headed for significant financial loss. In the example of householders' insurance, the insurance company may try to avoid adverse selection by avoiding the marketing of their lower cost insurance product in neighborhoods with rising rates of property crime. In the higher crime neighborhoods, the insurance company may attempt to market an insurance product with a higher FAP and a higher deductible that better reflects the local level of burglary risk—in effect creating a separate *insurance pool* for the purchasers living in the higher crime neighborhood. Specifically, an *insurance pool* refers to a set of insured individuals sharing the same estimated level of risk and cost as that used to calculate their common FAP price, with the FAP applied to offset the costs of any instances of an insured event occurring to any member of the insurance pool.

In sum, insurance companies are viable financial entities to the extent that they have capacity to: (1) accurately assess the risks and the costs of an array of events people are averse to having occur, (2) define and market insurance products that will attract people into appropriately priced insurance pools, and (3) accurately assess and pay the costs of claims they are legally liable for. The actual price of an insurance premium is in excess of the FAP, because the FAP does not incorporate the costs of overhead and profit. However, most forms of insurance function in highly competitive markets and the non-FAP portion of the insurance premium is typically quite small.

Risk and Insurance in the Context of Health Care Insurance

In a variety of ways, health care insurance violates a number of assumptions that are viable for other forms of insurance. As noted previously, unlike other forms of insurance, individuals who possess health care insurance are not always averse to the insured event—an episode of health care. While few people genuinely enjoy being ill (there are exceptions to everything of course), there are often aspects of receiving health care that if not enjoyable, are at least reassuring. Any parent of a sick child, even when the illness appears routine and probably self-resolving, can attest to the anxiety experienced and the desire to have a doctor present to dispel very normal albeit unrealistic fears. If mom or dad is more disposed towards a visit to the E.R. for what is likely a nonthreatening childhood illness *because the visit is substantially covered by their health care insurance*, this constitutes an instance of moral hazard. There are also aspects of health care that are either pleasurable or self-reinforcing that have no basis for the diagnosis given for an episode of care, such as visiting a clinic to dispel loneliness and isolation. Again, the moral hazard issue arises where, due to the fact of health care insurance coverage, the patient is at least less averse to receiving care. Although the problem of moral hazard is conceptualized as an issue pertaining to the motivation and behavior of the insured patient rather than the health care provider, health care providers are also significantly influenced in their treatment decisions and interventions by the extent of health insurance coverage (Fuchs, 2004).[5] In fact, the fundamental dilemma of health care insurance is that both the insured and the provider often have very strong incentives to promote the use of health care, while at the same time both are protected from the true costs (Starr, 1992).

The problem of adverse selection is also a significant dilemma in health care, the dynamic here being that health insurance products that are designed to attract one type of consumer at a given level of risk often attract higher risk consumers. This is a particular problem in health care policies that are marketed to individuals rather than groups, because for a variety of reasons persons who are not eligible for coverage under group insurance plans have higher levels of illness, injury, and disability and on average have higher rates of health care utilization (Harrington & Miller, 2002). It is also the case that when individuals are paying the costs of their own health care insurance premiums, as is typically the case with individual plans, they are more likely to drop the insurance when healthy and seek insurance health care coverage when ill or injured. This of course becomes the definition of adverse selection. It is also true that less healthy workers are more likely to work in low-end jobs as a function of their poor health, jobs that don't offer affordable health insurance—thus leaving them to the vicissitudes of the individual insurance plan market. In many insurance markets, even healthy individuals find the costs of health insurance to be prohibitive because of the impact of problems with adverse selection. Finally, for reasons that are explained in more detail in the discussion that follows, small employers employ a disproportionate share of the risk burden that is a function of the linkage between social class and health.

---

[5] Often this is either benign or benevolent, because the physician wants to provide optimal treatment irrespective of cost to the patient. There are of course a variety of economic incentives to providing more rather than less health care having little to do with what constitutes optimal care.

Things were not always so grim for individuals seeking health care insurance. Until the 1970s, the U.S. insurance market was dominated by health insurance plans that utilized *community rating* systems of premium pricing. Under the community rating scheme of health insurance pricing, "risk pool" for purposes of insurance pricing was defined as the community of residence—for historical reasons typically the county of residence. For most communities, this meant the calculations of health care risks and costs were based upon a large pool of heterogeneous individuals that differed by education, occupation and in effect overall state of health. However, as the health inflation escalated over the 1970s, employers began to balk at the rising costs of community-rated health care plans and a market for *employer-based rating* systems of health insurance gradually became dominant. As a parallel trend, many of the largest employers began to *self-insure,* in essence placing the health care benefit portion of labor costs in a fund earmarked to pay the cost of employee health insurance claims—with the role of health insurance company limited to claims processing and reinsurance.[6] In essence, employer-based rating systems worked well for those employers with more skilled, more educated, and ergo generally healthier workers because such employers were able to shed the higher costs of the less skilled, less educated, and less healthy workers (and their dependents) that they had previously subsidized through the community-rated health care plan. Because the labor market has become increasingly segmented by social class since the 1970s (Scott, Berger, & Black, 1989), lower skilled and less educated workers are ever less likely to work for the kinds of employers that offer health care benefits and are ever less likely to be able to afford the costs of their relatively higher health care risks. In simple terms, prior to 1970, health insurance access and pricing was, to a significant degree, a buffering mechanism that mitigated the effects of social class on health through a nearly universal mechanism of community rating–based health insurance. In the decades since the 1970s, the private health insurance market has devolved to an employer-based rating system that serves to *enlarge* the linkages between social class and health.[7]

---

[6] Reinsurance, also a form of stop-loss, refers to an insurance policy that applies to health care expenditures that significantly exceed those anticipated. Employers who self-insure typically allocate only the health care benefit funds that they expect to spend, and then purchase an insurance policy that covers the cost of health care claims that significantly exceed the funds set aside.

[7] There will be an extensive discussion of the socioeconomic gradient in health in chapters that follow. Briefly, individual socioeconomic characteristics (education, employment, occupation, and income) are all strongly linked to health through multiple pathways, e.g. higher levels of exposure to illness in childhood, poorer nutrition, access to health care, and by some accounts the deleterious effects of discrimination and lower social status. Because

Forms of Risk and Payment of Claims

Hopefully, it has been clear to this point that health care insurance does not insure against illness, but rather it assumes some specified level of risk for the costs of health care services. There are multiple ways to do this, but the dominant forms of health care insurance risk assumption are *indemnity* based, *benefit* based, and *capitation* based. In the case of indemnity insurance, the health care insurance product assumes the cost of care for a given claim up to a set amount that is explicitly stated in the insurance contract—no matter what the provider's fee or the ultimate cost. In contrast, benefit-based plans pay for a specified range of health care services or health care products without specifying the dollar amount of the costs covered—thus leaving the insured largely out of any pricing negotiations between the provider and the insurance company. The third form of insurance risk assumption, capitation, is best conceptualized as insuring not the specific costs for episodes of care, but rather agreeing to provide the totality of health care that the insurance carrier deems is prudent and/or necessary to sustain health and treat illness over the agreed-upon period of coverage. The latter form of health care risk assumption is the foundation of health maintenance organizations. In truth, these forms of insurance risk assumption no longer tend to exist as pure types; most health care insurance carriers combine different features of each in the complex array of insurance products that serve the preferences of different purchasers. However, it is also true that of these general forms of risk assumption, the once popular indemnity-based plans are the exception—largely as a function of rising health care costs, managed care and preferred provider networks.

Payments made to providers of health care take any one of five general forms: *fee-for-service, per diem payment, prospective payment, cost plus reimbursement* and *capitation* payment. All five forms of payment have played prominent roles in the structure of health care finance at different points in the history of the U.S. health care system. It is also the case that different forms of insurance payment arrangements offer very different incentives for health care providers and insurers, with related effects on the accessibility, quantity, and quality of health care delivered. Throughout most of the history of the health insurance industry, fee-for-service forms of payment have been both dominant and the preferred form of

lower socioeconomic status (SES) increases the risk of poorer health and lower SES is linked to the likelihood of employment in the small employer sector of the economy, small employers face a significant disadvantage in the insurance market due to the dynamics of adverse selection.

payment—consistent with the dominant ideal of medical free enterprise in American medicine (Starr, 1982). In essence the provider either sets or negotiates a fee for a given diagnostic or treatment procedure, and the provider's income is determined by the profit margin, service mix, and the overall volume of services provided. When claims are paid on a per diem basis, the health care provider is reimbursed at a daily rate for care that is a fixed amount for all health care services and products/procedures provided over the course of each day the patient is under the care of the provider. The prospective payment method of claims payment involves a set amount paid to the provider for a given episode of care that is typically defined in terms of a diagnosis or a combination of diagnosis and procedure. Finally, cost plus reimbursement guarantees the provider a small margin for profit or return on equity after the provider has justified the costs of providing care to the insurance carrier.

Obviously, each form of claims payment offers a different set of risks and incentives for the health care provider that ultimately affects the nature of the care provided. In fact, there is a large health care policy literature on the effects of alternative systems mechanisms of insurance payment on clinical decision-making by physicians, clinics, and hospitals. Figure 3.5 provides a simple illustration of the provider incentives to encourage more or fewer episodes of care (e.g. hospital admissions or physician visits) and higher or lower levels of care intensity under different regimes of insurance payment. The term "care intensity" is deliberately chosen to represent the quantity of care provided during a given episode of care without inferring with anything about quality—the point being that more procedures, tests, and medications are not in and of themselves suggestive of more quality (Anderson & Poullier, 1999). It should also be noted that the incentives shown in Figure 3.5 are assumed to operate where the knowledge pertaining to what constitutes "best practices"

| | Episodes of Care | |
	More	Fewer
High Care Intensity	Fee-for Service Cost Plus Reimbursement	
Low Care Intensity	Per Diem Prospective Payment	Capitation

Figure 3.5   Provider Incentives under Alternative Payment Mechanisms

is in dispute or ambiguous, as is often the case in clinical decision-making.[8]

As Figure 3.5 shows, both fee-for-service and cost plus mechanisms of insurance payment are the most inflationary, in the sense that providers have an economic incentive to both promote episodes of care and provide a more intensive level of care within each episode. The textbook example of this was the hospital reimbursement mechanisms during the first decades of Medicare (between 1965 and 1982), when hospitals were reimbursed on a cost plus basis for every procedure, item of supply, and hospital day utilized by each episode of care. Equally, under a fee-for-service regime of insurance payment, it is in the economic interest of the care provider to provide as much care as can be defended as "medically necessary." It is easy to see why these two forms of reimbursement functioned as the engines of the health care inflation growth that occurred as public and private health care insurance coverage dramatically expanded during the 1960s and 1970s. Per diem reimbursement and prospective payment regimes have similar "mixed" incentives in many respects, because providers have strong incentives to promote episodes of care, but then to reduce as much as possible the utilization of test, procedures, and supplies that contribute to the costs of care. This is because the dollars reimbursed for care are fixed on the basis of either a given amount paid for each day of care or a given amount based on the diagnostic/procedure code assigned to the episode of care. Both forms of reimbursement are extensively used by insurance carriers to control health care claims expenditures. The prospective payment approach has been a major form of inpatient hospital reimbursement mechanism since the early 1980s—a payment regime that yielded dramatic reductions in the growth of hospital care expenditures. Notably, the capitation-based system of insurance reimbursement offers providers the fewest incentives to provide care; in fact in contrast to the other forms of insurance payment the capitation system creates a strong *disincentive* to provide care—typically in absence of any clear long- or short-term benefits to health. This is because the under the capitation system the provider is paid a fixed amount per each person in the insurance plan pool, whether or not health care is provided during the period of coverage. In the parlance of Health Maintenance Organization, "lives" or person/years of health care expenditures are covered rather than specific episodes of health care.

---

[8] This assumption takes into account that patient care decisions typically involve subjective and objective components, and that provider economic incentives hold more sway where the level of subjectivity is high. This is a very benevolent assumption of course, but a fair one with respect to the far majority of health care providers.

How Private Health Insurance Operates

The conventional private health care market (as previously explained in chapter 2—The Historical Evolvement of the U.S. Health Care System) emerged as a partnership between local (typically county level) hospitals, physicians, employers and labor unions. In all respects it has been an employment-based system, with either the labor union or the employer acting as a sponsor of group health insurance plans. During roughly the first 4 decades of private insurance, employers would typically contract with the county-level Blue Cross and Blue Shield Insurance Plans, which as mentioned earlier functioned on the basis of community rating systems. This made contracting very straightforward, because health care benefits were a much smaller proportion of overall labor costs and health insurance premium prices were consistent across employers for whatever array of benefits was either offered by the employer or negotiated through collective bargaining. During this earlier period, health insurance premium prices were subject to a multiyear *insurance cycle* that permitted the insurance health care plan to both keep prices low and avoid irrecoverable losses. During the first period of the cycle, premium prices for a health insurance plan were based upon an actuarial estimate of the anticipated expenditures in claims. Because it takes time to properly process claims data and assess the claims expenditures for a given year of coverage, the second period of recalibration of premium prices to take account of true expenditures and recover losses occurred 2 to 3 years after the initial first year of premium pricing. In effect this created a fairly consistent fluctuation of profits and loss that typically encompassed 6 calendar years (Doran, Dobson, & Harris, 2001).

As mentioned previously in this chapter, by the early 1980s a decade of rampant health care inflation and ineffective cost controls pushed employers to seek more competitively priced health care plans that were based upon the employer's rather than the community's actuarial risk. This in turn spawned expansion in the insurance brokerage industry and various attempts by employers to pool their risk and purchasing power. As the private insurance market functions currently, how employers purchase health insurance is very much a function of the size of the employer's labor force and the industry sector in which the employer is located (e.g. manufacturing, mining, retail, service). Both labor force size and industry sector are key attributes of a "segmented labor market" (Dickens & Lang, 1992), meaning in essence that the labor market is comprised of distinct parts, each with different rules for the determination of wages and employment policies, and with different levels of employment opportunity (Dickens & Lang, 1992 p. 7). Although size and industrial sector both affect the dynamics of the health insurance availability and costs, the first attribute to be considered is employer size—in particular the distinction between the health insurance markets for small and large employers.

Small employers typically rely on an insurance broker, a function analogous to real estate that brings together the buyers and the sellers and charges the seller a commission—in the case of group health insurance typically 2–8% of the premium price (Conwell, 2002). Medium-sized employers, those with a labor force of 100 to 500 employees, tend to involve both brokers and health care benefits consultants (Marquis & Long, 2000). Large employers who don't self-insure tend to use a combination of insurance brokers and external benefits consultants, while self-insured large employers tend to rely more upon a combination of benefits consultants and third party administrators—the latter being a firm that contracts with the employer to act as the administrator of employee health care benefits (Marquis & Long, 2000).

An important consideration in the operation of health insurance markets is the extent to which the insurance broker acts as an agent of the employer seeking the affordable group health care coverage or the health insurance company seeking to find the "lowest risk" employers—in essence, employers that have employees who are the least likely to introduce an adverse selection problem. It is not uncommon in some health insurance markets for insurance carriers to use financial incentives that discourage brokers from bringing them higher risk business, sometimes in violation of state and federal laws that govern the health insurance market (Conwell, 2002).[9] The situation is akin to the problem of racial discrimination in housing, where real estate agents are given incentives by developers and lenders to "steer" minority home buyers away from desirable neighborhoods. While extensive regulations have been promulgated to promote small employer access to reasonably priced health insurance, there is a significant debate as to whether these reform efforts are effective or even counterproductive (Xirasagar et al., 2004). Ironically, other federal regulations contained in the Employee Retirement Income Security Act of 1974 (ERISA) don't appear to prohibit employers from engaging in various forms of risk selection, including finding ways to push higher risk employees out of their labor force (U. S. Court of Appeals Third Circuit,

---

[9] For example, the federal Health Insurance Portability and Accountability Act of 1996 (HIPAA) contains provisions against small employer discrimination. The origins of HIPAA and its sweeping impacts on health care insurance markets and patient care delivery will be discussed at a later point in this chapter.

2000; U.S. Court of Appeals Eleventh Circuit, 1993).[10] In fact, ERISA protects self-insuring employers who engage in risk selection practices from state level laws banning such activities.

Employer Size and Effects on Insurance Premium Costs and Expenditures

Health care insurance premiums are about $3700 per year for single coverage and about $9,950 per year if the insurance coverage extends to the employee's family (EBRI, 2005).[11] Although the premium prices are similar for small and large employers (GAO, 2001), the quality and extent of health care benefits are much more limited for the workers of small employers (businesses that employ less than 50 persons)—a difference that is largely explained by the higher proportion of premium costs that go to administrative overhead. According to the U.S. General Accounting Office, 20–25% of the premium costs for small employers is absorbed by administrative expenses (broker fees, claims processing, insurance carrier profit or return on equity), while only 10 percent of the premium costs of large employers are absorbed by administrative overhead (GAO, 2001).

To an extent, this is explained by volume efficiency and also the capacity of large employers to self-insure. However, a significant amount of this difference is accounted for by the costs of higher insurance broker's fees and insurance carriers spending more money on administrative processes needed to reduce the higher risks of adverse selection in the small-employer insurance market (GAO, 2001). Obviously, if the dollar costs for premiums are relatively the same between small and large employers and the administrative expenses 10–15% higher for small businesses, there is less money to be spent on the accessibility and quality of health care for workers in small firms.

Table 3.2 examines the comparative disadvantage in health care benefits encountered by workers in the small business sector, even if they are fortunate enough to have employer-based health insurance available

---

[10] The first of these referenced cases, Owens v. Storehouse, involved a $25,000 cap placed on care for AIDS for all employees. The second, DiFederico v. Rolm Company, involved allegations of wrongful discharge by an employee who contended that her employment termination was based upon her employer's desire to avoid health and disability insurance benefit obligations. In both of these cases, federal courts established legal precedent for a significant burden on the employee to establish a clear link between the employer's actions and selective abrogation of health care coverage obligations. The specifics of ERISA will be discussed in more detail at a later point in the chapter.

[11] See also the Henry Kaiser J. Foundation for updated estimates of health insurance coverage and costs.

Table 3.2   Employer Size Effects on Net Benefits of Health Insurance

	Large Employer	Small Employer	Net Disadvantage
		(Less Than 50 Employees)	
Hospital Care	$3,354	$2,888	−$466
Physician's & Clinical Services	$3,471	$2,989	−$482
Other Professional Services	$352	$303	−$49
Home Health Care	$138	$119	−$19
Retail Prescription Drugs	$1,567	$1,349	−$218
Misc. Benefits	$74	$63	−$10
Total Paid in Claims	$8,955	$7,711	−$1,244
Administrative Costs	$995	$2,239	$1,244
Total Premiums	$9,950	$9,950	_____
Administative Costs as Percent of Premium	10.0%	22.5%	_____

Note: The estimated proportion of health insurance premium allocated to adminstrative costs by employer size is based upon U.S. General Accounting Office estimates (see GAO 2001, Report 02-8). The estimated claims expenditures are based on Smith et al's (2005) analysis of Centers for Medicare and Medicaid Services data, as reported in *Health Affairs* 24 (1), "Exhibit 5 -Expenditures for Health Services and Supplies, by Type of Services and Source of Funds for Calendar Year 2003." In this example, it is assumed that the distribution of health care expenditures as a proportion of funds available for claims payment is the same despite differences in adminstrative overhead. In practice, this varies significantly by the structure of individual contracts and premiums and the preferences of purchasers.

(this is a separate issue that will be discussed shortly). Essentially, Table 3.2 provides an estimate of the pattern of health insurance claims expenditures by the type of health care provided that one would expect to see, given (a) the average annual premium price of an employer-based policy that provides dependent coverage, (b) the average amount of administrative overhead embedded in the price of the premium by the size of employer, and (c) the general pattern of private insurance expenditures that is observed nationally (see Smith et al., 2005). As noted previously, although the actual premium prices paid by large and small employers are nearly equal, the costs of administrative overhead relative to the funds available to pay benefits are far greater among small employers (GAO, 2001). These disadvantages derive in large part from costs associated with the risks of adverse selection, in effect meaning that small employers pay a significant "size" penalty in order to participate in the private health insurance market—a penalty that further places small employers at a competitive disadvantage. As shown in Table 3.2, unless the small employer were to absorb the full burden size penalty portion of the health insurance premium, the typical family dependent upon the health insurance policy of a small employer would have $1,244 less available from their policy to pay claims relative to a like family of a large employer. Given the typical distribution of private health care expenditures, a family of a small employer would then have $466 less in insurance coverage for hospital care, $482 less in coverage for physician and related clinical services, and $218 less available for coverage of pharmaceutical costs.

In actual practice, small employers tend to avoid providing dependent coverage and opt for the strategy of limiting health care insurance benefits to the individual employee rather than their dependents. Only about 1 in 5 smaller firms[12] offer family benefits to at least 75% of their employees, whereas family benefit coverage is available in 6 of 10 of larger employers (Kaiser Foundation, 2004). In addition, employees of small firms also wait longer for health care benefit coverage eligibility, pay more for dependent benefits where available, and typically have only one health insurance plan available (Kaiser Foundation 2004, pp. 52, 60, and 73).

Industry Sector Effects on Health Insurance Access and Cost

Consistent with segmented labor market theory (Dickens & Lang, 1992), different sectors of the economy clearly offer very unequal conditions of employment—the exemplar here being health insurance coverage by employers. Figure 3.6 shows dramatic differences in the proportion of workers covered by employer-provided health insurance by each major sector of the economy. Although across all employers of any size, industrial type, and regional location, the average proportion of workers covered by employer sponsored insurance is 67%, less than half of workers in the retail sector of the economy are covered by health insurance that is sponsored through their employer. Clearly the most advantaged sectors of the economy are in health care, government, utilities/transportation, and manufacturing. Although there are multiple explanations for the disparities in employment-based health insurance by industry, the major factors include the histories of collective bargaining specific to each industry, the gender composition of the industrial sector labor force, the prevalence of workers with lower levels of education and job skills within each industrial sector, and increasingly the susceptibility of each employment sector to global competitive pressure on wages and benefits—particularly to the extent that U.S. employers are confronted with the dilemma of ever-increasing health insurance premium prices (Battistella, Burchfield, & Fitzgerald, 2000).

---

[12] In this comparison, provided by the Henry J. Kaiser Foundation's *Employer Health Benefits: 2004 Summary of Findings*, small employers are defined as employers with a work force of fewer than 200 employees (see complete citation for further reference).

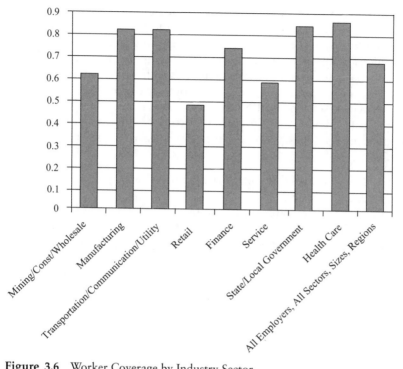

Figure 3.6 Worker Coverage by Industry Sector.
Source: Based on data from Survey of Employer Health Benefits: 2004. Exhibit 3.2 "Eligibility, Take-Up Rates, and Coverage in Firms Offering Health Benefits, by Firm Size, Region, and Industry, 2004." The Henry J. Kaiser Family. Menlo Park, CA.

Managed Care and Other Forms of Cost Control

Thus far, the brunt of the discussion pertaining to employment-based health insurance has concerned the problem of adverse selection and its effects on equity of health insurance access. However, the original dynamic that propelled the private health insurance market toward employer-based insurance pricing (from the community rating system) was the *moral hazard* problem discussed previously—the problem that arises when the effect of having insurance alters the risk behavior of the insured. To repeat a point made earlier in the chapter, under a variety of conditions individuals are more disposed toward seeking health care because they have health care insurance than they otherwise would be. To compound the problem, the availability of health insurance has fueled technological innovation in nearly every sphere of health care (e.g. drugs, diagnostic equipment) that lends its own inflationary pressures. Finally, providers have strong incentives to provide more health care at higher prices to the extent that insurance is available to assure them a profitable return for their services.[13]

In contrast to the incentives of the other three actors (the patient, the provider, and the technology innovator), employers and health insurance carriers have strong incentives to reduce health care utilization and the prices paid for health care. Further, in contrast to the interests of health care providers and the health care innovators, the employer and the insurance carrier have joint incentives to reduce the prices of health care products and services. There are a five very basic ways for them to do this:

1. Lower the level of health risk among the insured pool of health care consumers.
2. Make health care consumers more risk averse to seeking health care, in essence, impose penalties for health care utilization.
3. Reduce or reverse the incentives on the part of providers to provide care.
4. Reduce the prices/costs of health care services and products provided.[14]
5. Reduce utilization of care that falls outside explicit standards of efficacy and/or cost efficiency.

The first way to control the escalation of health care expenditures generally involves (as previously mentioned) various recruitment and retention strategies by the employer to develop a healthier pool of employees. Also, some employers pursue various health promotion strategies in the work place, particularly large employers who self-insure. Prominent among health promotion strategies are employer campaigns to eliminate smoking and other forms of tobacco addiction, although other avenues of employer-sponsored health promotion include weight loss campaigns, exercise programs, stress management, and education about the effective use of health care services. The evidence suggests that such efforts pay a return to employers in the reduced use of sick leave and avoidable health care expenditures that is three to four times their cost (Fries et al., 1993).

The remaining four strategies to reduce health care utilization and costs fall under the broad rubric of *managed care*. Although "managed

---

[13] The term profit is used broadly to refer to the difference between the costs of providing a service and the price paid. Not-for-profit organizations refer to this difference as a return on equity.

[14] The terms prices and costs are both used here, to note the distinction between prices that are paid by an insurance underwriter to a given provider and the costs of providing care if the care is provided by the insuring organization—as in the case of an HMO.

care" is defined in multiple ways, it commonly encompasses various activities by health care underwriters to control health care costs, quality, and access (Baily, 2003). In contrast to the passive stance of traditional insurance companies that merely estimate risk, set insurance premium prices, and then process the payment of claims, managed care organizations engage in a variety of activities aimed at influencing the process of health care decision making—both by the providers and the consumers of health care (Baily, 2003, p. 36). Managed care can also be thought of as referring to *provider structures* (i.e. specific forms of organizational arrangements between the providers and underwriters of health care), and a repertoire of tactics pertaining to the control of health care utilization and pricing. Because all managed care provider structures, to a greater or less extent, rely upon a similar set of utilization and pricing tactics, it makes sense to describe the main types of provider structures first.

Although there are multiple variations within each type, employment-based health care plans rely on three main kinds of managed care organization provider structures: *HMOs, PPOs* and *POS* providers (Robinson, 1999). In contrast to other provider structures, HMOs (health maintenance organizations) combine the functions of health care underwriting and health care provision within a single organization through the mechanism of capitated financing. As explained earlier in this chapter, instead of insuring against the costs for specific services and episodes of care, capitation insures against the costs of totality of health care that the insurance carrier (HMO) deems is prudent and/or necessary to sustain health and treat illness over the agreed-upon period of coverage. The term "capitation" is derived from the idea that the insurance financing is on a per member–per month (or per capita) basis rather than on the basis of episodes of care, or services/products furnished. Among HMOs, a distinction is made between HMOs that provide health care services through a network of provider contracts such as with Independent Practice Associations (IPAs),[15] and HMOs that principally provide care through health care professionals they employ and facilities that they own and operate. Preferred provider organizations (PPOs) are networks of providers

---

[15] An Independent Practice Association (IPA) is an association of providers, most typically physicians, who contract with the HMOs and other managed care organizations to provide care for managed care plan members. The contracts typically involve some level of "risk sharing" by the IPA, meaning that the IPA agrees to furnish some level of care on a capititated basis rather than a fee-for-service basis. Obviously, if the IPA provides care that exceeds that covered by the capitation rate, the IPA membership assumes the financial loss. IPAs permit a member physician to maintain ownership and control over his or her individual practices while providing the physician with the advantages of a corporate structure for the negotiation and administration of managed care contracts (Grumbach, Coffman, Vranizan, Blick, & O'Neil, 1998).

(e.g. physician groups, hospitals, pharmacies) that contract with health insurance underwriters to furnish an array of health care services and products at a discounted price. Providers that are a part of a PPO network are also generally required to follow procedures set by the insurance underwriter that serve to monitor and control health care utilization and quality, and they often must meet specified benchmarks in each to avoid financial penalties. Finally, point-of-service (POS) provider structures are a particular form of the preferred provider arrangement that permits the health care consumer to choose their own primary care provider, who then functions as the "gatekeeper" for other health care services—or more benevolently as the provider responsible for coordinating all other aspects of the consumer's health care. Many consumers prefer the POS provider structure because they perceive that they are able to exercise more personal choice in the health care they utilize, including referral to specialists (Forrest et al., 2001). It should be noted that POS arrangements are often included as a higher cost option within HMO health plans, and that such "hybrid" provider structures have become increasingly common as consumers have sought alternatives to more rigid forms of managed care (Mechanic, 2004).

According to the most recent survey of health care plans published by the Henry J. Kaiser Foundation, only about 5% of workers in the United States who are covered by employer health insurance are enrolled in health care plans that don't have a managed care provider structure (Kaiser Foundation, 2004). Of the remaining 95% of covered workers, 25% are enrolled in HMOs, 55% in PPOs, and 15% in POS plans (Kaiser, 2004, p. 70). Table 3.3 provides a general overview of how each type of managed care organization provider structure employs various methods that serve the four previously discussed "managed care" strategies for the reduction of health care utilization and cost. The strategies and methods that are shown are those that tend to be more prevalent within each type of organizational structure.

Many of the cost containment mechanisms displayed in Table 3.3 are generally familiar and don't require special explanation. Others may be less familiar and require brief explanation. Under the first column, selective wait-listing refers to imposing longer waits on some forms of care where urgent attention is not critical. Gatekeeping triage refers to information and referral processes that have as a central goal diversion of the patient from clinical services that are deemed nonessential, such as requiring primary care visits be scheduled through a clinic nurse. High copays for use of non-PPO providers require the patient to pay more out of pocket if the patient selects the use of a health care provider that is outside the PPO provider network. Under the second column, "utilization review" refers to the auditing of clinic records for the purposes of identifying

Table 3.3 Managed Care Cost Containment Methods by MCO Provider Structure

Managed Care Organization Structure	Managed Care Cost Containment Strategy I	Managed Care Cost Containment Strategy II	Managed Care Cost Containment Strategy III	Managed Care Cost Containment Strategy IV
	Make health care consumers more risk averse to seeking health care, in essence, impose penalties for health care utilization	*Reduce or reverse the incentives on the part of providers to provide care*	*Reduce the prices and costs of health care services and products provided*	*Reduce utilization of care that falls outside explicit standards of efficacy and/or cost efficiency.*
HMO	Modest co-pays for selected services Selective wait-listing Gatekeeping Triage	Salaried Providers Utilization Review and sanctioning of provider outliers Risk pool-based incentives/profit sharing	Bulk purchasing and competitive bidding Selective outsourcing/carve-outs Selective case management Discounted contracts for outside providers	Utilization Review and Care Process Improvement Selective Pre-review Selective case management Widespread use of clinical protocols
PPO	Significant to modest co-pays for broad range of services. Significant deductibles High co-pays for use of non-PPO providers	Utilization Review and sanctioning of outliers Payment denial for services deemed unnecessary	Bulk purchasing and competitive bidding Selective case management	Utilization Review and Care Process Improvement Selective Pre-review Selective case management Widespread use of clinical protocols
POS	Significant to modest co-pays for broad range of services. Significant deductibles High co-pays for referrals to specialists	Close monitoring of utilization of services, sanctioning of provider outliers Payment denial for services deemed unnecessary	Discounted provider fees Referral within PPO network Primary care gatekeeping	Utilization Review and Care Process Improvement Selective Pre-review Primary care case management Widespread use of clinical protocols

care delivery by providers that fails to meet explicit standards of care established by the insurance underwriter, and "sanctioning of outliers" refers to actions by the insurance carrier that have negative consequences for the provider—including at the extreme terminating the contract with the provider, and identifying providers who deliver care outside of the established practice. The positive incentive method identified in the second column involves the mechanisms of profit sharing or higher provider reimbursements for meeting patient risk pool-based outcomes, such as achieving a benchmark for a reduced incidence of hospital admissions among the pool of the HMO members assigned to the HMO physician's practice.

The cost-reducing method of "selective outsourcing/carve outs" shown in the third column, involves the selective use of either subcontracting the management and provision of a segment of the benefits package to a specialty provider or making some benefits available on a discounted fee-for-service basis through an external provider contract. These kinds of arrangements are made where the HMO determines it is less able to manage a certain type of benefit on a capitation basis and contracting with an external provider is more cost efficient—the typical example being the carve-out of benefit obligations for mental health care. Also under the price and cost control strategy (the third column) is selective case management. Case management has a variety of definitions and approaches, but for the purposes here it means assignment of a care coordination specialist to a patient with a difficult-to-manage disease profile or one that involves high utilization of resources, such as a patient dually diagnosed with Type I diabetes and bipolar disorder. Depending on a variety of factors, the case manager may be a clinical nurse specialist, social worker, or a licensed physician's assistant.[16]

Under the fourth column, the strategy to reduce utilization of care that falls outside explicit standards of efficacy and/or cost efficiency, key methods include selective pre-review for some categories of health care service, and utilization review for care process improvement. The former is familiar to most patients having employer-based insurance that have needed either surgery, an expensive diagnostic procedure, or specialized treatment—and it involves review by an agent of the insurer (typically a nurse specialist or physician) and preapproval as a condition of insurance coverage. The justification usually entails criteria related to clinical necessity and cost efficiency, though many patients and providers view and have experienced this method as a bureaucratic obstacle that serves a

---

[16] Case managers are in some cases selected from other disciplines as well, but for the purposes stated here the three disciplines identified are more prevalent.

penalty function (per Cost Containment Strategy I). Utilization review for purposes of process improvement involves retrospective review of clinical practice processes to discover opportunities for improvement either in cost savings/clinical outcomes or both. It is often the case that more efficient care is also care that yields direct clinical benefits to the patient: unnecessary care is often not only costly but also detrimental—the classic example being the risks to the patient imposed by needlessly prolonged hospital stays.[17] The final method shown in column four that is worthy of highlighting, widespread use of clinical protocols, refers to the delivery of care in accordance to pre-established standards of care for a given profile of disease symptoms, stage of disease, and/or patient characteristics in combination with a given diagnosis. In simple terms clinical protocols generally involve doing what the evidence suggests is most effective and cost efficient for a given type of case—in some situations substituting the clinical practitioner's and or the patient's independent judgment or preference concerning what is best or most effective in the individual situation.[18]

Although the strategies and methods shown in Table 3.3 fall far short of an exhaustive review of the full range of managed care strategies and methods for the control of health care utilization and costs, those shown encompass the prevalent approaches. Aggressively pursued, most have proved very effective as mechanisms of cost reduction and control under a variety of contexts. In fact, managed care utilization mechanisms employed by insurance companies as well as by the federal government largely accounted for the temporary plunge in health care cost inflation that occurred during the first half of the 1990s decade (Altman & Levitt, 2002). It is also clear that the insurance market has shifted away from aggressive forms of managed care over the most recent years—much to the detriment of health care cost containment. According to the widely accepted narrative of medical sociologist David Mechanic,[19] the use of

---

[17] There is an extensive literature pertaining to the iatrogenic risks (risk arising from medical treatment rather than underlying disease processes) of hospital care. See in particular the Institute of Medicine report *To Err is Human: Building a Safer Health Care System*, issued in 1999 and available through the National Academy Press, Washington, DC.

[18] In the pejorative sense, this can be seen or referred to as "assembly line medicine" that discounts the unique nature of each clinical encounter and the autonomous exercise of informed clinical judgment. On the benevolent side, use of clinical protocols reduces the incidence of arbitrary decision making and biased preferences by individual practitioners that ultimately reduce the quality of care. Clinical protocols often entail explicit cost justifications for the probability of achieving a given clinical outcome, which can be viewed as good or bad depending upon the ethical framework of the practitioner.

[19] Aptly titled "The Rise and Fall of Managed Care," published in the *Journal of Health and Social Behavior* 2004 (Vol. 45).

many of these utilization and cost control mechanisms have been on the wane in the face of a widespread "managed care backlash" that gained momentum as the insurance industry consolidated and a larger share of middle class Americans experienced reduced exercise of preferences and access to health care firsthand (Mechanic, 2004). However, even in Mechanic's analysis, there are many promising aspects of managed care that will remain in the U.S. health care system to the extent that they contribute to better management of chronic diseases and to health care quality rather than solely to reductions in utilization or cost (Mechanic, 2004, p. 82). Given the short life of the more aggressive forms of managed care, the employer-based health insurance system has more recently turned to other avenues of cost containment, specifically reductions in employee coverage, *health savings accounts* (HSAs), and *defined contribution plans*.

Each of these forms of cost containment will be discussed in depth in a later chapter on health care reform. However, a brief explanation of each is in order at this point to round out the understanding of the private insurance market. As noted previously, reductions in employer-based coverage have primarily shown up in the reduced tendency of many (particularly small) employers to offer dependent coverage and the simultaneous decline in the proportion of employers providing health insurance as a benefit (Kaiser Foundation, 2004). Health savings account plans have two parts, a conventional health insurance plan with a high deductible and a tax sheltered savings account that is dedicated to an array of Internal Revenue Service (IRS) approved health care expenditures. This insurance approach works as a mechanism of utilization and cost containment because the worker has a financial incentive to avoid unnecessary health care expenditures: under IRS rules funds not spent for health care in qualified HSA accounts are retained by the worker. While this approach has some distinct advantages with respect to the management of moral hazard as well as exercise of individual preferences for health care, it also introduces a significant adverse selection problem to the extent that healthier employees abandon conventional health insurance plans for HSAs.[20] The third "non-managed care" approach to health insurance cost containment, defined contribution plans (DCPs), vary in structure but commonly limit upfront the employer's overall contribution to the cost of employee health insurance by either (a) specifying a set contribution toward the

---

[20] It should be intuitively clear that HSAs have high potential to "cream off" or favorably select healthier workers, thus raising the average level of insurance risk and costs to workers left in other plans. Since health is highly correlated with SES, it is widely believed that over time the increased prevalence of HSAs will contribute further to the social stratification of health care.

purchase of an array of employer-approved health insurance plans or (b) setting up an employer sponsored HSA that is linked to a high deductible policy (Christianson, Parente, & Taylor, 2002). In the Kaiser Foundation's 2004 survey of employer health benefits, one-quarter of small employers and one-half of the largest employers surveyed anticipate they will offer a DCP form of health insurance coverage within the next 2 years (Kaiser Foundation 2004, p. 66).

Regulation of the Employment-Based System

Extensive regulation of the employer-based health insurance system takes place at both the state and the federal level. At the federal level, regulation largely comes through the tax code and three omnibus acts of legislation, the Employee Retirement and Income Security Act of 1974 (ERISA), the Consolidated Omnibus Budget Reconciliation Act of 1985 (COBRA), and the Health Insurance Portability and Accountability Act of 1996 (HIPAA). At the state level, regulation occurs through the oversight of state insurance commissioners and state laws that govern insurance industry practices. State insurance commissioners serve as advocates for insurance consumers and to some extent as mediators between the interests of the public and the interests of the insurance industry. Insurance commissioners also function as the state government's official expert on various insurance markets within their respective states. Although state legislatures vary greatly in the extent to which they aggressively regulate the health insurance industry and pursue reform (Xirasagar et al., 2004), they play a central role in setting the basic conditions for participation of insurers in the state insurance market; conditions that generally include the array of required benefits, requirements of disclosure of costs and limitations in coverage, and procedures for the adjudication of insurance claim disputes. However, states do not have carte blanche in the governance of the local health insurance industry. In fact, there are very key limitations imposed by the federal government through ERISA that have been used to "eviscerate state attempts to regulate both health care financing and health care delivery" (Chirba-Martin & Brennan, 1994, p. 152).

As originally conceived, the Employee Retirement and Income Security Act of 1974 (ERISA) was intended to protect employee pension and benefits plans from abuses by employers and pension and benefits plans administrators and fiscal managers (Chirba-Martin & Brennan, 1994). As pointed out previously, ERISA was also designed to protect workers from employer discrimination on the basis of benefit utilization. In order to assure that workers in different states enjoyed uniform protections against pension and benefit plan abuses and pension and benefit plan underwriters could operate across state lines without encountering different rules pertaining to the protection of workers or management of benefits, ERISA was passed with provisions that preclude states from imposing regulations on pension and benefit plans that fall under ERISA regulation—a preclusion that extends to self-insured health care benefit plans. In effect, these provisions of ERISA undermine the capacity of states to reform their local employer-based health insurance markets and moreover, promote segmentation of employer-based health insurance coverage and benefits. Although the details are complex, employers can avoid a wide array of state regulations aimed at enhancing or even protecting minimum health insurance coverage protections because self-insured plans are sheltered under ERISA from state level health care reforms. Because of the favorable treatment of self-insuring employers under ERISA, employers that are in the best position to self-insure (in essence large employers with a healthier work force) exit the conventional health insurance market—thus deepening the adverse selection problem among small employers. ERISA has also been used by opponents of state level health care reform efforts to block the implantation of employer mandates, the development of state-sponsored strategies to cross-subsidize the benefit costs of workers confined to high risk insurance pools, and even regulate key aspects of the way HMOs and PPOs do business (Chirba-Martin & Brennan, 1994, p. 152). Under ERISA, the segment of the health insurance market comprised of larger self-insuring employers is sheltered from the central features of state level health insurance regulation (consumer protection, coverage provisions, and minimum benefits) that applies to all other health care benefit plans—without the reciprocal oversight of equally relevant federal regulations (Hall, 2000). Thus reform of ERISA is ultimately essential to any significant progress health care reform, whether initiated by states or at the national level.

In contrast to ERISA, the health insurance regulations spelled out in the Health Insurance Portability and Accountability Act of 1996 (HIPAA) primarily affect the segments of the health insurance markets that are unable or unwilling to self-insure (Hall, 2000). The insurance regulation provisions of HIPAA added a new title to the Public Health Service Act that essentially complemented and made more uniform various insurance market reforms that had been undertaken at the state level in the early 1990s (Hall, 2000). Included in these reform provisions are guarantees of the availability of coverage for small employers, the ability to renew coverage for both small and large employer groups, limitations on preexisting condition exclusion periods, and prohibitions against discrimination against individual insurance participants based on health status (CMS, 2004b).

Like most budget bills, the Consolidated Omnibus Budget Reconciliation Act of 1985 (COBRA) contains a wide array of provisions affecting multiple sectors of the government and economy. The health care provisions in COBRA[21] that directly affect the health care insurance market provide protections for workers and dependents against losing health care insurance coverage through such events as loss of employment, divorce, bankruptcy, and even reduction in work hours below the maximum required for inclusion in employment coverage (Cabral, 2003). Under COBRA regulations, the worker or dependent that loses eligibility for coverage under the group plan of a private or public employer is allowed the option of continuing the coverage for a specified period (that ranges from 18 to 36 months depending on a variety of specifics) at a cost that is no more than 102% of the full premium cost.[22] The critical protection that COBRA provides is the ability of the worker or affected dependent to extend the advantages of the group insurance rate for a period that is often sufficient to gain other health insurance coverage, such as through reemployment.

AN OVERVIEW OF HEALTH CARE SYSTEM FINANCE PART II: PUBLIC FINANCING OF HEALTH CARE

Approximately 45% of health care expenditures in the United States are publicly funded, and as explained at the beginning of the chapter, the largest proportion of public funding of health care is through two programs: Medicare (17.5% of all expenditures) and Medicaid (16.6% of all expenditures) (Smith et al., 2005). In addition, a large share of public health care expenditures occur through the Veterans Administration health care system—about $20 billion annually (Hadley & Holahan, 2003). Of all public programs, Medicare has by far been the most influential in building the infrastructure of the health care system and currently enjoys the most political support. As noted in chapter 2 on the history of the U.S. health care system, Medicare has also been the most inflationary of all public health care programs. For all of these reasons, Medicare will be the first of the three major public finance programs to be described.

---

[21] COBRA also has provisions that impose serious sanctions on health care facilities that transfer indigent or underinsured patients for reasons that appear to be financial. In the jargon of hospitals this is referred to as "patient dumping."

[22] The full premium cost under COBRA refers to the sum of both the employer and the employee contribution.

The Basics of Medicare

Medicare and Medicaid were jointly enacted by the U.S. Congress in 1965, with Medicare designed as a health insurance program for persons ages 65 and older and Medicaid designed as a state and federal partnership to fund health care for the poor. The enactment of Medicare was seen by many advocates and opponents of a federally sponsored system of universal health insurance as an intermediate step toward a system of universal entitlement to health care, and on that basis the profession of medicine vigorously resisted Medicare's creation (Starr, 1982). In order to counter this resistance, the Medicare program as originally structured lacked any mechanisms of cost control, and left the discretion of what was medically necessary to the judgment of medical providers that were being paid on a noncompetitive, fee-for-service basis. Although effective cost control mechanisms were introduced in the early 1980s that for a time reined in runaway hospital care expenditures,[23] the fee-for-service system of reimbursement for physician providers remains the cornerstone of Medicare's approach to medical provider reimbursement.

Currently Medicare covers approximately 42 million Americans, of whom 85% qualify under old-age entitlement, 14% qualify on the basis of disability, and just under 1% on the basis of the end-stage renal disease eligibility criteria (CMS, 2005; Office of Research Development and Information, 2002). Although the ratio between Medicare enrollees that qualify under age and disability criteria are expected to remain stable over the coming decades, the actual enrollment of Medicare beneficiaries is expected to expand to 77 million Americans by the year 2030 under current eligibility criteria (ORDI, 2002, Section III.B.1, p. 4). This growth trend in enrollment is projected to place the Medicare Hospital Insurance Trust Fund (Medicare Part A) in financial insolvency by the year 2018 (CMS, 2005), which actually precedes by many years the projected insolvency of the Social Security retirement trust fund. The second major component of the Medicare program that covers physician services (Medicare Part B) is also presenting a major fiscal challenge because its ever-increasing bite on general tax revenues (CMS, 2005). There are a

---

[23] The central feature of this cost control legislation was the Prospective Payment System (PPS) to hospitals, which changed hospitals from an inherently inflationary fee-for-service form of reimbursement to a system of reimbursement based on a patient's assignment to any one of roughly 450 Diagnosis Related Groups (DRGs). DRGs are categories of patient characteristics that include such factors as discharge, diagnosis, sex, age, complicating conditions, and procedures performed. The fact that reimbursement is based on a DRG rather than the number of days of hospital care provided, procedures performed, or services used reduces the incentives of doctors and hospitals to provide unnecessary or unbeneficial care.

number of proposals on the table averting this financial crisis, including transforming Medicare from a defined benefit program to a defined contribution program or imposing an annual global budget with mandatory spending caps similar to the cost control policies of other OECD countries with universal health insurance programs (Marmor & Oberlander, 1998).[24] These issues are discussed in more depth at a later point in this chapter.

Medicare is a highly complex program that links together different parts (A, B, C, and D) with various levels of coverage for hospital care, physician's services, outpatient diagnostic and therapy services, nursing home care, home health care, and most recently outpatient prescription drugs. In place of an tedious narrative, Table 3.4 provides a general overview of the essentials. Although Table 3.4 serves well as a general reference for the Medicare program's main features, it is not an exhaustive guide to all current benefits and eligibility criteria.

What Medicare Doesn't Cover: Gaps in Coverage and the Role of Supplemental Insurance

Even with the addition of limited coverage for prescription drugs in 2006, it should be apparent from Table 3.4 that the out-of-pocket hospital deductibles and coinsurance requirements under Part A and the high levels of coinsurance under Part B leave any Medicare beneficiary with a severe acute illness or chronic illness in serious financial jeopardy, even leaving aside such uncovered services as dental care. In fact, the Medicare program covers slightly less than one-half of all the health care expenditures of Medicare beneficiaries (KFF, 2005). For this reason, most Medicare program beneficiaries either directly purchase supplemental insurance or receive coverage as a part of their employer's retiree benefit package and a minority of the poorest elderly (14%) qualify for Medicaid assistance for expenses that are not covered by Medicare (KFF, 2005).

Supplemental insurance for Medicare (so-called Medicap insurance) varies substantially in premium prices and in coverage. Since the reforms enacted by the Omnibus Budget Reconciliation Act (OBRA) of 1990, Medigap insurance policies that are sold to Medicare recipients are required to conform to any one of 10 standardized benefit packages and (in contrast to the abusive insurance industry practices prior to OBRA 1990) insurance companies are not permitted to sell duplicate policies or engage in a variety of other unethical marketing practices. Low-end Medigap policies cover only a part of Medicare Part A coinsurance costs,

---

[24] The leading contenders among Medicare reform alternatives will be discussed in greater depth in a later chapter devoted to the general topic of health care system reform.

Table 3.4 Overview of Medicare Program Services, Coverage, and Eligibility Criteria

---

Medicare Part A–The Hospital Insurance Program

Financing: Provider's payments and expenditures are drawn from a trust fund created by a 2.9% tax on earnings, paid in equal parts by employer and employee.

Program Eligibility Criteria: Persons ages 65 and older who are otherwise eligible for Social Security Old-Age and Survivors Insurance (OASI) benefits, persons under age 65 who have received Social Security Disability Insurance payments for 2 years, and persons with end-stage renal disease.

The applicable coverage period for Part A benefits is defined as a "spell of illness," which begins at the point the beneficiary enters hospital care and ends at the point the person has been out of the hospital or skilled nursing facility for 60 days.[a]

Services	Scope of Coverage[b]	Coverage Eligibility Criteria
Hospital Care	100% after a $912 deductible for hospital stays of 1–60 days. All but $228 per day in days 61–90 of a hospital stay. All but $456 per day for days 91–150 of a hospital stay.	Hospital admissions certified by the hospital utilization review committee as "medically necessary" under Medicare program criteria for acute care.
Skilled Nursing Facility Care	Nothing for the first 20 days. $114 per day for days 21–100.	Care in Medicare certified Skilled Nursing Facility that is certified as skilled, "non-custodial" care.
Home Health Care	100% of "part-time or intermittent skilled nursing or home health aide services" and/or specific therapies (physical, occupational, speech) 20% of the Medicare-approved amount for durable medical equipment.	Plan of care signed by physician Beneficiary must be "home-bound" meaning unable to leave home without considerable effort and assistance. Need for intermittent skilled nursing care or specific therapies (physical, occupational, or speech)

Table 3.4   (*Continued*)

Services	Scope of Coverage[b]	Coverage Eligibility Criteria
Hospice Care	In general, 100% of in-home hospice services and in-patient hospice services where determined medically necessary or for purposes of caregiver respite. There is a $5 copayment for outpatient prescription drugs.	Physician certification that the beneficiary is suffering from a terminal illness and the beneficiary's acceptance of hospice care.

Medicare Part B–The Medical Insurance Program

Financing: 25% of the estimated Part B insurance premium actuarial cost is deducted from the OASI recipient's Social Security benefit ($78.20 in 2005), and the balance is financed from general tax revenues.

Program Eligibility Criteria: Predicated on eligibility for Medicare Part A plus voluntary enrollment in the Part B premium cost deduction option.

Services	Scope of Coverage	Coverage Eligibility Criteria
Physician Services	80% of approved charges after $100 deductible for Part B services and supplies	Based on physician order.
Rehabilitative Therapies[d]	As above	As above
Diagnostic Tests/Procedures	As above	As above
Durable Medical Equipment	Varies by type of equipment	As above
Preventative Care	80–100% of approved charges	As above, some exceptions

Medicare Part C–Medicare Advantage Plans

Financing: Medicare "Advantage Plans" (prior to 2005 referred to Medicare + Choice options) combine the funds from Medicare Part A and Part B into an array of coverage alternatives to the traditional Medicare fee-for-service program. These options include Medicare sponsored HMOs, Preferred Provider Organizations (PPOs), Provider Sponsored Organization's (PSOs), alternative private fee-for-service (PFFS) plans, Medical Savings Account (MSAs) and specialty plans (e.g., special disease management plans). Medicare Advantage plans are essentially local (county and regional level) health care plans that contract with the Medicare program (CMS) on a capitated basis to provide the equivalent of Medicare Parts A and B services to enrolled beneficiaries. Differences between Medicare payments to such plans and the costs of services provided are returned to the plan enrollees in the form of additional benefits, lower Part B premiums, and/or lower copayments.

(*continued*)

Table 3.4 (*Continued*)

Program Eligibility Criteria: Predicated on eligibility for Medicare Part A, plus voluntary enrollment in the Part B premium cost deduction option, plus voluntary enrollment in a locally available Medicare Advantage plan.

Services	Scope of Coverage	Coverage Eligibility Criteria
At minimum the equivalent of Medicare Parts A and B	Typically at minimum the equivalent of Parts A and B, with enhanced coverage (e.g., outpatient prescription drugs or reduced co-payments) a component of some plans.	Medicare Part C plans that are managed care plans (HMOs, PPOs, PSOs and specialty care plans) have similar eligibility criteria to traditional fee-for-service Medicare, but constrain the beneficiary's choice of providers to those within the plan network. In addition, such plans (like most managed care plans) impose restrictions on access to specialty care and services.

Medicare Part D–Outpatient Drug Benefit (Beginning 2006)

Financing: Medicare Part D is financed through a combination of drug coverage premiums paid directly by Medicare program beneficiaries to prescription drug insurance plans, premium subsidies from general tax revenues, and fund transfers from states for coverage costs of former Medicaid program enrollees.[f] Medicare beneficiaries either pay premiums to private plans that contract with Medicare to provide the Part D prescription drug benefit, or they are able to enroll in Medicare Part C (Medicare Advantage) plans that are enhanced with a prescription drug benefit.

Program Eligibility Criteria: Predicated on eligibility for Part A, plus voluntary enrollment in Medicare Part D program.

Services	Scope of Coverage	Coverage Eligibility Criteria
Outpatient prescription drug restrictions through subsidized and Medicare approved private sector insurance plans.	75% annual prescription drug costs after a $250 deductible, to a cap of $2,250. Annual prescription drug costs in excess of $2,251 are excluded from coverage, until out-of-pocket costs reach $3,600.	Enrollment is required during the "initial enrollment" period (November 15, 2005 through May 15, 2006) to lock-in the initial premium costs to beneficiaries. Enrolled beneficiaries will be required to pay a monthly premium (estimated average of $37.37 for 2006).[g]

Table 3.4 (*Continued*)

Services	Scope of Coverage	Coverage Eligibility Criteria
Approved plans can employ formularies and tiered cost sharing, but must provide at least two drugs within each therapeutic class of drugs.	When out of pocket costs reach $3,600 in any year, 95% of prescription drug costs for the balance of the calendar year.	

[a]It is possible for Medicare beneficiaries to exhaust their benefits during a single spell of illness and not be eligible again unless and until their care has been able to be sustained outside of a hospital or skilled nursing facility for at least 60 days. Such instances are rare but they do occur, e.g. a case of severe burns and multiple skin grafting surgeries that requires more than 150 continuous days of hospital care.

[b]The deductible amounts and benefit coverage limits are those that were in effect for 2005, recent updates can be obtained at the CMS website: www.medicare.gov/publications.

[c]Medicare does not provide coverage for ordinary or custodial nursing home care. This is a limitation that is often confusing to consumers because state licensing regulations can identify nursing homes as "skilled nursing facilities" despite the "custodial" level of care being provided under Medicare program criteria.

[d]Including but not limited to physical therapy, occupational therapy and speech therapy, although coverage can vary by the type of rehabilitative therapy.

[e]The past 15 years have seen an enormous volatility in the demand for alternatives to traditional Medicare among beneficiaries, the availability of non-traditional Medicare options in various parts of the country, and the solvency of plans.

[f]According to recent CMS estimates (CMS 2005), during the first five years of the Medicare Part D benefit program 11.3% of the program's expenditures will be funded through beneficiary premium payments, 77.6% through general tax revenues, and 11.1% through transfers from states for coverage of Medicaid eligible clients that will qualify for Medicare Part D. Given the history of wildly incorrect estimates of the Medicare Part D programs costs, it is difficult to argue for a great deal of confidence in these projections.

[g]This is the estimated average premium provided by the *2005 Annual Report of the Boards of Trustees of the Federal Hospital Insurance and Federal Supplementary Medical Insurance Trust Funds* (see CMS 2005, Table V.C2.—SMI Cost Sharing and Premium Amounts). This report projects a premium price increase to Medicare beneficiaries that participate in the Part D option that is in excess of 70% by the year 2014.

while high-end Medigap benefit packages include an array of protections including coverage of Medicare Part A and B coinsurance costs, coverage of medical expenses during foreign travel, preventative medical care and generous prescription drug benefits (Fox, Snyder, & Rice, 2003). Other factors that go in to the prices of Medigap premiums include the Medicare recipients' age, gender, and geographic location and whether the Medicap policy is part of a group or an individual coverage plan.[25] Although the

[25] According to the Henry J. Kaiser Foundation's 2004 Survey in Retiree Health Benefits, the average health insurance premium costs per Medicare eligible recipient at the point of retirement was $262 per month (Kaiser Family Foundation and Hewitt Associates, 2004).

enactment of the Medicare Part D drug benefit will eliminate high-end Medigap policies that include coverage for prescription drugs, there will still be a need for medium and lower-end Medigap policies that provide protections for the gaps in Medicare coverage represented in deductibles and other coinsurance costs.

The Medicare Funding Crisis and Alternatives to Medicare Reform

As of 2006, the expenditures of the Medicare Hospital Insurance Trust fund (Medicare Part A) were above revenues, leading a trend of deficits that are projected to exhaust the trust fund's assets by the year 2018 (Social Security and Medicare Boards of Trustees, 2006). In addition, the other major Medicare benefit programs, both the voluntary Supplementary Medical Insurance Program (Medicare Part B) that pays for physician services and outpatient diagnostic services and the new prescription drug benefit program (Medicare Part D) are projected to require substantial increases over time, such as financing from general tax revenues and beneficiary premium charges (Social Security and Medicare Boards of Trustees, 2006). There are a variety of factors that converged to create this crisis, but most are tied to health care inflationary pressures arising from both advancements in health care technology and the growing population of Medicare beneficiaries—especially those in the medically intensive advanced years of aging. Congress and successive presidential administrations have delayed taking more than incremental actions on the so-called "impending Medicare funding crisis" for years, and now the word "impending" must in all honesty be dropped from the phrase. The Medicare funding crisis has arrived.

Medicare Reform Options. At this point, there are six general policy alternatives that have either been implemented to a limited extent or at least seriously debated. These policy alternatives include:

1. Creating incentives to move Medicare beneficiaries out of the inherently inflationary traditional fee-for-service program to Medicare benefit options that either entail managed care or health savings account plans that encourage selective use of health care.
2. Unilaterally reducing payments to physicians and hospitals.
3. Raising beneficiary co-payments and premiums.
4. Reducing the scope of Medicare program coverage.
5. Raising Medicare Trust Fund payroll taxes.
6. Transforming Medicare from a defined benefit to a defined contribution program.

The policy alternatives that don't involve draconian cuts to hospitals and physicians entail strategies that either the elderly or younger wage earners thus far have balked at.

The first alternative is the basis of the much touted "Medicare Advantage Plan" options, which prior to 2005 were referred to Medicare + Choice options. Although the central intent of these plan options was move both high- and low-cost Medicare beneficiaries into less inflationary Medicare benefit plans, the Medicare options plans have been plagued with enrollment difficulties and unintended policy consequences, including the excessive complexity of plan options and the confusion created among the elderly, the tendency of Medicare private plans to attract healthier, lower-cost beneficiaries, extreme geographic variations in plan options, and significant instabilities in benefits, out-of-pocket costs, and provider participation (Biles, Dallek, & Nicholas, 2004). Efforts to implement the second alternative, reducing payments to providers, have provoked a political firestorm from hospitals and physician groups that for the foreseeable make this alternative unviable. Both alternatives (3) and (4) thus far have proved equally politically unviable, particularly in the current highly polarized Congress where each party vies to be viewed as the true guardian of Medicare entitlements. Alternative (5), raising Medicare payroll taxes, is equally alienating to the under-50 age group of wage earners—an alternative that neither major political party is likely to risk in the foreseeable future. Finally, because alternative (6) fundamentally alters the nature of the Medicare social contract (from benefit entitlement to a defined contribution), it encounters a politically formidable coalition of elderly and progressive wing Democrats. These political realities not withstanding, Congress will eventually have to converge on a compromise that the various key stakeholders in Medicare (elderly, wage-earners, providers) will have to live with.

A notable new direction for Medicare reform has been suggested by health policy scholar Edward Lawlor,[26] in his (2003) *Redesigning the Medicare Contract* (University of Chicago Press). In essence, Lawlor suggests that the design and purpose of the Medicare bureaucracy be reframed in accordance with agency theory, a well-established paradigm in economics that resolves a number of thorny issues pertaining to the mediation of public goals and stakeholder incentives. Briefly stated, Lawlor argues that the Medicare bureaucracy should function as an agent of two

[26] Edward Lawlor is founding editor of the *Public Policy and Aging Report*. He has served as Dean of School of Social Service Administration, Director of the Center for Health Administration Studies, and Professor of Public Policy at the Irving B. Harris Graduate School of Public Policy Studies, all at the University of Chicago.

principals: the broad public citizenry and Medicare program beneficiaries. For the broad public, the Medicare bureaucracy is charged with the
task of representing the public's intent that the elderly be offered an entitlement program that meets certain goals encompassing cost, quality,
and outcomes. For the Medicare beneficiaries, the agency obligations entail ensuring that there is adequate access to health care through a range
of health care contracts that meet evaluative criteria pertaining to process and outcome. Thus, the central task of the Medicare bureaucracy
is to represent both principals (the broad public and Medicare beneficiaries) in the negotiating and monitoring of an array of health care contracts with health care providers (Lawlor, 2003). Reframed in this way,
Congress is removed from its frequently duplicitous role as pseudo agent
for the public and de facto agent for Medicare health care providers, and
is constrained instead to return to its constitutionally intended function
as the deliberative body for the formulation and enactment of demo-
cratically determined health care policy. While the arguments and policy
variations offered in Lawlor's book are complex, the central idea is a re-
freshing and provocative departure from the prior directions in Medicare
reform that have thus far led the Medicare Trust Fund to the edge of
bankruptcy.

The Basics of Medicaid

As originally designed, Medicaid was a state and federal partnership to
meet the costs incurred in providing health care for the poor. Essentially,
Medicaid functions as a federal program that is administered by states
under a strict set of rules pertaining to state participation in funding, eligible recipients, and covered services. Depending on the state's per capita
income, the federal share of Medicaid program expenditures range from
a statutory minimum of 50 percent to a maximum of 83 percent. In fiscal year 2004, the average federal share of Medicaid expenditures was
60.2 percent (CMS, 2004a). At the time that Medicaid was enacted into
law (1965), other sources for funding health care for the poor existed
through such sources as the Hill–Burton program[27] and widespread use
of cost-shifting mechanisms that allowed hospitals to recover uncompensated care costs through higher prices to privately insured patients. In the
decades since, however, Medicaid has evolved to a program that is the
principal source of care for both the low-income recipients and also

[27] The Hill–Burton Act, previously discussed in chapter 2 on the history of the U.S. health
care system, is a federal program which requires "obligated facilities" (health care facilities
including hospitals) that have used federal money for facility reconstruction or modernization to provide free or low cost health care services to local medically indigent patients.

the largest single source of funding for elderly in need of nursing home care.

Although various modifications and expansions of the Medicaid program coverage have occurred over the 40 years of its existence, the key expansions in recent years have targeted low-income children. Since the Omnibus Budget Reconciliation Act of 1990, Medicaid has expanded its mandatory coverage to children under age 5 in families with income at or below 133% of the federal poverty level and to older children living in families with income at or below 100% of the poverty level. In order to expand Medicaid eligibility further plus allow states some flexible alternatives to the funding of health care for children, in 1997 Congress enacted the State Children's Health Insurance Program (SCHIP). SCHIP is essentially a block grant program that provides an enhanced federal match to state expenditures on Medicaid and other forms of state-subsidized health insurance coverage for children. The most important feature of the SCHIP program is the capacity of states to expand Medicaid and other vehicles for publicly subsidized health insurance to children in families with income in excess of 200% of the federal poverty level.[28] In contrast to the Medicaid program as a whole, the SCHIP program has enjoyed significant bipartisan support at both the state and federal levels, and most states appear to look for ways to expand SCHIP's enrollment as yearly economic circumstances allow (Hill, Courtot, & Sullivan, 2005). However, a significant barrier to SCHIPs enrollment of many eligible children in low-income families appears to be related to the stigma the program inherits through its close association with conventional Medicaid.

Unlike Medicare, Medicaid is a means-based program rather than a social insurance program that includes all gradients of wealth. In that sense the distinction between Medicaid and Medicare mirrors the differences between public assistance (Temporary Assistance to Needy Families) and Social Security. That is, Medicaid is politically a much less popular program and its recipients are burdened with program-based stigma.[29] Among health care providers, Medicaid recipients are generally regarded as dependents, whereas Medicare program participants are seen as beneficiaries. Despite these negative aspects of Medicaid, many of the provisions of Medicaid are significantly more expansive than Medicare. In

[28] A recent estimate of state SCHIP programs found that a nationally representative sample of states expanded SCHIP eligibility to an average family income threshold at 227% of the federal poverty line (see Hill et al. 2005).

[29] Some of this stigma is introduced directly through the means-based nature of Medicaid, but Medicaid also brings with it the twin disincentives of bureaucracy and low fees to providers—thus adding further impetus to the stigma experienced by Medicaid patients.

Mandatory Medicaid Services, Applicable to All States as a Condition of Medicaid Program Participation:

- Inpatient hospital services.
- Outpatient hospital services.
- Prenatal care.
- Vaccines for children.
- Physician services.
- Nursing facility services for persons aged 21 or older.
- Family planning services and supplies.
- Rural health clinic services.
- Home health care for persons eligible for skilled-nursing services.
- Laboratory and X-ray services.
- Pediatric and family nurse practitioner services.
- Nurse-midwife services.
- Federally qualified health-center (FQHC) services, and ambulatory services of an FQHC that would be available in other settings.
- Early and periodic screening, diagnostic, and treatment (EPSDT) services for children under age 21

Exemplars of Optional Medicaid Services, Determined by States but Qualified for the Federal Share of Medicaid Expenditures[a]:

- Diagnostic services.
- Intermediate care facilities for the mentally retarded (ICFs/MR).
- Prescribed drugs and prosthetic devices.
- Rehabilitation and physical therapy services.
- Home and community-based care to certain persons with chronic impairments.

[a] See *Medicaid: A Brief Summary* available at www.cms.hhs.gov/publications.

Figure 3.7   Mandatory and Optional Medicaid Services.

contrast to Medicare, Medicaid provides coverage for prescribed drugs, custodial nursing home care, and an array of in-home support services for low-income elderly and disabled. Figure 3.7 provides a general overview of Medicaid program eligibility criteria and services that are universal among states, and examples of optional eligibility criteria and services

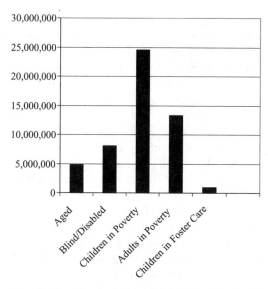

Figure 3.8 Number of Medicaid Beneficiaries by General Eligibility Status: FY 2002. (Source: *National MSIS Tables by State–2002*, Table 4-Medicaid Eligibles by Basis of Eligibility Centers for Medicaid and Medicare, last updated 2/14/2005.)

that states may add at their discretion. However, states must absorb as much as 50% of whatever Medicaid expenditures are incurred by more generous eligibility criteria and services—thus Medicaid programs differ widely from one state to the next depending on local economic resources and the prevailing political context.

There are abundant policy questions that surround the Medicaid program, most pertaining in one way or another to its sustainability as limited state resources are increasingly strained by competing demands and the costs of the Medicaid program escalate. Clearly though, Medicaid plays dual crucial roles in providing funds for health care to the most vulnerable segments of society, in particular children in poverty and the most fragile of the aged and disabled (see Figure 3.8). Further, Medicaid has been called upon to subsidize the failures of the employer-based insurance system to a degree that was never anticipated at the inception of the program in 1965. For example, during 2003 over 25 million children were enrolled in Medicaid, and the SCHIP program expanded coverage to an additional 4 million children (Kaiser Commission on Medicaid Facts, 2005). Although Medicaid and SCHIP have managed to increase health insurance coverage to just over 70% of uninsured children in families at or below 200% of the federal poverty level,[30] the problem of health care coverage for the parents in low income families remains unresolved. According to current Medicaid eligibility criteria, the far majority of low income parents (68%) that do not have insurance through an employer are also ineligible for Medicaid coverage (Families USA, 2004). While those affected by these dual failures of the employment-based system of health insurance and the public safety net are largely comprised of the working poor, the current political climate does not suggest there is sufficient commitment at either the state or the federal level to expand Medicaid eligibility as a fix. On the right side of the political spectrum, the reluctance to expand Medicaid coverage to more working poor adults arises in significant part from a belief that the solution lies with a fix of the employer-based system (e.g. subsidized premium vouchers) rather than further expansion of what is viewed as a wasteful, inefficient and increasingly expensive government welfare program. On the left side of the body politic, Medicaid is generally regarded as a poor stop-gap substitution for a publicly sponsored program of universal health care coverage. The tragedy of the Medicaid program is that it is both of these things, an issue that will be taken up in chapter 8 on health care reform.

The Department of Veterans Affairs Health Care System

The Department of Veterans Affairs health care system has it roots in the special obligations the U.S. government has historically assumed on behalf of its military veterans, beginning with those of the Revolutionary War. At various points in national history and typically at the conclusion of major wars, Congress has extended and enlarged upon special provisions and compensations created on behalf of the nation's veterans, including homes for aged and disabled veterans, veteran's pensions, survivor's benefits, special loan programs, educational benefits, and the provision of health care. The Department of Veterans Affairs (VA) health care systems beginning can be traced to an action by Congress in 1917 that amended the War Risk Insurance Act to include medical benefits to veterans with service-connected disabilities. In the World War Veterans Act of 1924, Congress expanded benefits to include hospital services to all war veterans. During this same period Congress also enacted laws that transferred several hospitals that had been a part of the U.S. Public Health Service to the Veterans Bureau—the early predecessor to the Department

---

[30] Estimate calculated from Figure 1 in *Health Coverage for Low-Income Children September 2004*, The Henry J. Kaiser Foundation. Menlo Park, CA.

of Veterans Affairs (Kizer, Demakis, & Feussner, 2000). Through various reorganizations and expansions, the VA health care system now operates a system of 163 hospitals, 859 clinics, and 134 nursing homes serving just over 4 million of the nation's 26 million veterans (Ashton et al., 2003; Department of Veterans Affairs, 2004a).[31] Throughout most of its history the VA health care system operated as a hospital-based system with a highly centralized and rigid bureaucracy. Since 1997, however, the VA system has been radically transformed from a hospital-based system with utilization-based financing to an enrollment-based system of 22 regional networks financed principally by capitation (Ashton et al., 2003). As such, the VA health care system exists as the only federally sponsored and operated system of comprehensive capitation-based care. Unlike the Medicare and Medicaid programs, both of which are primarily fee-based programs, the VA has the capacity to directly negotiate favorable pricing of drugs with the pharmaceutical industry.[32]

Although all veterans are eligible for enrollment in the VA health care system, eligibility for care in the system is determined by the year-by-year balance between utilization and congressional appropriations, and the veteran's standing in a system of prioritized eligibility criteria. The only veterans that are automatically eligible for VA system care are those that have an established service-connected disability that is rated as at least 50% disabling, or veterans that have been recently discharged from military service with a service-connected disability that has not as yet been rated. Other higher priority groups for VA care includes veterans with service-connected disabilities that are rated as 30 to 40% disabling, former POWs, and recipients of the Purple Heart.[33] The VA health care system's eligibility criteria also include a means-based qualifier for low-income veterans that do not have a service-connected disability— as it happens an eligibility criterion that has proved critical to countless veterans.

Aside from the VA health care system's central mission to provide health care to disabled veterans and its role as a health care safety net

---

[31] These VA system utilization statistics are from FY 2002, prior to the enrollment of veterans of the Iraq War. As of mid-year 2005, there is a significant partisan debate raging on the effect of the Iraq War on the VA health care system utilization. As a matter of historical irony, the major party that has been the most critical of the war (the Democratic Party) has been the party advocating for an expanded VA budget for the health care of Iraq War veterans.

[32] At the behest of the powerful pharmaceutical industry lobby, the "Medicare Prescription Drug, Improvement and Modernization Act," passed by Congress in 2003, precludes the Medicare program using purchasing power to negotiate more favorable drug pricing.

[33] A complete listing of the VA system's eight-level priority system can be accessed at http://www.va.gov/healtheligibility/eligibility.

for low-income veterans, the VA health care system supports an extensive array of medical school residency programs and has long been on the cutting edge of research on trauma, substance abuse, mental illness, and aging. More recently the VA has made significant inroads in the development of health care system quality assessment and improvement methods that are both innovative and applicable to the improvement of health care quality among nongovernmental health care systems (Kizer et al., 2000). Although evidence of the benefits of military service on lifetime earnings and education is mixed and appears to differ significantly by historical period (Teachman, 2005), there is little question that the VA health care system plays a critical role as the health care safety net for low-income veterans. In fiscal year 2002, the low-income veterans without a service-connected disability accounted for 36% of VA health care system expenditures—a proportion of expenditures that was actually larger than expenditures for service-connected veterans (Department of Veterans Affairs, 2004b). In other words, in a very real sense the VA health care system functions as much as a safety net for the poor as it does as a health care system for those disabled during military service.

Federally Funded Community Health Centers

Though small relative to Medicare, Medicaid, and the VA health care system, federally funded Community Health Centers (CHCs) serve as a critical safety net provider in low-income communities. CHCs are a diverse group of not-for-profit and public health care clinics that are federally funded under provisions of the Public Health Service Act to provide an array of primary health care services to low income and medically underserved communities.[34] The essential elements that are required of all CHCs as a condition of federal funding include location in a high-need community, the provision of comprehensive primary care services, availability of transportation and language translation services that promote access to health care, a community- and consumer-based governance structure, and fees that are adjusted for patients' ability to pay (HRSA, 2005a). Despite an infinitesimal annual budget (by federal standards) of under $2 billion, during fiscal year 2005 the Health Resources and Services Administration estimates that 15 million uninsured and underserved individuals will receive primary care through 3,800 CHCs (HRSA, 2005b).

---

[34] Section 330 of the Public Health Service (PHS) Act, as amended by the Health Centers Consolidated Act of 1996 (P.L. 104-299) and the Safety Net Amendments of 2002.

CONCLUDING COMMENTS—THE LARGE PRESENCE OF PUBLIC DOLLARS IN THE FINANCING OF HEALTH CARE

The public role in the financing and provision of health care is not limited to direct care. Public health expenditures exceed $50 billion annually (Smith et al., 2005), the brunt of it going to research and training of the health professions. For example, in the 2004 fiscal year, the National Institutes of Health and its subordinate agencies (e.g., the National Institute of Mental Health, National Institute on Drug Abuse, the National Institute on Aging) were appropriated $27.9 billion—most of these funds for basic and applied research on health and health care. During the same recent fiscal year the Centers for Disease Control and Prevention, another key destination of public health expenditures, was appropriated $6.9 billion (CDC, 2005). These expenditures underscore further the reality that the U.S. health care system, at least in its system of finance, is as much a public system of health care as a private one. The next chapter, which addresses the organization of health care services, will further illustrate the private/public interdependence that characterizes the U.S. health care system.

REFERENCES

Altman, D. E., & Levitt, L. (2002). The sad history of health care cost containment as told in one chart. *Health Affairs (W-2)*, 83.

Anderson, G., & Poullier, J. (1999). Health spending, access, and outcomes: trends in industrialized countries. *Health Affairs, 18*(3), 178–192.

Anderson, G. F., Reinhardt, U. E., Hussey, P. S., & Petrosyan, V. (2003). It's the prices, stupid: Why the United States is so different from other countries. *Health Affairs, 22*(1), 90–105.

Ashton, C. M., Souchek, J., Petersen, N. J., Menke, T. J., Collins, T. C., Kizer, K. W., et al. (2003). Hospital use and survival among Veterans Affairs beneficiaries. *New England Journal of Medicine, 349*(17), 1637–1646.

Baily, M. A. (2003). Managed care organizations and the rationing problem. *The Hastings Center Report, 33*(1), 34–42.

Battistella, R., Burchfield, D., & Fitzgerald, J. W. (2000). The future of employment-based health insurance. *Journal of Healthcare Management, 45*(1), 46–55.

Biles, B., Dallek, G., & Nicholas, L. H. (2004). Medicare Advantage: Déjà vu all over again? *Health Affairs (W-4)*, 586–697.

Cabral, A. B. (2003). COBRA for state and local governmental plans. *Employee Benefits Journal, 28*(4), 34–38.

CDC. (2005, February 2). *FY 2005 CDC budget request—Detail of increases/decreases financial management office.* Retrieved July 1, 2005, from http://www.cdc.gov/fmo/fmofybudget.htm

Chirba-Martin, M. A., & Brennan, T. A. (1994). The critical role of ERISA in state health reform. *Health Affairs, 13*(2), 142–156.

Christianson, J. B., Parente, S. T., & Taylor, R. (2002). Defined-contribution health insurance products: Development and prospects. *Health Affairs, 21*(1), 49–64.

CMS. (2004a, December 3, 2004). *Medicaid: A brief summary.* Retrieved June 28, 2005, from http://www.cms.hhs.gov/publications/overview-medicare-medicaid/default4.asp

CMS. (2004b). *Requirements for the group health insurance market; non-federal governmental plans exempt from HIPAA Title I requirements. Final rule.* Washington, DC: Centers for Medicare & Medicaid Services (CMS), HHS.

CMS. (2005). *2005 Annual Report of the Boards of Trustees of the Federal Hospital Insurance and Federal Supplementary Medical Insurance Trust Funds.* Washington, DC: Centers for Medicare and Medicaid Services.

Conwell, L. J. (2002). *The role of health insurance brokers: Providing small employers with a helping hand (No. 57).* Washington DC: Center for Studying Health Policy Change.

Department of Veterans Affairs. (2004a, March 26). *Program statistics: FY 2002 Annual accountability report statistical appendix Table 1.* Retrieved July 1, 2005, from http://www.va.gov/vetdata/ProgramStatics/index.htm.

Department of Veterans Affairs. (2004b, March 26). *Program statistics: FY 2002 Annual accountability report statistical appendix Table 10.* Retrieved July 1, 2005, from http://www.va.gov/vetdata/ProgramStatics/index.htm

Dickens, W. T., & Lang, K. (1992). *Labor market segmentation theory: Reconsidering the evidence.* Unpublished manuscript, Cambridge, MA.

Doran, P. A., Dobson, R. H., & Harris, R. G. (2001). *Financial management of health insurance: Forecasting, monitoring and analyzing health plan experience*: Seattle, WA: Milliman USA.

EBRI. (2005). *What do workers and employers pay for employment-based coverage?* Retrieved June 13, from http://www.ebri.org/benfaq/hlthfaq6.htm.

Families USA. (2004). *Working without a net: The health care safety net still leaves millions of low-income workers uninsured.* Washington DC.

Forrest, C. B., Weiner, J. P., Fowles, J., Vogeli, C., Frick, K. D., Lemke, K. W., et al. (2001). Self-referral in point-of-service health plans. *JAMA, 285*(17), 2223–2231.

Fox, P. D., Snyder, R. E., & Rice, T. (2003). Medigap reform legislation of 1990: A 10-year review. *Health Care Financing Review, 24*(3), 121–137.

Fries, J. F., Koop, C. E., Beadle, C. E., Cooper, P. P., England, M. J., Greaves, R. F., et al. (1993). Reducing health care costs by reducing the need and demand for medical services. *N. Engl. J. Med., 329*(5), 321–325.

Fuchs, V. R. (2004). Perspective: More variation in use of care, more flat-of-the-curve medicine. *Health Affairs,* var. 104.

GAO. (2001). *Private health insurance: Small employers continue to face challenges in providing coverage-GAO-02-8*. Washington, DC: General Accounting Office.

Grumbach, K., Coffman, J., Vranizan, K., Blick, N., & O'Neil, E. H. (1998). Independent practice association physician groups in California. *Health Affairs*, *17*(3), 227–237.

Guest, A., Almgren, G., & Hussey, J. (1998). The ecology of race and socioeconomic distress: Infant and working-age mortality in Chicago. *Demography*, *35*(1), 23–35.

Hadley, J., & Holahan, J. (2003). How much medical care do the uninsured use, and who pays for it? *Health Affairs*, (W-3),66.

Hall, M. A. (2000). The geography of health insurance regulation. *Health Affairs*, *19*(2), 173–184.

Harrington, S., & Miller, T. (2002). Perspective: competitive markets for individual health insurance. *Health Affairs*, w2.359.

Hill, I., Courtot, B., & Sullivan, J. (2005). *Ebbing and flowing: Some gains, some losses as SCHIP responds to third year of budget pressure* (Series A, No. A-68,). Washington DC: The Urban Institute.

HRSA. (2005a). *Bureau of primary care: Community health centers*. Retrieved July 1, 2005, from http://bphc.hrsa.gov/chc/.

HRSA. (2005b). *FY 2005 budget in brief—Health Resources and Services Administration*. Retrieved July 1, 2005, from http://www.hhs.gov/budget/05budget.

Kaiser Commission on Medicaid Facts. (2005). *Enrolling uninsured low-income children in Medicaid and SCHIP*. Menlo Park, CA: The Henry J. Kaiser Family Foundation.

Kaiser Family Foundation and Hewitt Associates. (2004). *Kaiser/Hewitt 2004 Survey in retiree health benefits*. Menlo Park, CA: Henry J. Kaiser Family Foundation.

Kaiser Foundation. (2004). *Employer health benefits: 2004 summary of findings*. Menlo Park, CA: The Henry J. Kaiser Family Foundation.

KFF. (2005). *Medicare fact sheet: Medicare at a glance*: The Henry J. Kaiser Foundation.

Kizer, K., Demakis, J., & Feussner, J. (2000). Reinventing VA Health Care: Systematizing quality improvement and quality innovation [VA's Quality Enhancement Research Initiative]. *Medical Care, 38*(6 (Special Supp)), 7–16.

Lawlor, E. (2003). *Redesigning the Medicare contract: Politics, markets, and agency*. Chicago: University of Chicago Press.

Marmor, T., & Oberlander, J. (1998). Rethinking Medicare reform. *Health Affairs, 17*(1), 52–68.

Marquis, M. S., & Long, S. H. (2000). Who helps employers design their health insurance benefits? *Health Affairs, 19*(1), 133–138.

Mechanic, D. (2004). The rise and fall of managed care. *Journal of Health and Social Behavior, 45*(1), 76–86.

OECD. (2003). *Health at a glance: OECD indicators for 2003*. Paris, France: Organisation for Economic Co-Operation and Development.

OECD. (2004a). *Health data:*. Paris, France: Organisation for Economic

Co-Operation and Development. Table 11: Public expenditure on health, % total expenditure on health.

OECD. (2004b). *Health data.* Paris, France: Organisation for Economic Co-Operation and Development Table 10: Total expenditure on health, % GDP.

Office of Research Development and Information. (2002). *Program Information on Medicare, Medicaid, SCHIP, and other programs of the Centers for Medicare & Medicaid Services.* Washington, DC: Centers for Medicare and Medicaid Services.

Robinson, J. C. (1999). The future of managed care organization. *Health Affairs,* 18(2), 7–24.

Scott, F. A., Berger, M. C., & Black, D. A. (1989). Effects of the tax treatment of fringe benefits on labor market segmentation. *Industrial and Labor Relations Review,* 42(2), 216–229.

Smith, C., Cowan, C., Sensenig, A., & Catlin, A. (2005). Health spending growth slows in 2003. *Health Affairs,* 24(1), 185–194.

Social Security and Medicare Boards of Trustees. (2006). *Status of the Social Security and Medicare Programs: A summary of the 2006 annual reports.* Washington DC: Social Security Administration.

Starr, P. (1982). *The social transformation of American medicine.* New York: Basic Books.

Starr, P. (1992). *The logic of health care reform.* Knoxville, TN: Whittle Direct Books.

Teachman, J. (2005). Military service in the Vietnam era and educational attainment. *Sociology of Education,* 78(1), 50–69.

U.S. Census. (2005). *File 1. Interim State Projections of Population by Sex: July 1, 2004 to 2030.* Washington, DC: U.S. Census Bureau, Population Division,Projections Branch.

U. S. Court of Appeals Third Circuit. (2000). *DiFederico v. Rolm Company, 201 F.3d 200.*

U.S. Court of Appeals Eleventh Circuit. (1993). *Owens v. Storehouse, Inc.*

World Health Organization. (2005a). *Annex Table 6 national health accounts indicators: Measured levels of per capita expenditure on health, 1998–2002.* Geneva, Switzerland: World Health Organization.

World Health Organization. (2005b). *World Health 2005. Annex Table 1 Basic Indicators for All Member States.* Geneva, Switzerland: World Health Organization.

Xirasagar, S., Samuels, M., Stoskopf, C., Shrader, W., Hussey, J., Saunders, R., et al. (2004). Small group health insurance: Ranking the states on the depth of reform, 1999. *Journal of Health and Social Policy,* 19(1), 1–35.

CHAPTER FOUR

The Contemporary Organization of Health Care: Health Care Services and Utilization

THE MIXED PUBLIC /PRIVATE STRUCTURE OF THE U.S. HEALTH CARE SYSTEM

The U.S. health care system is a highly complex and often volatile mixture of free enterprise, philanthropy, and public sector health care. It is also the most expensive health care system in the world both in per capita dollars spent and in the proportion of national economic output spent on health care. The purpose of this chapter is to provide a general overview of the organizational structure of the U.S. health care system, in particular what the dollars allocated to health care purchase in terms of the facilities, services, technologies, and human resources that compose the resources of the health care system. Significant attention will also be devoted to the structure of the health care "safety net"—generally defined as the clinics, hospitals, and individual health care providers that care for a disproportionate share of the poor, the uninsured, those afflicted by stigmatizing health conditions, and persons otherwise isolated from the mainstream health care system.

A good beginning point to a general grasp of the organization of the U.S. health care system is a brief comparison between the U.S. health care system and the health care systems of other democracies with market economies. Undertaking even a very basic comparison yields some surprising findings. For example, although it is widely known that the United States allocates more of its economic output to health care than all other countries, the United States is significantly below the OECD[1] average in the hospital and physician resources available to provide health care to its citizens (see the first and final two columns of Table 4.1).

Another nonintuitive finding from the OECD comparisons pertains to pharmaceutical expenditures. Despite the escalating controversy that surrounds rising prescription drug prices in the United States and the pricing practices of the pharmaceutical industry, relative to all other OECD countries the *share* of the health care dollar spent on prescription drugs is actually below that of the OECD average. However, this comparison does not adjust for the large difference in the total dollars spent per capita on health care by U.S. citizens relative to all other OECD countries. When this is considered it is indeed the case that U.S. citizens *spend more dollars* on prescription drugs than citizens from the other OECD countries. This example illustrates the point that when considering how a health care system is organized, both the total amount of expenditures allocated to different parts of the health care system and the distribution of those expenditures should be taken into account.

More consistent with common perceptions of the U.S. health care system is the magnitude of the gap between the share of health care costs that are publicly financed in the United States and the publicly financed share in other countries. That is, only about 44 cents of the U.S. health care dollar comes from government programs like Medicare and Medicaid, while the OECD average is 72 cents of every dollar. Among the OECD member states, only the United States, Korea, and Mexico have less than half of health care expenditures funded by public dollars. In the case of the United States, the larger share of health care system expenditures is assumed by a combination of the private health care insurance market (37.2 cents of the health care dollar) and out-of-pocket expenditures by health care consumers (14.3 cents of the health care dollar).[2]

An additional distinctive feature of the U.S. health care system is that, in contrast to the general pattern among OECD member states, the United States does not ensure health care coverage for all of its residents. Although several OECD member states have a mixture of public and private insurance funds for the coverage of health care, the United States is one of the few OECD countries that does not provide access to publicly funded health care for persons that lack other sources of health insurance. The other exceptions among OECD member states are countries that are considerably less affluent than the United States, for example Mexico

Table 4.1 Brief Comparative Overview of Expenditures and Resources: The U.S. vs Other OECD Countries*

OECD Country	Health Care as Percent of GDP	Percent Expenditures Publicly Financed	Health Expenditures Per Capita USD PPP	Percent Expenditures for Pharmaceuticals	Acute Care Hospital Beds/ 1000 Persons	Practicing Physicians/ 1000 Persons
Australia	9.3	67.5	2699	14	3.6	2.5
Austria	7.6	69.9	2280	16.1	6	3.4
Belgium	9.6	–	2827	16.6	4	3.9
Canada	9.9	69.9	3003	16.9	3.2	2.1
Czech Republic	7.5	90.1	1298	21.9	6.5	3.5
Denmark	9	83	2763	9.8	3.4	2.9
Finland	7.4	76.5	2118	16	2.3	2.6
France	10.1	76.3	2903	20.9	3.8	3.4
Germany	11.1	78.2	2996	14.6	6.6	3.4
Greece	9.9	51.3	2011	16	—	4.4
Hungary	7.8	70.2	1115	27.6	5.9	3.2
Iceland	10.5	83.5	3115	14.5	—	3.6
Ireland	7.3	75.2	2386	11	3	2.6
Italy	8.4	75.1	2258	22.1	3.9	4.1
Japan	7.9	81.5	2139	18.4	8.5	2
Korea	5.6	49.4	1074	28.8	5.9	1.6
Luxembourg	6.1	85.4	3190	11.6	5.7	2.7

(continued)

Table 4.1 (Continued)

OECD Country	Health Care as Percent of GDP	Percent Expenditures Publicly Financed	Health Expenditures Per Capita USD PPP	Percent Expenditures for Pharmaceuticals	Acute Care Hospital Beds/ 1000 Persons	Practicing Physicians/ 1000 Persons
Mexico	6.2	46.4	583	21.4	1	1.5
Netherlands	9.8	62.4	2976	11.4	3.2	3.1
New Zealand	8.1	78.7	1886	14.4	-	2.2
Norway	10.3	83.7	3807	9.4	3.1	3.1
Poland	6	72.4	677	-	5.1	2.5
Portugal	9.6	69.7	1797	23.4	3.1	3.3
Slovak Republic	5.9	88.3	777	38.5	5.9	3.1
Spain	7.7	71.2	1835	21.8	3.1	3.2
Sweden	9.2	85.3	2594	13.1	2.4	3.3
Switzerland	11.5	58.5	3781	10.5	3.9	3.6
Turkey	6.6	62.9	452	24.8	2.3	1.4
United Kingdom	7.7	83.4	2231	15.8	3.7	2.2
United States	15	44.4	5635	12.9	2.8	2.3
OECD Member Average	8.62	72.08	2306.87	17.73	4.14	2.89

*Most estimates are pertain to 2003, though some OECD estimates for specific countries are derived from the most recently available data in prior years.

Source: OECD Health Data 2005, OECD, Paris, 2005. Data from Table of Health, Spending and Resources.

and Turkey (Colombo & Tapay, 2004). One consequence of the lack of universal health insurance coverage is the reinforcement of a *two-tiered* system of health care in the United States; one system for the segment of the population with adequate health care insurance coverage and another for those dependent upon either inadequate public subsidies for health care or "charity care" from the limited number of health care providers willing to provide it.[3] Although almost all countries have some semblance of a two-tiered health care system that privileges the more affluent and influential, in the United States the two-tiered structure of the health care system is particularly pronounced.

THE RESOURCES OF THE U.S. SYSTEM: FACILITIES, TECHNOLOGY, AND HUMAN RESOURCES

Facilities

Hospitals and Hospital Systems

As mentioned in the previous chapter, the American hospital and hospital system industry[4] (HHSI) is divided into three distinct ownership sectors: the public sector, the voluntary sector, and the proprietary sector. Public hospitals are those that are owned and operated by local, state, and federal government agencies. They include hospital and hospital systems operated by the county and municipal governments, state universities, state and federal prison hospitals, the Veterans Administration, the various branches of the military, and the Indian Health Service. The voluntary sector of the HHSI is comprised of hospitals and hospital systems that are owned and operated as not-for-profit organizations by religious, civic, and philanthropic organizations for the broad purpose of providing benefits to the community. The proprietary sector of the HHSI operates its facilities to make profit that is returned to investors, which may be a small group of investors or a publicly traded corporation.

---

[3] Charity care is generally defined as care that is provided both without payment and without obligation to pay for persons unable to afford it. This is distinct from the other form of uncompensated care, bad debt, which represents a provider's decision to write off fees for health care that are deemed uncollectible. Both forms of uncompensated care compose a significant source of the financing for health care delivered to the poor and the uninsured.

[4] The term "hospital and hospital system industry" is used to denote the fact that hospitals may be owned and operated as independent institutions, or as a component of an integrated health care system comprised of multiple hospitals and clinics.

Statistics on Hospital Ownership. Of the 5,759 hospitals in the United States in 2004, there were 239 hospitals operated by the federal government (AHA, 2005b). Most of the remaining hospitals (4,919) are classified as *community hospitals*, that is, nonfederal, short-term general and specialty hospitals that provide services to the general public (Shi & Singh, 2001).

As Figure 4.1 shows, the voluntary sector of the hospital industry in the United States dominates the industry, despite growth over the past two decades in the proportion of hospitals owned by the proprietary sector. The state and local government sector, although it is it slightly less than a quarter of the hospital industry, is crucial because local and state government hospitals serve a much higher relative proportion of the poor and uninsured than either the voluntary or the proprietary sectors of the hospital industry (GAO, 2005b).

The for-profit sector of the hospital industry is the smallest nationally, however, in some parts of the United States investor-owned hospitals and hospital systems have a large market share. This tends to be a regional phenomenon among states in the South and Southwest. The state with the highest proportion of investor-owned hospitals is Florida, where 46.8%

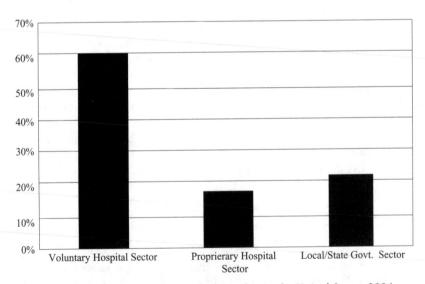

Figure 4.1 Distribution of Hospital Ownership in the United States, 2004. Source: Data from the 2004 annual survey of hospitals, *Fast Facts on U.S. Hospitals from AHA Hospital Statistics.* 2005, American Hospital Association, Chicago, IL.

of hospitals belong to the proprietary sector (Kaiser Family Foundation, 2006c). Although many Americans are strongly opposed to the idea that hospitals should exist for the purpose of generating profits to investors, there is no question that in large parts of the country the idea is firmly entrenched. It is also the case, when it comes to dollars returned in the form of tangible community benefits like uncompensated care for the poor and uninsured, that the not-for-profit hospitals in the voluntary sector do not behave in ways that appear to clearly justify their tax-exempt status. For example, in a recent analysis of the relationship between hospital ownership and the proportion of operating expenses allocated to uncompensated care in five representative states, the U.S. Government Accountability Office found that there was a relatively small difference between the voluntary and the proprietary sector in the dollars contributed to care for the poor and the uninsured (GAO, 2005b).[5] In fact, during recent years a large number of lawsuits have been filed against not-for-profit hospitals, contending that they have failed to fulfill their charitable obligations (Horowitz, 2005).

Types of Hospitals. Hospitals can be classified and made distinct from one another in a variety of ways, but the most common classifications applied pertain to acute short-term vs. long-term care, acute specialty care versus acute general service hospitals, the level of care provided (secondary versus tertiary care hospitals), teaching versus nonteaching hospitals, number of licensed beds, and urban versus rural location. Of the specialty care hospitals, the most common are psychiatric hospitals (according to the American Hospital Association's 2004 survey there are 466 nonfederal psychiatric hospitals nationwide). Nonpsychiatric long-term care hospitals tend to provide care that is too complex and intensive for custodial long-term care facilities like nursing homes, for example hospitals that provide care for patients that are dependent upon artificial respirators. General service hospitals are the most common type, and these hospitals provide medical and surgical services that include an array of highly utilized surgical specializations, internal medicine subspecialties (e.g. gastroenterology, cardiology, and pulmonary medicine), obstetrics and gynecology, and emergency medicine. Not all general service hospitals provide the full array of medical and surgical services, in fact what any hospital provides is determined by such factors as market demand for particular services, local competition among hospitals, and the decisions of state and community health planning authorities.

[5] This finding is examined more closely later in this chapter.

Hospitals are also differentiated by the *level* of care provided. Most community hospitals in the United States provide what is termed *primary care* and *secondary care*, and a minority of hospitals provide what is termed *tertiary* care. Primary care, broadly speaking, refers to the routine care that is provided for the common health care needs that make up the brunt of clinical encounters between doctor and patient. Examples include short-term respiratory infections, small injuries, well-baby care, and control of hypertensive disease. Secondary care refers generally to the health services provided by a specialist and the use of more advanced diagnostic and treatment technologies. However, secondary care also typically involves the diagnosis and treatment of a relatively common array of both serious (life threatening or disabling) and ordinarily nonserious health conditions or events (e.g. childbirth, tonsillectomy). Tertiary care on the other hand, typically involves diagnosis and treatment of more rare and complex diseases or injuries that require highly specialized practitioners and technologies (e.g. neonatal intensive care, organ transplantation).[6]

Hospital Systems. Over the past 25 years the hospital industry in the United States has been in a consolidation trend that favored the emergence of multihospital systems over the survival of independently operated hospitals. The definition of a multihospital system employed by the American Hospital Association involves provider relationships where "two or more hospitals are owned, leased, sponsored, or contractually managed by a central organization" (Shi & Singh, 2001, p. 290). Historically, most multihospital systems have existed in either the government or not-for-profit sectors of the industry. It is also the case that over the last decade, most of the consolidation of the hospital industry has taken place in the not-for-profit sector. This is not to suggest that for-profit hospital corporations are not large players among hospitals systems—they are. For example, the Tenet Healthcare Corporation operates 73 acute care hospitals with 18,445 licensed beds in 13 states and Healthcare Corporation of America operates 182 hospitals with 41,852 licensed beds in 23 states[7] (Hospital Corporation of America, 2004; Tenet Healthcare Corporation, 2006).

Historically, the earliest hospital systems were created primarily through expansion into communities that did not have hospitals, an example being the Sisters of Providence hospital system on the West Coast that emerged in the latter half of the 19th century. In more recent decades

---

[6] Sometimes the term "quaternary care" is used to denote an even higher level of care than tertiary. However, the term "tertiary care" is the more typically used to refer to the highest level of hospital care.

[7] The data for Tenet Corporation are as reported in the corporate Web site as of 2006 and the data for Columbia HCA are as of year end 2005.

hospital systems developed through mergers and acquisitions (Cuellar & Gertler, 2003). Mergers are transactions in which separate hospitals come together under a shared license, whereas acquisitions involve the acquired hospitals' retention of their individual licenses under a common governing body (Cuellar and Gertler, 2003, p. 77). The hospitals that merge into a multihospital system generally involve facilities within the same community. Hospitals merge with each other to pursue survival and competitive advantage through such mechanisms as consolidation of purchasing power, reductions in duplication, and the pooling of capital essential to modernization. Hospitals that are acquired may become a part of an existent local hospital system, or they may be acquired by an outside multihospital system that is seeking expansion into a new health care market (Cuellar & Gertler, 2003). Although it is too soon to sound the death knell of the independent community hospital, during the last decade solo hospitals did slip into the minority (Cuellar and Gertler, 2003, p. 79).

For a variety or reasons, it seems safe to assume that the consolidation trend toward multihospital systems will continue. Aside from the reasons just cited, multihospital systems have the advantage of "vertical integration"—providing the complete array of health care services from prevention to chronic illness management and long-term care under a single organizational umbrella. Aside from the competitive advantages gained in purchasing of supplies, equipment, and services, multihospital services are also in a better position than solo hospitals in the negotiation of favorable contracts with the insurance plans and employer groups that are primary purchasers of their services. Finally, larger multihospital systems also have better capacity to accommodate or even play a direct role in sponsoring an array of health insurance products capable of capturing different segments of the health insurance market.

Recent Trends in Hospital Resources. Table 4.2 provides a general overview of the hospital facility resources over the most recent ten-year period for which federal data on hospitals available are available (National Center for Health Statistics, 2005). National trends are shown in three areas: the number of hospitals, the number of hospital beds, and the occupancy rate (the percentage of staffed beds that are occupied). As the last column on Table 4.2 shows, there is a general downward trend in the number of hospitals and the number of hospital beds in the United States, but a general rise in occupancy rates. These trends reflect a broad shrinkage of the hospital industry that has occurred over the past 25 years due to two major, highly interactive factors: advances in medicine and the advances in systems of managed care. In simplified terms, advances in medicine permitted more of health care to be provided on an

Table 4.2 Hospitals, Beds, and Occupancy Rates, According to Type of Ownership and Size of Hospital: United States, Selected Years 1993–2003

(Data Are Based on Reporting by a Census of Hospitals)

Type of Ownership and Size of Hospital Hospitals	1993	1994	1995	1996	1997	1998	1999	2000	2001	2002	2003	Change in Percent
All hospitals	6,467	6,374	6,291	6,201	6,097	6,021	5,890	5,810	5,801	5,794	5,764	−10.9%
Federal	316	307	299	290	285	275	264	245	243	240	239	−24.4%
Non-Federal[1]	6,151	6,067	5,992	5,911	5,812	5,746	5,626	5,565	5,558	5,554	5,525	−10.2%
Community[2]	5,261	5,229	5,194	5,134	5,057	5,015	4,956	4,915	4,908	4,927	4,895	−7.0%
Nonprofit[2]	3,154	3,139	3,092	3,045	3,000	3,026	3,012	3,003	2,998	3,025	2,984	−5.4%
For profit	717	719	752	759	797	771	747	749	754	766	790	10.2%
State-local government	1,390	1,371	1,350	1,330	1,260	1,218	1,197	1,163	1,156	1,136	1,121	−19.4%
6–24 beds	227	235	278	262	281	293	299	288	281	321	327	44.1%
25–49 beds	894	900	922	906	890	900	887	910	916	931	965	7.9%
50–99 beds	1,181	1,157	1,139	1,128	1,111	1,085	1,082	1,055	1,070	1,072	1,031	−12.7%
100–199 beds	1,337	1,331	1,324	1,338	1,289	1,304	1,266	1,236	1,218	1,190	1,168	−12.6%
200–299 beds	730	746	718	692	679	644	642	656	635	625	624	−14.5%
300–399 beds	402	377	354	361	367	352	365	341	348	358	349	−13.2%
400–499 beds	205	210	195	196	185	183	161	182	191	174	172	−16.1%
500 beds or more	285	273	264	251	255	254	254	247	249	256	256	−10.2%
Beds												
All hospitals	1,163,460	1,128,066	1,080,601	1,061,688	1,035,390	1,012,582	993,866	983,628	987,440	975,962	965,256	−17.0%
Federal	87,847	83,823	77,079	73,171	61,937	56,698	55,120	53,067	51,900	49,838	47,456	−46.0%
Non-Federal[1]	1,075,613	1,044,243	1,003,522	988,517	973,453	955,884	938,746	930,561	935,540	926,124	917,800	−14.7%
Community[2]	918,786	902,061	872,736	862,352	853,287	839,988	829,575	823,560	825,966	820,653	813,307	−11.5%
Nonprofit[2]	651,272	636,949	609,729	598,162	590,636	587,658	586,673	582,988	585,070	582,179	574,587	−11.8%
For profit	98,964	100,667	105,737	109,197	115,074	112,975	106,790	109,883	108,718	108,422	109,671	10.8%

State-local government.....	168,550	164,445	157,270	154,993	147,577	139,355	136,112	130,689	132,178	130,052	129,049	−23.4%
6–24 beds.....	4,323	4,388	5,085	4,770	5,128	5,351	5,442	5,156	4,964	5,629	5,635	30.3%
25–49 beds.....	33,711	33,635	34,352	33,814	33,138	33,510	32,816	33,333	33,263	33,200	33,613	−0.3%
50–99 beds.....	84,950	83,018	82,024	81,185	79,837	78,035	78,121	75,865	76,924	76,882	74,025	−12.9%
100–199 beds.....	189,234	187,369	187,381	189,630	182,284	186,118	181,115	175,778	174,024	171,625	167,451	−11.5%
200–299 beds.....	178,864	182,111	175,240	168,977	165,197	156,978	155,831	159,807	154,420	152,682	152,487	−14.7%
300–399 beds.....	138,473	129,300	121,136	123,822	126,307	120,512	126,259	117,220	119,753	123,399	119,903	−13.4%
400–499 beds.....	91,389	93,415	86,459	86,913	82,250	81,247	71,580	80,763	84,745	77,145	76,333	−16.5%
500 beds or more.....	197,842	188,825	181,059	173,241	179,146	178,237	178,411	175,638	177,873	180,091	183,860	−7.1%

Occupancy rate in Percent[3]

All hospitals.....	67.3	66.0	65.7	64.5	65.0	65.4	66.1	66.1	66.7	67.8	68.1	1.2%
Federal.....	76.0	74.9	72.6	71.4	79.1	78.9	74.4	68.2	69.8	66.0	64.8	−14.7%
Non-Federal[1]	66.6	65.3	65.1	64.0	64.1	64.6	65.6	65.9	66.5	67.9	68.3	2.6%
Community[2]	64.4	62.9	62.8	61.5	61.8	62.5	63.4	63.9	64.5	65.8	66.2	2.8%
Nonprofit.....	66.4	64.8	64.5	63.3	63.6	64.2	64.9	65.5	65.8	67.2	67.7	2.0%
For profit.....	51.1	50.1	51.8	51.6	52.0	53.2	54.8	55.9	57.8	59.0	59.6	16.6%
State-local.....	64.5	63.5	63.7	61.7	62.3	62.7	63.4	63.2	64.1	64.9	65.3	1.2%
government.....												
6–24 beds.....	30.8	31.7	36.9	33.2	35.4	33.2	33.0	31.7	31.3	32.4	31.9	3.6%
25–49 beds.....	41.4	40.9	42.6	40.0	40.3	41.2	41.5	41.3	42.5	44.0	44.6	7.7%
50–99 beds.....	53.2	53.1	54.1	53.1	54.2	54.7	54.5	54.8	55.5	56.7	57.2	7.5%
100–199 beds.....	59.3	58.2	58.8	57.8	58.2	58.4	59.3	60.0	60.7	61.7	62.6	5.6%
200–299 beds.....	64.3	62.9	63.1	62.0	61.8	62.9	64.1	65.0	65.5	66.7	67.0	4.2%
300–399 beds.....	66.9	65.5	64.8	63.6	63.2	64.7	66.1	65.7	66.4	68.2	68.5	2.4%
400–499 beds.....	69.9	68.9	68.1	67.4	68.0	67.3	68.3	69.1	68.9	70.5	70.7	1.1%
500 beds or more.....	74.6	71.8	71.4	69.7	69.8	70.9	71.7	72.2	72.8	74.0	74.2	−0.5%

[1] The category of non-Federal hospitals comprises psychiatric, tuberculosis and other respiratory diseases hospitals, and long-term and short-term general and other special hospitals.

[2] Community hospitals are non-Federal short-term general and special hospitals whose facilities and services are available to the public.

[3] Estimated percent of staffed beds that are occupied.

Source: Health, United States 2005 Edition. National Center for Health Statistics. Table 112 (spreadsheet version): Hospitals, beds and occupancy rates, according to types of ownership and size of hospital: United States selected years 1973–2003.

outpatient basis, and the evolvement of managed care provided the health care information systems and financial incentives that were the essential preconditions and impetus necessary for such widespread institutional change. It should also be appreciated that advances in medicine and the evolvement of managed care are interactive. In essence, advances in managed care information and financing create knowledge and incentives for advancements in medicine, which in turn lead to further adaptation in systems of managed care.

Although the inpatient care side of the hospital industry has contracted significantly in the past decade (a 10.9% reduction in hospitals and a 17% reduction in the number of hospital beds), Table 4.2 also shows some areas of growth. For example, the for-profit sector of the hospital industry has grown by 10.2 percent in the number of hospitals and nearly 11 percent in the number of hospital beds.

Another trend over the most of the past decade has been a gradual rise in hospital occupancy rates after a long period of significant declines. The rise in occupancy rates among hospitals in the for-profit sector has been particularly vigorous, underscoring the observation from hospital industry analysts that the for-profit sector is better able to hone its marketing strategies to profitable use of resources (Horowitz, 2005). The sole exception to this pattern is the dramatic decline in the occupancy rates of federal hospitals, which reflects a significant and (what many would argue is a belated) shift toward ambulatory health care management of both acute and chronic diseases among the Veterans Administration system.[8]

Geographic Distribution of Hospital Resources. The conventional statistic for describing the distribution of hospital resources is the number of community hospital beds per 1,000 persons in a given geographic entity, such as cities, metropolitan areas, counties, states, and sovereign nations. Within the United States, there is wide variation in the number of hospital beds per thousand persons no matter what geographic unit is considered. In large part, the hospital resources in a given geographic area are as much a matter of local history, politics, and the socioeconomic distribution as they are a matter of population characteristics that are more predictive of the need for hospital care, such as the age distribution and prevalence of disease. Other factors that have influenced geographic variation in

---

[8] This shift toward ambulatory care in the VA system reflects a recent restructuring of the system to a population-based model of health care, as opposed to the VA system's traditional hospital-based system of caring for veterans. (see chapter 3 on Health Care Finance).

the number of hospital beds/1000 persons are geographic variations in the diffusion of alternatives to hospital care (e.g. outpatient diagnostic and surgical centers) and variations in standards of medical practice that impact hospital utilization.

In order to offer a general idea of the degree to which there are significant geographic variations in hospital resources and utilization of hospital services, Table 4.3 shows the state-by-state comparison of the number of hospital beds/1000 persons and the average length of hospital stays within each state. For example, the two states with the highest number of beds/1000 are North Dakota and South Dakota (6.1 beds/1000) and the state with the fewest is Washington (1.9/1000). Differences in average length of stay among states are also quite dramatic, ranging from a high of 6.6 days per hospital stay in New York to a low of 4.0 days in Wyoming. In general, the trend nationally over the past couple of decades has been a dramatic decline in the average length of hospital stays, which in turn has contributed to the decline in the number of hospitals and hospital beds shown previously on Table 4.2.

For the most part, these trends in the decline of hospital resources reflect advancements in the delivery of health care. However, in many parts of the United States communities with the highest level of population morbidity (disease and injury) have the fewest hospital beds/1,000 persons available. This problem is has long been known to be common to low-income rural communities, but more recent analysis also highlights this issue among low-income suburban areas (Andrulis & Duchon, 2005). As Figure 4.2 shows, the distribution of hospital utilization and resources is very much a function of a given suburban area's poverty level. Were the number of hospital visits, admissions, and staffed beds an exact function of the size of the local population, all of the bars shown in Figure 4.2 would be in perfect alignment with the lowest bar—that showing the percentage of the suburban population living in low, medium, and high poverty suburbs. Instead, what the pattern reveals is a strongly disproportionate representation of hospital visits, hospital admissions, and hospital beds in the suburbs that have lower levels of poverty.

Specific to hospital resources, the suburbs with the lowest level of poverty contain 26% of the population but account for 42% of the hospital beds. Generally similar patterns are shown for hospital emergency department visits, outpatient visits, and hospital visits. Given the well-documented higher prevalence of disease and premature death among the poor, it is hard to escape the conclusion that, to a large extent, the distribution of hospital resources in the United States is a matter of population wealth rather than population health.

Table 4.3 Average Length of Hospital Stays and Hospital Beds/1,000 Persons, by State, 2002

State	Average Length of Stay	Rank	Beds/1000 Persons	Rank
ALABAMA	4.8	36	3.6	13
ALASKA	5.8	3	2.1	41
ARIZONA	4.4	46	2.0	46
ARKANSAS	5.0	24	3.7	11
CALIFORNIA	4.9	30	2.1	42
COLORADO	4.4	44	2.1	43
CONNECTICUT	5.5	6	2.2	40
DELAWARE	5.7	4	2.5	34
FLORIDA	5.0	26	3.1	20
GEORGIA	5.3	12	2.9	23
HAWAII	6.4	2	2.6	30
IDAHO	4.2	48	2.5	35
ILLINOIS	4.9	31	2.9	24
INDIANA	5.3	11	3.1	21
IOWA	4.8	38	3.8	9
KANSAS	4.9	34	4.0	7
KENTUCKY	5.0	25	3.7	12
LOUISIANA	5.4	7	4.0	8
MAINE	5.0	27	2.9	25
MARYLAND	4.5	42	2.1	44
MASSACHUSETTS	5.3	9	2.5	36
MICHIGAN	4.9	33	2.6	31
MINNESOTA	4.7	41	3.3	16
MISSISSIPPI	5.4	8	4.6	5
MISSOURI	4.9	28	3.3	17
MONTANA	4.7	40	4.7	3
NEBRASKA	5.6	5	4.7	4
NEVADA	5.3	14	2.1	45
NEW HAMPSHIRE	5.0	22	2.3	38
NEW JERSEY	5.2	15	2.8	26
NEW MEXICO	4.7	39	1.9	47
NEW YORK	6.6	1	3.4	15
NORTH CAROLINA	5.2	18	2.8	27
NORTH DAKOTA	5.1	19	6.1	1
OHIO	4.9	32	3.0	22
OKLAHOMA	5.0	23	3.2	19
OREGON	4.1	49	1.9	48
PENNSYLVANIA	5.3	13	3.3	18
RHODE ISLAND	5.2	16	2.3	39
SOUTH CAROLINA	5.3	10	2.7	28
SOUTH DAKOTA	4.8	35	6.1	2
TENNESSEE	5.1	21	3.5	14
TEXAS	5.1	20	2.6	32

Table 4.3   (*Continued*)

State	Average Length of Stay	Rank	Beds/1000 Persons	Rank
UTAH	4.3	47	1.9	49
VERMONT	4.8	37	2.6	33
VIRGINIA	5.2	17	2.4	37
WASHINGTON	4.4	45	1.9	50
WEST VIRGINIA	4.9	29	4.3	6
WISCONSIN	4.5	43	2.7	29
WYOMING	4.0	50	3.8	10
Average for United States	**5.1**		**2.8**	

Note: Data pertain only to community hospitals.
Sources: Data from Oregon Association of Hospitals and Health Systems. (2005). State Comparisons: Average Length of Stay Community Hospital Units by State–2004 and Kaiser Family Foundation. (2005). Statehealthfacts.org.
Beds per Thousand Population 1999–2002.

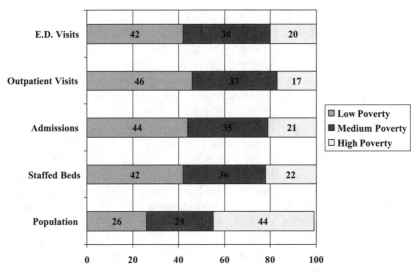

Figure 4.2   Percentage Distribution of Hospital Visits, Admissions, and Staffed Beds in Suburbs of 100 Largest Cities by Suburban Poverty Level, 2002. (Source: Data from Andrulis, D. P., & Duchon, L. M. (2005). *Hospital Care in the 100 Largest Cities and Their Suburbs, 1996–2002: Implications for the Future of the Hospital Safety Net in Metropolitan America.* New York, NY: SUNY Downstate Medical Center. Chart 4: Suburbs of 100 Largest Cities by Poverty Level: Distribution of 2000 Population Compared with Distribution of Hospital Beds and Utilization, 2002.)

Hospital Utilization. Nationwide, there are 120 hospital admissions per 1000 persons annually to community hospitals (Kaiser Family Foundation, 2006b).[9] However, admission rates vary dramatically by geographic location due to a number of factors, all of which can be considered either demand side factors or supply side factors. On the demand side are population health factors including the age distribution, socioeconomic status distribution, the prevalence and distribution of disease, health insurance coverage, and cultural norms that influence the demand for health care. On the supply side are such factors as hospital beds and related staffing resources, physicians who specialize in hospital care, and diagnostic and treatment technology capable of yielding health benefits. Notably, a significant component of hospital utilization pertains to local area standards of practice pertaining to the diagnosis and management of injury and disease. Among the states, the rates of hospital admission vary from a low of 71/1000 persons annually in Alaska, to a high of 163/1,000 persons in West Virginia. Patterns of hospital utilization are also reported and analyzed in a variety of ways, including by discharge diagnosis, by procedure(s) performed, by year, and by demographic characteristics such as age, sex, race, and nativity.

As implied by the decline in hospital beds over the past decade shown previously in Table 4.2, hospital utilization rates have also declined over the same period. One way of accounting for the reasons for the decline is to examine changes over time in the utilization of hospital diagnostic and surgical procedures. Shown in Table 4.4 are the changes in relatively common diagnostic and surgical procedures that occurred in U.S. hospitals during the recent decade ending in the year 2003.

As the table shows, the annual rates of hospitalizations for all diagnostic and surgical procedures performed on adults declined by 9.57%, with the largest declines in radiology and ultrasound diagnostic procedures. In contrast, there was a dramatic rise in the rate (per 10,000 persons) in hospital stays for joint replacements of the hip and the knee. To a large extent, the downward trend in hospital stays for the diagnostic procedures represent the shift of these technologies over time to ambulatory care settings. On the other hand, the rise in hospital stays for hip and knee joint replacements suggests more prevalent use of these procedures to counter the degenerative effects of aging.[10]

---

[9] Estimate based on data compiled by the American Hospital Association for the year 2003.
[10] The rates shown are age adjusted, meaning that the change in rates shown are net of the effects of changes in the age distribution of the adult population that occurred between 1992–93 and 2002–03. This suggests that the increasing prevalence of such procedures as total knee replacement is not explained by the aging of the population per se, but the way the effects of aging are countered by changes in standards of practice.

Table 4.4 Hospital Stays With At Least One Procedure, per 10,000 Persons Age 18 and Over, According to Selected Procedures: United States, Average Annual 1992–93 and 2002–03*

(Data Are Based on a Sample of Hospital Records)

	Number per 10,000 Persons		Change in Rate
	1992–1993	2002–2003	
Hospital stays with at least one procedure.............	992.3	897.3	−9.57%
Cardiac catheterization............................	54.6	58.8	7.69%
Insertion, replacement, removal, and revision of pacemaker leads or device........................	8.8	10.4	18.18%
Incision, excision, and occlusion of vessels............	40.3	64.1	59.06%
Angiocardiography using contrast material.............	45.6	47.5	4.17%
Operations on vessels of heart.......................	37.0	43.1	16.49%
Removal of coronary artery obstruction and insertion of stent(s).....................................	21.0	30.2	43.81%
Insertion of coronary artery stent(s).............	...	25.0	
Coronary artery bypass graft......................	16.9	13.2	−21.89%
Diagnostic procedures on small intestine.............	44.8	47.1	5.13%
Diagnostic procedures on large intestine.............	28.7	26.7	−6.97%
Diagnostic radiology...............................	78.0	35.1	−55.00%
Computerized axial tomography....................	54.9	28.4	−48.27%
Diagnostic ultrasound..............................	66.1	32.7	−50.53%

(continued)

Table 4.4 (*Continued*)

(Data Are Based on a Sample of Hospital Records)

	Number per 10,000 Persons 1992–1993	2002–2003	Change in Rate
Joint replacement of lower extremity..........	22.6	35.6	57.52%
Total hip replacement..........	6.8	9.5	39.71%
Partial hip replacement..........	4.9	5.0	2.04%
Total knee replacement..........	8.9	17.7	98.88%
Reduction of fracture and dislocation..........	27.5	24.2	−12.00%
Excision or destruction of intervertebral disc..........	17.3	14.4	−16.76%
Cholecystectomy..........	27.2	19.7	−27.57%
Laparoscopic cholecystectomy..........	18.1	14.5	−19.89%
Lysis of peritoneal adhesions..........	18.0	15.2	−15.56%

*See NCHS, Health, United States 2005, Table 100 and related appendices for qualitifiers and a more complete explanation of reported statistics.

Notes: Up to four procedures were coded for each hospital stay.

If more than one procedure with the same code (e.g., a coronary artery bypass graft) was performed during the hospital stay, it is counted only once. Procedure categories are based on the *International Classification of Diseases, Ninth Revision, Clinical Modification (ICD-9-CM)*. See Appendix II, Procedure; and Table X for ICD-9-CM codes. Rates are based on the civilian population as of July 1. The rates shown are extracted from an age adjusted table, to compare 2002–2003 rates with prior years see the complete source table.

Source: Health, United States 2005 Edition, National Center for Health Statistics. Table 100 (spreadsheet version) Hospital stays with at least one procedure, according to sex, age, and selected procedures: United States, average annual 1992–93 and 2002–03.

To a significant extent, the prospects for future increases or decreases in hospital utilization will be an outcome of two opposing trends: the rise in the general demand for health care that accompanies the aging of the population and a countertrend that is driven by innovations in health care technology and other advances in medicine that reduce the demand for hospital care. Another important trend that might influence prospects for hospital utilization involves reductions in Medicare program funding undertaken during the second term of the George W. Bush administration, which if implemented over time may propel the Medicare program toward a significant transformation of the program's benefits and risk structure. Given the large role of Medicare as a payment source for hospital care, any broad changes in this program will in one way or the other significantly influence hospital utilization.[11]

Ambulatory Care Facilities

The largest sector of the U.S. health care system is that committed to various forms of ambulatory care. Ambulatory care is health care that is delivered to persons who are classified as outpatients (not confined to a hospital or classified as an inpatient) at the time care is provided. As such, ambulatory services include the offices of such licensed health care practitioners as physicians, dentists, physical therapists, chiropractors, optometrists, and various kinds of mental health care professionals (e.g., psychologists, social workers, and psychiatric nurse practitioners). The ambulatory care sector of the health care industry also includes diagnostic laboratories, diagnostic imaging centers (e.g., CT and MRI scanners), radiation therapy centers, family planning clinics, and the entire home health care industry. Although the term "ambulatory" implies the capacity to move about rather than being bedridden, as applied to the organization of the health care industry "ambulatory care" refers to care other than that provided to inpatients of institutions like hospitals, nursing homes, and inpatient hospices.

Table 4.5 provides a general overview of the ambulatory care sector of the U.S. health care system. The table delineates the facilities, annual revenue, and paid staffing by six major areas: physician's offices, non-physician provider offices, outpatient care centers, medical laboratories, and diagnostic imaging centers, and a general category for all other health care services (e.g. ambulance services, blood banks).

---

[11] Medicare financing and reform issues are discussed at length in later chapters.

Table 4.5 Ambulatory Care Sector of the Health Care System: Facilities, Annual Revenue and Paid Employees (Year 2002)

	Facilities	Revenue (in $1000)	Paid Employees
Ambulatory health care services	**488,511**	**$493,192,661**	**4,938,069**
Offices of physicians	**202,982**	**$250,449,190**	**1,918,393**
Offices of physicians (mental health specialists)	10,400	$4,315,946	42,862
Offices of physicians (non-mental health specialists)	192,582	246,133,244	1,875,531
Offices of non-physician practitioners	**222,437**	**$109,368,547**	**1,240,049**
Offices of dentists	118,024	$71,258,064	744,478
Offices of chiropractors	34,359	$9,390,288	112,367
Offices of optometrists	18,701	$8,392,137	93,193
Offices of mental health practitioners (except physicians)	13,452	$3,855,119	61,024
Offices of physical, occupational and speech therapists, and audiologists	19,661	$10,763,007	162,541
Offices of podiatrists	8,671	$3,154,287	34,133
Offices of all other Miscellaneous Health Practitioners	9,569	$2,555,645	32,313
Outpatient care centers	**25,556**	**$55,905,403**	**584,152**
Family planning centers	1,920	$1,198,356	18,639
Outpatient mental health and substance abuse centers	7,772	$9,085,605	163,280
HMO medical centers	430	$3,748,369	29,690
Kidney dialysis centers	3,135	$8,741,239	63,551
Freestanding ambulatory surgical and emergency centers	3,373	$8,664,024	63,383
All other outpatient care centers	8,926	$24,487,810	245,609
Medical laboratories and diagnostic imaging centers	**11,090**	**$28,860,583**	**205,631**
Medical laboratories	5,513	$17,214,888	135,589
Diagnostic imaging centers	5,577	$11,645,695	70,042
Home health care services	**17,666**	**$30,574,989**	**775,933**
Other ambulatory health care services	**8,820**	**$18,033,949**	**213,911**
Ambulance services	3,933	$6,747,602	113,656
All other ambulatory health care services	4,887	$11,286,347	100,255
Blood and organ banks	1,291	$6,533,260	54,208
All other miscellaneous ambulatory health care services	3,596	$4,753,087	46,047

Source: Data extracted from U.S. Census Bureau. (2004). 2002 Economic Census: Ambulatory Health Care Services (No. EC02-62I-01). Washington D.C.: U.S. Department of Commerce. Table 1 Summary Statistics for the United States 2002.

Nursing Homes and Other Long-Term Care Facilities

Although the hospital and ambulatory care components of U.S. health care system provide services to the chronically ill and disabled populations, for the most part hospital and ambulatory health care resources are organized around an acute care paradigm. In essence, this means that the organization of the hospital and ambulatory services sectors of the health care system is dominated by an implicit assumption that the diagnostic and treatment process is immediate problem–focused and short term. In contrast, the long-term care component of the health care system is organized around the provision of health care over a sustained period of time for health conditions that are chronic and disabling in nature (Kane, Kane, & Ladd, 1998). In addition, long-term facilities, services, and funding mechanisms are primarily focused on optimal functioning as opposed to cure.

For a variety of historical reasons, the dominant mode of provision of long-term care services has been institutional care. That is, over much of U.S. history care for persons with functional limitations that strain the resources of family and community (or significantly challenge prevailing notions of acceptable appearance and behavior) has been the province of long-term psychiatric hospitals (asylums), nursing homes, and residential care facilities. Despite the progress that has been made over the past 50 years in the "de-institutionalization" of long-term care services,[12] nursing homes and other types of residential care facilities remain central to the provision of long-term care in the United States and a significant component of the U.S. health care system. For example, the most recent estimates of the number of certified nursing facilities by the Henry J. Kaiser Family Foundation places the number of these facilities in the United States at 15,209, and the number of their residents at 1,351,159 (Kaiser Family Foundation, 2005).[13] The far majority of the residents of these facilities are elderly adults, estimated to compose 3.8% of the population of Americans age 65+ (Kaiser Family Foundation, 2005). It should be noted, however, that throughout most of the United States the criteria for admission to these facilities are the level of functional disablement and need for nursing assistance—thus certified nursing facilities also provide care for persons that are disabled primarily by injury, chronic disease, retardation, or mental illness.

---

[12] Meaning the substitution of community-based long-term services for institutional care.

[13] Estimate is for the year 2003. The term "certified nursing facility" applies to nursing homes and other residential care facilities that are licensed by states to provide nursing care, and in most cases qualify for either Medicare or Medicaid funding for services.

A brief statistical summary of the resources allocated to the nursing home and residential care component of the health care system is shown on Table 4.6. Clearly, nursing homes account for the largest share of the institutional long-term care services shown on the table ($73.8 billion dollars in revenue), followed by the dollars spent on community care facilities for the elderly ($26.6 billion). By contrast, the dollars allocated to in-home residential care for the retardation, mental illness, and substance abuse sum to 19.5 billion annually—or about 15% of the total dollars allocated for all forms of nursing home and residential care.

Compared with the other institutional component of the health care system, hospitals, the nursing home and residential care component has a much higher proportion of its facilities owned and operated by for-profit partnerships and corporations. This is particularly the case for nursing homes and retirement homes (the latter shown on Table 4.6 as "homes for the elderly"). Of all the nursing homes in the United States, approximately two-thirds are owned and operated as for-profit entities (Kaiser Family Foundation, 2006a). It is also worth noting that within the for-profit

Table 4.6 Nursing Home and Residential Care Sector of the Health Care System: Facilities, Annual Revenue and Paid Employees (2002)

	Facilities	Revenue (in $1000)	Paid Employees
Nursing and residential care facilities	69,136	$127,828,065	2831835
Nursing care facilities	16,479	$73,806,163	1594290
Residential mental retardation, mental health and substance abuse faciliities	28,448	$19,560,834	500582
Residential mental retardation facilities	22,328	$13,375,703	370322
Residential mental health and substance abuse facilities	6,120	$6,185,104	130260
Community care facilities for the elderly	17,929	$26,603,295	572372
Continuing care retirement communities	3,936	$15,220,057	316112
Homes for the elderly	13,993	$11,383,238	256260
Other residential care facilities	6,280	$7,907,773	164591

Source: Data extracted from U.S. Census Bureau. (2004). 2002 Economic Census: Nursing Home and Residential Care Facilities (No. EC02-62I-03). Washington D.C.: U.S. Department of Commerce. Table 1 Summary Statistics for the United States 2002.

sector of the industry, ownership is fairly concentrated. That is, about 20% of all facilities are owned by the eight largest firms in the industry (U.S. Census Bureau, 2004).

Technology

Health care technology can be broadly defined as the practical application of knowledge gained from shared experience and scientific research to the delivery of health care (Shi & Singh 2001, p. 155).[14] Thought of in this way, health care technology encompasses both "hard technologies" in the form of material devices like CT scanners, laser knives, and kidney dialysis machines and "soft technologies" in the form of procedures, protocols, and ways of organizing, disseminating, and applying large volumes of complex information to the delivery of health care. Although not completely inclusive, one way to conceptualize health care technology is to delineate the forms that it takes by information systems, diagnostic technology, and treatment technology.

Information Systems

Health care information systems involve the procedures and devices that are employed to collect, organize, store, analyze, and disseminate health care information. Although there has been a historic distinction between health care information systems that have been dedicated to administrative management information and those dedicated to clinical information, these lines have become increasingly blurred as health care providers assume an ever larger share of the financial risk for health care that is costly relative to its clinical benefits. Moreover, there is a central trend in the health care industry toward consolidation into large multihospital provider systems that integrate traditionally independent components of the health care system—which in turn demands a high level of information system integration. The hardware and software components of health care information system technology are essential to the ultimate accomplishment of three forms health care provider system integration: *functional integration, physician–system integration,* and *clinical integration* (Conrad & Shortell, 1996). Functional integration refers to the extent to which key support functions and activities are efficiently coordinated across

---

[14] Shi and Singh's (2001) definition of medical technology refers more narrowly to the "application of the scientific body of knowledge produced by biomedical research." The more broad definition here takes into account the nonscientific sources of information that contribute to the accepted body of knowledge in health care, for example, the diffusion of conventions in diagnosis and treatment that, when closely examined, have no scientific basis.

different parts of the provider system. Physician–system integration brings physicians into an increased level of engagement with the provider system in terms of exclusive utilization and system governance. Finally, clinical integration involves the coordination of health care decision-making and services across providers, functions, and settings within the system to maximize patient benefits relative to cost (Conrad & Shortell, 1996, pp. 5–6). A short list of the information system technologies that this level of integration involves includes electronic medical records, hardware networks that link diagnostic labs and imaging services with physician clinics, and software that links clinical decision makers with utilization management and quality improvement data.

As key as these information system technologies have been, the most significant source of technological innovation in health care information systems in recent years has been the Internet (Shi & Singh, 2001). In addition to shrinking the information gap between the health care consumer and health care providers, the Internet is assuming an ever larger part of the patient care management infrastructure of health care provider systems and serving as an important source of information for clinical decision making, for example, through connections between physicians' offices and the information databases of medical libraries located at top research universities.

Diagnostic Technology

Diagnostic technology primarily refers to the devices and procedures employed to detect and differentially diagnose disease processes and injuries. As such, diagnostic technology includes such things as the equipment used in clinical laboratories to process body fluid and tissue samples and diagnostic imaging devices like ultrasound machines, CT (computerized tomography) scanners, MRI (magnetic resonance imaging) scanners, and PET (positron emission tomography) scanners. The three latter devices are examples of extremely sophisticated and expensive technologies that, while they represent significant advancements in the application of physics and computer science technology to health care, also require enormous investments by the hospitals/hospital systems that seek to acquire them—and thus retain their competitiveness as a health care provider.

Treatment Technology

In contrast to diagnostic technology, the definition of treatment technology encompasses devices and procedures that have been developed for

the purposes of curing injury and disease, promoting optimal independence, functioning in the face of chronic illness and disability, alleviating
suffering, and preventing disease. A partial list of treatment technologies
includes pharmaceutical products, auxiliary devices like pacemakers and
hearing aids, "big ticket" devices like linear accelerators, the full range
of surgical procedures from the routine to the highly technical (e.g. her-
nia repair vs. organ transplant), clinical protocols for the treatment of
specific diseases (e.g. adjuvant chemo and radiation therapy for treatment of breast cancer), and specialized facilities like neonatal intensive
care units. Some treatment technologies, just like diagnostic technologies, require similarly enormous investments by the hospitals/health care
systems motivated to acquire them. Also like highly expensive diagnostic technologies, expensive and sophisticated treatment technologies also
serve fodder for "capital based competition" between different hospitals,
hospital systems, and provider groups.

The Diffusion of Health Care Technology

The broad scale diffusion and utilization of very expensive health care
technology (whether categorized as diagnostic or treatment technology)
is a point of significant distinction between the organization of health care
in the United States and that found elsewhere. In the United States much
of increased investment in highly sophisticated and expensive technology
is driven by the phenomenon of "capital based competition" between
hospitals and hospital systems vying against one another to attract and
retain a limited pool of insured patients. This is very distinct from either
price-based competition or outcome-based competition, where the consumer chooses the provider based on either price or a higher likelihood of
delivering a desirable outcome. In most other OECD countries, where the
health care technology is pitted much more directly against other kinds
of public dollar expenditures, the diffusion of technology is driven far
more by a cost–benefit orientation. The result, from a systemwide standpoint, is less investment in the most sophisticated and expensive health
care technologies and more selective utilization.

An illustrative example is the contrast between the system of health
care technology assessment and acquisition in France and the general process of technology assessment acquisition in the United States offered by
Rosenau (2000). The process of technology assessment is in essence a
process for determining the benefits, applications, and costs of new innovations in health care technology for the purpose of guiding decisions
pertaining to technology acquisition, distribution, and appropriate utilization. Although the federal government is the largest single purchaser

of health care (principally as a function of the Medicare and Medicaid programs), the technology assessment functions of the federal government are quite weak relative to the power of the medical technology industry in the United States. Several federal agencies assume important technology assessment functions (e.g. the National Institutes of Health, the Centers for Medicaid and Medicare Services, and the Agency for Health Care Research and Quality), but no particular agency either coordinates the health care technology assessment process or assumes a lead role in making specific recommendations pertaining to the best use of public dollars (Rosenau, 2000). This not an example of government inefficiency, but rather a sustained pattern of political decisions reflecting an entrenched belief among many American politicians and policy makers that the free market functions as the most efficient mechanism for identifying the optimally efficacious health care technologies.

In France, where the national government both directly regulates various health care insurance funds and assures universal coverage, health care technology assessment is a highly centralized function that involves a nonprofit agency sanctioned and funded by the French government to both carry out the technology assessment function and guide appropriate use. Of equal importance, the French government plays a very direct role in determining the geographic distribution of medical technology in accordance with such factors as population need and disparities in access (Rosenau, 2000). As stated by Rosenau (p. 625), health care technology is generally regarded as public good rather than a commodity.

The results of these two different approaches, predictably enough, are that in the United States there is a significant pattern of overinvestment in very expensive health care technologies relative to France. Using MRI units as an illustrative example, the OECD health statistic estimates for 2003 put the number of MRI units in France at 2.8 MRI units per million persons, while in the United States the OECD estimated there were 8.6 MRI units (OECD, 2005b). It should be noted that the OECD considers the actual number of MRI units in the United States to be much higher, because the OECD estimate excludes enumeration of MRI units that are not located in hospitals. Although some might take issue with the notion that such differences represent an example of overinvestment, the population health indicators in the United States relative to France fail to make the case that there is a discernable population health benefit yielded by having at least three times the number of MRI units available.[15] The

---

[15] According the most recent OECD estimates available (OECD, 2005a), life expectancy at birth in France exceeds U.S. life expectancy by 2.2 years—a gap that has increased significantly in recent decades. While national investments in health care technology are one

arguments against overinvestment become even more tenuous when other potential health care investment priorities are added to the equation, such as making health care insurance coverage accessible to the working poor.

Human Resources

According to the U.S. Department of Labor (Bureau of Labor Statistics, 2005), there were 13 million Americans employed in health care in the United States in 2004, a figure expected to grow by 27.3% over the next decade. Table 4.7 provides a general overview of the distribution of the health care labor force by health care occupation, along with a forecast of employment growth within each occupation over the next decade. Several of the health care labor force statistics on Table 4.7 are worthy of comment. First, it can be seen that physicians and registered nurses, generally considered the core health occupations, actually compose less than a fifth of the health care labor force (18.4%). Second, it is evident that the areas of greatest expansion in the health care labor force over the next several years involve occupations that provide services that are extension of roles and tasks that at one time were largely the exclusive province of physicians and nurses, such as physician's assistants in place of physicians and home health aides in place of registered home care nurses. A third interesting observation is that the growth that is expected in health care service occupations is expected to outpace that in the health care professions, particularly those service occupations that involve the ambulatory and home care sectors of the health care industry.

In significant part, both the second and the third trend represent a shift in the organization of health care to services and occupations tied to the management of chronic illness and disability, rather than diagnosis and cure of acute conditions. During the next decade the so-called baby boom generation will join the ranks of the nation's aged population, exacerbating further a significant gap between the demands of an aging population and the human resources essential to the provision of adequate health care. Within the service occupation sector of the health care industry (home care aides, nurses aides, and orderlies), it is highly likely that the adequacy of the human resource pool over the next decade will in large part be determined by immigration policy—given the skewed age distribution of the native U.S. population. Within the professional sector of the health care industry, the human resource pool will likely be determined by the interplay between immigration policy and the level of domestic investment by professional schools in the health sciences and

source of influence on life expectancy among many, the arguments for increased investments in highly expensive technology typically claim significant benefits to population health.

Table 4.7 Employment of Workers in Health Services by Occupation, 2004 and Projected Change, 2004–2014. (Employment in Thousands)

Occupation	Number	Percent	Percent Change: 2004–2014
Total, all occupations	13,062	100	27.3
Management, business, and financial occupations	574	4.4	28.3
Top executives	101	0.8	33.3
Medical and health services managers	175	1.3	26.1
Professional and related occupations	**5,657**	**43.3**	**27.8**
Psychologists	33	0.3	28.1
Counselors	152	1.2	31.8
Social workers	169	1.3	29.3
Health educators	17	0.1	27
Social and human service assistants	99	0.8	38.6
Chiropractors	21	0.2	47.8
Dentists	95	0.7	18.5
Dietitians and nutritionists	32	0.2	20.1
Optometrists	18	0.1	29.6
Pharmacists	63	0.5	17.3
Physicians and surgeons	417	3.2	28.7
Physician assistants	53	0.4	54.8
Podiatrists	7	0.1	22.2
Registered nurses	1,988	15.2	30.5
Therapists	358	2.7	32.8
Clinical laboratory technologists and technicians	257	2	22.7
Dental hygienists	153	1.2	43.7
Diagnostic related technologists and technicians	269	2.1	26.4
Emergency medical technicians and paramedics	122	0.9	27.8
Health diagnosing and treating practitioner support technicians	226	1.7	18
Licensed practical and licensed vocational nurses	586	4.5	14.2
Medical records and health information technicians	134	1	30
Service occupations	**4,152**	**31.8**	**33.2**
Home health aides	458	3.5	66.4
Nursing aides, orderlies, and attendants	1,230	9.4	22.2
Physical therapist assistants and aides	95	0.7	41
Dental assistants	257	2	43.6
Medical assistants	361	2.8	53.7
Medical transcriptionists	81	0.6	22.1

Table 4.7   (*Continued*)

Occupation	Number	Percent	Percent Change: 2004–2014
Food preparation and serving related occupations	462	3.5	12.6
Building cleaning workers	365	2.8	20.6
Personal and home care aides	312	2.4	60.5
Office and administrative support occupations	**2379**	**18.2**	**16.2**
Billing and posting clerks and machine operators	179	1.4	10.9
Receptionists and information clerks	353	2.7	31.3
Medical secretaries	347	2.7	17.3

Source. U.S, Bureau of Labor Statistics Career Guide to Industries, Table 2, Employment of wage and salary workers in health services by occupation, 2004 and projected change, 2004–14. (Employment in thousands). U.S. Department of Labor, 2005.

in their affiliated clinical training sites (e.g., teaching hospitals and community clinics). While human resource issues loom across a broad range of health care occupations in the coming decade, those pertaining to the supply of physicians and nurses will be highlighted. In the case of both professions, issues emerge in both overall labor supply and in specialization.

Physicians

As previously shown in Table 4.1, the United States has about 2.3 practicing physicians per thousand persons, considerably below the OECD average of 2.9 practicing physicians per thousand (OECD, 2005c). Although at various points over the last 50 years policy makers has identified either an oversupply or undersupply of physicians, the number of physicians in the United States has increased as a nearly perfect linear function of the nation's gross domestic product (GDP; Cooper, Getzen, McKee, & Laud, 2002). That is, as the economy has produced more across all sectors, demand for health care services from physicians has also expanded—and for the most part the supply of physicians has increased sufficiently to accommodate it. This simple demand model of physician supply does not in and of itself suggest what mechanisms are employed to accommodate the demand, but in reality only three options are available: expanding the number of medical school slots, recruiting graduates of foreign medical schools, and preventing the attrition of trained physicians (e.g., delaying retirement). In a departure from prior projections of a physician oversupply, in its most recent appraisal of physician supply trends the Council on Graduate Medical Education (COGME) predicts the emergence of a significant undersupply of physicians by the year 2020. Among the factors that the COGME cites is the aging of the population, changes in the lifestyle preferences of physicians toward fewer hours of work, and continued growth in the GDP (Council on Graduate Medical Education, 2005).

Supply of Specialists. Relative to other countries with advanced health care systems, the United States has a higher proportion of its physician labor force allocated to specializations in medicine, namely physicians who are trained to diagnose and treat a defined subset of health conditions that generally are specific to a system of the body. Examples include endocrinology, orthopedic medicine, cardiology, and pulmonary medicine. In contrast, primary care physicians are trained to treat a wide range of routine health conditions and attend to the patient's overall health needs. The dominant primary care domains of medicine include family practice, pediatrics, general internal medicine, and obstetrics/gynecology. Where health care by a specialist tends to be shorter term and disease focused, care by a primary care physician is by nature longer term and holistic (Shi & Singh 2001, p. 122).

In the United States, the ratio between specialists and primary care physicians is about 2:1, whereas in Canada the ratio between specialists and primary care physicians is almost exactly 1:1(Bodenheimer & Grumbach, 2002; Canadian Labour and Business Centre, 2003). Fifty years ago, the specialist–primary care ratio in the United States was essentially same as that observed in Canada today, but the combined forces of a specialist-oriented culture in U.S. medical schools and a health care finance system that provides superior income opportunities for specialists ultimately yielded a physician labor force that is dominated by specialists (Bodenheimer & Grumbach, 2002, p. 196). Although it might appear that a physician labor force that is dominated by specialists with in-depth expertise in a wide range of debilitating and deadly health conditions should yield better population health outcomes, there are reasons to suggest that the opposite is true. For example, the more extensive training requirements of specialists take dollars out of the health care system that might have been spent on prevention or the direct provision of health care, and further, retain already highly trained physicians in training settings for a longer period (Grumbach, 2002). In fact, there is evidence that, to the extent that an emphasis on the training of specialists decreases the supply of primary care physicians, both population mortality levels and health disparities may increase (Starfield, Shi, Grover, & Macinko, 2005).

At this point, it is difficult to predict what direction the trend in the specialist–primary care mix will take over the next decade. Forces that are pushing toward a sustained emphasis on specialization include the aging of the population, the recent retreat from the aggressive growth of managed care that characterized the 1990s, and continued growth in the domestic economy. On the other hand, the reemergence of significant health care inflation in the current decade and the continued rise in the proportion of employed Americans without health insurance may signal a shift toward health care financing solutions that are less favorable to specialists, such as the resurgence of population-based health care insurance plans that are more affordable to a broad range of the labor force or more widespread use of health savings accounts.[16]

Registered Nurses

Just over one person out of every seven that is employed in the health care industry is a registered nurse (see Table 4.7). Nationally, there are 7.8 registered nurses for every 1,000 persons, although there is wide geographic variation in the supply of registered nurses relative to the population (Kaiser Family Foundation, 2006d). The basic level of credentialing for a Registered Nurse is completion of either a 2-year college degree, or a 3- or 4-year degree from an accredited school of nursing, followed by qualification for state licensure via passage of a state-sanctioned written examination.[17] Registered nurses are also credentialed in a wide range of advanced clinical specializations, including pulmonary care, intensive care, geriatrics, psychosocial nursing, and obstetrics—to name a few. In recent decades there has been enormous growth in the training and employment opportunities for nurse practitioners, generally defined as nurses with an advanced academic degree and the requisite clinical experience to diagnose and manage a wide range of common health conditions and chronic diseases. In most parts of the country nurse practitioners are sanctioned to practice as primary care providers. That is, they may diagnose disease, order diagnostic tests, prescribe medications, and otherwise fulfill all other essential functions of a primary care provider.

---

[16] Although population-based health insurance plans (i.e. Health Maintenance Organizations) became wildly unpopular during the latter half of the 1990s, they were effective in both constraining the rise in the cost of health care insurance coverage and reducing out-of-pocket expenditures for their enrollees. As American workers confront increased co-pays and premium cost sharing, it is plausible that HMO enrollment may resurge. Health Savings Accounts, the health care reform vehicle favored by the Bush administration, generally rewards more prudent use of health care services by health care consumers.

[17] Over the past 50 years, the 3-year hospital-based schools of nursing have largely disappeared and have been replaced by 2-year and 4-year programs sponsored by community colleges and universities.

In contrast to the debate that is raging among health care policy analysts pertaining to the prospects for a shortage of physicians, there is little debate about the basic reality of a nationwide shortage of registered nurses (RNs). Although projections vary, one particularly rigorous analysis (Buerhaus, Staiger, & Auerbach, 2000) suggests that the supply of the nursing labor force by the year 2020 will fall short of the demand by about 20%. Much of the projected nursing shortage has to do with demand-side factors (population growth, the aging of the population, and continued economic expansion). However, key supply-side factors include the aging of the nurses currently in the work force (by 2010 the average age is projected to be just over 45 years old, Buerhaus et al., p. 2952), declines in the number of women choosing nursing as a career, and declines in preferences for full-time employment among more recent cohorts of RNs.

To a significant extent, the nursing shortage in the United States and other developed countries is being mitigated by the influx of RNs trained in other countries (Ross, Polsky, & Sochalski, 2005). The U.S. proportion of foreign-trained RNs has risen dramatically in recent years, rising from 6 percent in 1999 to just over 14% in 2003 (Brush, Sochalski, & Berger, 2004). Aside from whatever challenges might be encountered in language, culture, and training differences between domestically trained RNs and those educated outside the United States, a larger question is raised about the role of the U.S. health care system as an agent of international social and economic exploitation. Although many foreign-educated RNs migrate from countries that have achieved levels of economic development and population health at least similar to that of the United States, every year there are increased numbers of RNs imported by the United States that leave countries and regions of the world that can ill afford to lose them, such as Southeast Asia, the Philippines, and sub-Saharan Africa (Brush et al., 2004). For example, in contrast to the 7.8 RN/1,000 person ratio in the United States, many the nations of Africa that are targets of recruitment by the United States and other developed countries (most notably Australia and the U.K.) have nurse-to-population ratios that are less than 1 RN/1,000 persons (Brush et al., 2004). To make matters even worse, the nurses that are the prime targets of recruitment are those with the highest levels of technical training, for example those having specialized skills in neonatal care, critical care, and surgery (Brush et al., p. 81).

All of this suggests that as a matter of international social justice as well as prudent domestic policy, the United States faces significant and immediate challenges in nursing recruitment and training. Solutions must involve considerable national investments at all levels of nursing education, ranging from the training of Ph.D.-level nursing educators to greatly expanded tuition subsidies to community college level schools of nursing. Although some might argue that the rise in the RN wages as the labor market tightens will ultimately accomplish much of the needed recruitment of RNs with little need for government leadership—thus far the evidence suggests that this will occur largely to the detriment of the poorest nations in the world.

THE HEALTH CARE SYSTEM SAFETY NET

The health care safety net is conventionally defined as the health care providers that care for those without health insurance, those on Medicaid and populations that face "special conditions," such as those with tuberculosis, AIDS, or serious and persistent mental illness (Hegner, 2001; IOM, 2000). As noted by the Institute of Medicine's comprehensive assessment of the nation's health care safety net published in 2000,[18] health care safety net providers can be distinguished from other providers of health care by two features: (1) either by mission or by legal mandate they are committed to the acceptance of any and all patients regardless of the patient's ability to pay and (2) their patient base is largely comprised of the uninsured, those on Medicaid, and those who have the special illnesses and conditions that often carry the burden of stigma and marginalization (IOM, 2000, pp. 3–4). This latter feature of safety net providers is particularly critical, because by definition it acknowledges that the burden of care for the poor and the marginalized in the U.S. health care system is not distributed uniformly across providers— but rather that safety net providers absorb a disproportionate share of care for the poor and the stigmatized. Put another way, the very existence of the health care safety net establishes the two-tiered nature of health care in the United States: one system for those having the ability to pay and another system for those relying on various forms of government subsidized programs. As will be shown in the discussion that follows, the magnitude of the burden of publicly financed and uncompensated care on the health care safety net reflects the extent to which the U.S. health care system is both segregated and hierarchical along lines of race and social class.

The Provider Composition of the Health Care Safety Net

Generally speaking, health care safety net providers include public and private not-for-profit community hospitals, publicly funded community

---

[18] *Americas Health Care Safety Net: Intact but Endangered*, full citation in list of references.

health clinics, local health departments, and individual physicians and other providers that for various reasons have a high level of commitment to caring for a disproportionate share of the poor and medically indigent.[19] Due to the mandates of the Emergency Medical Treatment and Labor Act of 1986 (EMTALA), a significant part of the health care safety net includes hospital emergency departments, since the provisions of EMTALA require that hospitals with emergency departments provide a medical screening examination for any individual who comes to the hospital and requests such an examination, regardless of ability to pay.[20] In practical terms, this means that hospital based emergency departments function not only as the primary provider of emergency care for the poor and medically indigent, but also as the provider of care for ordinary illnesses and minor injuries for those unable access the conventional primary care system.

A remarkable feature of the health care safety net is its existence as a loosely knit and in general ad hoc system of care—despite its crucial role as the care provider of last and only resort for many of the nation's poor, uninsured, and otherwise marginalized. As noted by the IOM's *America's Health Care Safety Net: Intact but Endangered* report (IOM, 2000), the safety net is at best a "patchwork of institutions, financing and programs that vary dramatically across the country as a result of a broad range of economic, political, and structural factors." These factors include the local tax base, each state's particular eligibility rules for Medicaid, and each community's historical commitment to the adequate provision of health care to the poor (IOM, 2000, p. 4).

Because the patchwork nature of the safety net system precludes an accurate and simple description that includes all of the nation's safety net providers, the approach taken here will involve a systematic description of the safety net's core providers—as identified by the Institute of Medicine. These core providers of the safety net include public hospitals, community health centers, local health departments, community hospitals, teaching hospitals, some categories of private providers (rural physicians, rural pharmacists, inner-city minority physicians), school-based clinics, Veterans Administration hospitals and clinics, and the Indian Health Service.

---

[19] The term "medically indigent" generally refers to those that lack sufficient insurance, income, or savings to pay for essential health care. Although medically indigent persons are more often either unemployed or in low-wage jobs, under a variety of circumstances the medically indigent can include persons of middle and even high income.

[20] Sanctions for violations of EMTALA are quite severe, and can include both direct fines and even the termination of the hospital's status as a provider of care to federally funded patients—which for almost all hospitals would result in financial ruin.

Public Hospitals

Excluding federal hospitals and hospitals serving special categories of illness and disability, as of 2005 there are 4,895 hospitals in the United States, of which 22.9% are owned by state and local governments (Kaiser Family Foundation, 2005). The remainder of the industry is divided between nonprofit hospital ownership (61%) and for-profit ownership (16.1%). Although public hospitals have the smallest share of the health care market, they carry the largest share of the burden for care that is broadly classified as "uncompensated"—that is, care that is either classified as charity care or bad debt. The graph shown in Figure 4.3, extracted from a recent research report prepared by the United States Government Accountability Office (GAO, 2005b), illustrates the pattern of uncompensated care by hospital ownership in five states that were selected as a representative sample of the United States. With the exception of Indiana, where nonprofit hospitals provide a slightly higher proportion of uncompensated care, the public hospitals function provide two to three times the uncompensated care than is provided by either the not-for-profit sector or the proprietary (for profit) sector of the hospital industry. In the states sampled by the GAO in this report, the for-profit sector of the industry devotes an average of 4.0% its patient care expenses to uncompensated care, while the public sector average level of commitment to uncompensated care is 11.7%. This difference represents the very different patient populations of public and for-profit hospitals, as well as their quite opposite fiduciary mandates The fiduciary mandate of public hospitals pertains to the accessibility of essential health care for all, while the boards and administrators of for-profit hospitals are obligated to place the interests of the hospital's investors ahead of the interest of the public. From this perspective, the gap in relative dollars devoted to uncompensated care between public hospitals and private ones is pretty much as one might expect.

However, what is less intuitive is the low level of commitment to charitable care on the part of not-for-profit hospitals, which on average have only a marginally higher proportion of their patient care dollars devoted to uncompensated care than for-profit hospitals (5.4% on average as opposed to 4.0% in the for-profit ownership sector). As noted by the GAO in the narrative that accompanies Figure 4.3, there are no clear standards to hold not-for-profit hospitals accountable for providing community benefits that are commensurate with the favored tax benefits of being a not-for-profit entity (GAO, 2005b, p. 19). Thus for the most part, nonprofit hospitals and for-profit hospitals behave very much like each other in terms of the kinds of patients each competes to serve—and competes not to serve.

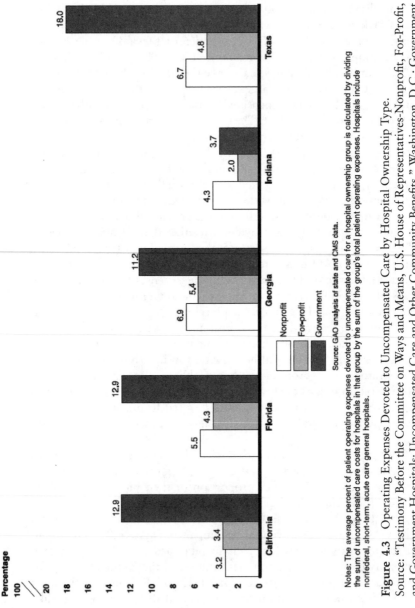

Figure 4.3 Operating Expenses Devoted to Uncompensated Care by Hospital Ownership Type.

Source: "Testimony Before the Committee on Ways and Means, U.S. House of Representatives-Nonprofit, For-Profit, and Government Hospitals: Uncompensated Care and Other Community Benefits." Washington, D.C.: Government Accountability office: May 26, 2005.

Among public hospitals there is a core of large institutions that, while they represent less than 4% of the staffed hospital beds in the United States, account for almost one-quarter of uncompensated care (AHA, 2005a; National Association of Public Hospitals and Health Systems, 2005).[21] These hospitals and health care systems represent such names as the Cook County Hospital system in Chicago, Bellevue Hospital in New York, the Los Angeles County Hospital system, and Charity Hospital in New Orleans—the latter totally destroyed in the wake of Hurricane Katrina.

Community Health Centers

Originally founded during the Lyndon Johnson administration as a partial measure to counter Medicare and Medicaid's inability to close the universal coverage gap (Hegner, 2001), community health centers and clinics provide primary care and preventative health services in communities characterized by high rates of poverty, low rates of health care insurance coverage, and limited access to health care services (IOM, 2000, pp. 59–60). Although local government financing, charitable support, and in-kind contributions are important sources of support for community health centers, federal funds are a large and essential source of support for the many community health centers that qualify for federally funding under Section 330 of the Public Health Services Act (IOM, 2000). As noted elsewhere (see chapter 3, Health Care Finance), though small relative to Medicare, Medicaid, and the VA health care system, federally funded Community Health Centers (CHCs) serve as a critical safety net provider in low-income communities. As a condition of federal funding, CHCs must be located in a high-need community, provide comprehensive primary care services, must ensure availability of transportation and language translation services, must have a community and consumer based governance structure, and finally must adjust fees in accordance with patients' ability to pay (HRSA, 2005a). Other common characteristics of CHCs include more extensive use of physician's assistants, midwives, and allied health professionals like social workers than is typically found in private sector primary health care practices, as well significant commitments to teaching, training, and entry level employment opportunities

---

[21] According the American Hospital Association's most recent annual survey of hospitals there are 955,578 staffed hospital beds in the U.S. (AHA, 2005b). The hospitals and health care systems belonging to the National Association of Public Hospitals and Health Care Systems, composing only 32,515 of the nation's staffed hospital beds (as counted in the year 2003), provided 24% of uncompensated care during 2003 (National Association of Public Hospitals and Health Systems, 2005).

for community residents (Waitzkin, 2005). Although the federal sponsorship of CHCs was less than $2 billion during fiscal year 2005, the
Health Resources and Services Administration estimates that 15 million
uninsured and underserved individuals will receive primary care through
3,800 CHCs (HRSA, 2005b).

Local Health Departments

As noted by the Institute of Medicine (2000), the more than 3,000 local city and county health departments are an essential source of health
care for those that are the least advantaged and often the most at risk
for disease and death from preventable causes: such as homeless persons, immigrants, the working poor, and those without health insurance
or a regular source of medical care (IOM, 2000, p. 64). Even so, local health departments function under an ongoing historical tension between the provision of those services that are critical to disease prevention
and preventable mortality and ongoing close scrutiny from the politically
dominant private practice sector of medicine—the primary concern being the incursion of public medicine into areas that are potentially profitable for the private practitioner (Starr, 1982). Thus, there is a significant discrepancy between what the federal government defines as the
core public health functions of local health departments (e.g., population health status monitoring, health regulation enforcement, birth and
death registration, and public health education) and a broader agenda endorsed by the far majority of Local Health Department (LHD) directors
that extends to the provision of direct health care services to vulnerable
populations (IOM, 2000). In addition to such direct services as maternal and child health care, screening and treatment for sexually trans-
mitted diseases and tuberculosis, and immunizations, LHDs often venture into a broader scope of direct primary care for populations that
are poorly served and of little interest to private sector medicine (Shi
& Singh, 2001). Although the rise of Medicaid-managed care programs
and the shifting of some Medicaid-mandated services to conventional
health care providers during the last decade reduced the direct health care
role of many LHDs, it appears that the most progressive LHDs can continue to provide some essential specialized services that are less likely to
be directly provided by conventional managed care organizations (IOM,
2000).

Teaching Hospitals

Although many teaching hospitals are also public hospitals with a mandated role as a safety net provider, many teaching hospitals that fall

within either the private not-for-profit sector or the private for-profit sector also provide health care to the poor, the uninsured, and the chronically ill and disabled by default. This occurs for several reasons, of which two are primary. The first is a historical relationship between clinical training and health services for the poor, where those unable to afford access to needed health care through private providers resort to teaching hospitals and affiliated clinics that have some willingness to provide free or heavily subsidized care in return for the patient's illness and treatment serving as an exemplar for teaching (Starr, 1982). Although on its face this appears (and some times is) an exploitive relationship, it is also the case that teaching hospitals often offer superior care. A second reason is that teaching hospitals are often the sole community or even regional providers of highly specialized and technologically advanced health care, such as trauma care, burn units, organ transplants, rare infectious diseases, and spinal cord injury (IOM, 2000). The patients that are in need of these specialized services are often without health care insurance coverage that is adequate, are made poor through the effects of their health conditions on their employment and savings, or are at higher risk for these conditions as a function of poverty (e.g., as in the relationship between housing conditions and severely burned children). An important source of funding for the care of the poor in teaching hospitals comes from both Disproportionate Share Medicaid and Medicare Indirect Medical Education payments.

Community Hospitals

Despite the disproportionate burden of care for the uninsured assumed by large public hospitals, it also the case that not-for-profit community hospitals and their affiliated clinics furnish the brunt of uncompensated care (IOM, 2000). Even though community hospitals typically provide a much smaller individual share of uncompensated care relative to public hospitals, they are by far the largest sector of the hospital industry in the number of hospitals and thus have a very large collective contribution. Community hospitals are generally defined as hospitals that are nonfederal and whose services are open to the general public (Shi & Singh, 2001), and they typically provide a broad array of the most commonly needed acute care medical and surgical services. The prevalent origins of community hospitals include establishment by religious organizations and ethnic communities, and through the joint efforts of civic leaders, local medical societies, and local philanthropists. However, by far the largest source of development and growth for community hospitals originated with the federal government's Hill–Burton Act of 1946,[22] which provided funding for the largest expansion of hospitals and hospital bed capacity in U.S. history. Because funding from the Hill–Burton Act carried with it the obligation to make an annual repayment of the federal debt in the form of uncompensated care, through most of the latter half of the 20th century the term "community hospital" implied a significant commitment to provision of uncompensated care to the poor and the uninsured. Another reason that community hospitals play such a key role in the health care safety net, aside from the faith-based commitments or the long-term impact of Hill–Burton funding obligations, is that they are also often the sole local provider of hospital and emergency services—thus necessitating a certain burden of care to the poor and uninsured that cannot be shifted elsewhere. In rural communities in particular, this poses a significant burden on the financial solvency of small community hospitals (Stensland & Milet, 2002).

The Veterans Administration System

The Veterans Administration System has long served as the core provider of health care services to disabled veterans, and historically as the health care provider of last resort for veterans who were unable to afford health care through the conventional employer-based insurance market. More recently, as more working Americans lack health insurance and as states have imposed greater restrictions on access to Medicaid for low-income adults, the VA system has become an even more essential source of health care for low-income veterans. Aside from those veterans receiving care from the VA for service-connected disabilities, over a third of those treated in the VA system meet low-income–based eligibility (Hughes, 2003). As discussed in chapter 3 (Health Care Finance), beginning in 1997 the VA system has gone through a radical transformation from primarily an inpatient-based system with a centralized bureaucracy to a more outpatient intensive system of 22 regional networks with independent budgets that are based on capitation (Ashton et al., 2003). Under the new system of organization, the VA is accessible to veterans on the basis of an ordered set of seven priorities, of which low-income status is ranked fifth. Under the current scheme, the extent to which any of the 22 regional VA networks is able to serve as a safety net for low-income veterans appears in large part to be a function of the local proportion of veterans who are among the ranks of the uninsured.

---

[22] Also known by its official title as The Hospital Survey and Reconstruction Act of 1946 (see chapter 2 on the history of the U.S. Health Care System).

The Indian Health Service

The Indian Health Service (IHS) is an agency within the U.S. Department of Health and Human Services responsible for the provision of health services to American Indians and Alaska Natives. Thus, the IHS is supposed to serve as the principal health care safety net for the indigenous peoples of the lower 48 states and Alaska. At the present time, the IHS serves approximately 1.5 million of the 2.5 million Americans who identified their race as American Indian or Alaska Native in the 2000 census (IHS, 2005). The Native Americans and Alaska Natives receiving health care services from the IHS services are members of one of 557 tribes in 35 different states (IHS, 2005), so from that perspective it must be acknowledged that the IHS has limited geographic coverage as a safety net. For the tribal members that the INS is able to serve, it acts as not only a primary care provider but also as the principal public health agency for indigenous peoples. Prevention and treatment initiatives undertaken by the IHS address (among other priorities) the disproportionate rates of injury, alcoholism, diabetes, and mental health problems among Native Americans (Shi & Singh, 2001). Nationally, the IHS is divided into 12 geographic area offices responsible for program operations that generally deliver direct health care services through IHS-funded hospitals, health centers, and health stations (GAO, 2005a). As a recent Government Accountability Office report points out, the Native Americans and Alaska Natives dependent upon the IHS for health care encounter a variety of barriers to adequate access to primary health care services. These barriers include waiting periods in some clinics of between 2 and 6 months, limited access to transportation, and endemic shortages in staff, equipment, and contract care funds for services IHS hospitals and clinics could not provide directly (GAO, 2005a). Although the Indian Health Care Improvement Act of 1976 had as its central goal a systematic effort to raise the level of Native Americans to parity with the U.S. general population (Shi & Singh, 2001), it is clear that the agency has never been funded to achieve anything like parity in health care services—let alone parity in population health.[23] However the IHS, to its credit, continues to pursue an aggressive and often innovative public health and health care safety net

---

[23] It should be emphasized here, as it is elsewhere in this volume, that population health is only partially a function of public health interventions and optimal access to high-quality health care services. The disproportionate incidence of infant mortality, adult onset diabetes, injuries, suicides, pneumonia, and renal disease among Native Americans is a function of historic and contemporary racial oppression, poverty, and enduring sources of structural disadvantage that cannot be overcome by even radical improvements in the health services available to native peoples.

agenda despite the limited fiscal support it receives from the U.S. Congress and successive administrations.

Other Safety Net Providers

Other safety net providers highlighted by the IOM report on the safety net system include school-based health clinics, some private health care practitioners, and in particular some groups of private health care practitioners. While it is the case that some private physicians and other allied health care providers such as dentists, psychologists, and social workers in private practice often discount or provide uncompensated health care, it is difficult to quantify their contributions or identify their criteria for determining the recipients of uncompensated care. However, the IOM report identifies three practitioner groups that tend to provide a disproportionate share of care to the poor, disabled, and/or the uninsured. These are physicians that practice in rural communities, rural pharmacists, and minority physicians serving inner-city populations.

Federal Support for the Health Care Safety Net

Federal support for the health care safety net comes in two primary forms. The first form of support is legislation that requires some health providers to ensure essential care for an array of medical emergencies, health conditions, and special populations with or without adequate reimbursement. One example of federal supportive legislation is the previously mentioned Emergency Medical Treatment and Labor Act of 1986 (EMTALA), which requires that hospitals with emergency departments provide a medical screening examination for any individual who comes to the hospital and requests such an examination, regardless of ability to pay. A second example is the Consolidated Omnibus Reconciliation Act of 1985 (COBRA),which precludes hospitals from "patient dumping," i.e. transferring patients in need of care to other less appropriate facilities for financial reasons. The second source of support for the health care safety net is funding through Medicaid direct care programs that fund health care for low-income children and adults living in poverty, indirect supports like Medicaid and Medicare Disproportionate Share payment adjustments that provide limited subsidy to providers with a large share of the poor, tax benefits to not-for-profit private sector providers that provide the brunt of safety net health care (although there is some debate as to whether the tax benefits are given their full value in charity care and other community benefits), funding community health care clinics in low-income communities, and systems of the health care for special populations—most notably the VA system and the Indian Health Service. The most recent estimate of federal spending on the health care safety net, compiled by the Kaiser Commission Medicare and the Uninsured, estimates that the U.S. government spent a total of 22.8 billion dollars on the health care safety net in 2004—which in relative terms is less than 1 percent of the overall federal expenditures (Kaiser Commission on Medicaid and the Uninsured, 2005b). This expenditure is also about one-half of the 41 billion dollars that the Kaiser Commission estimates providers contributed in 2004 to care for the uninsured (KCMI, 2005a, p. 2). The take-home message from these estimates is that while the federal plays a crucial role in the financing of the health care safety net, the fiscal commitment at the federal level is neither adequate to the task nor generous.

Threats to the Health Care Safety Net

Due to both its patchwork nature and the year-to-year financial solvency problems of its core providers, the stability of the health care safety net in America has long existed in a state of ongoing jeopardy. However, the Institute of Medicine's comprehensive report on the status and prospects of the health care safety net (IOM, 2000) identifies three major challenges to America's care safety net that places core safety net providers even at more risk than in the past (IOM, 2000, p. 209):

- The rising numbers of uninsured individuals.
- The full impact of mandated Medicaid managed care among core safety net providers in a more competitive health care marketplace.
- The erosion and uncertainty of major direct and indirect subsidies that have helped to support safety net functions.

In the 5 years since this comprehensive report was published, all three areas of threat have grown and merit a brief summary of the main concerns.

The Rising Tide of the Uninsured: An Old Threat Growing Worse

At the time of the IOM report on the health care safety net, in the year 2000, the numbers of Americans without health insurance had at last leveled off at just under 40 million after several years of disconcerting growth—about one million more persons every year without health insurance coverage (Kaiser Commission on Medicaid and the Uninsured, 2005a). Between the years 2000 and 2004, the nation added another 6 million persons without health insurance and there is no reason to assume these trends will abate in the absence of a major shift in national health care policy. As the 1990s demonstrated, even sustained improvements in the national economy and the labor market are insufficient to offset rising global pressures on employers to reduce health care benefit costs and a weakening level of commitment among even very large employers to the provision of affordable health care for their employees. Not all of this reflects global competition either. In the face of competitive pressures from employers that are particularly willing to engage in aggressive practices to avoid the provision of health care insurance to their employees, even employers with a historically significant commitment to the viability of the employer-based insurance market may be forced to participate in a so-called "race to the bottom" in terms of even minimal health care insurance benefits (Altman, Shactman, & Eilat, 2006). The national poster child for this trend is the Wal-Mart Corporation, which as the largest employer in the United States may also become the standard setter for the typical wages and benefits available to at least the retail sector of the economy—if not in all economic sectors. Although claims and counterclaims abound concerning Wal-Mart's labor practices, a recently published well-documented analysis of Wal-Mart's health care benefits estimated that Wal-Mart covered only 38.3% of its employees—in contrast to a national average for other large employers of 66% (West, 2005).[24] For good or for bad, the extent to which Wal-Mart indeed assumes the role as national trend setter in health benefits and other labor practices in large part will be a function of consumer preferences. As observed health policy scholar Stuart Altman, "... We might not like the pay and benefit package Wal-Mart provides to its employees, but many are content to shop there and pay lower prices." (Altman et al., 2006, p. 20).

Federal Budget Deficits and Cutbacks in Medicaid

Also at the time of the IOM report of the health care safety net in year 2000, the U.S. budget was running a significant surplus—leading many to offer an optimistic appraisal of more generous federal support for the expansion of Medicaid to cover a larger share of the working poor. However, in the years since the fiscal and political climate has turned 180 degrees, and at this point in the first decade of the 21st century the federal budget is deeply in the red and the Medicaid program is facing

[24] The Center for a Changing Workforce (CFCW), the publisher of this report, is a nonprofit research and policy organization that examines issues affecting what it terms "low-wage and nonstandard workers" (West, 2005, p. 1). The CFCW's analysis of the Wal-Mart's health benefit expenditures is based upon corporate documents, Internal Revenue Service filings, and health and welfare benefit trust filings with the U.S. Department of Labor.

significant reductions. Contained in the provisions of the Deficit Reduction Act of 2005[25] are rather drastic cuts to the Medicaid program. As estimated by the Congressional Budget Office, the Deficit Reduction Act of 2005 reduces the federal Medicaid expenditures by 26.4 billion over the 2006–2015 period (Congressional Budget Office, 2006). The central cost reduction strategy of this legislation permits states to both reduce benefits and impose additional cost sharing requirements on persons eligible for Medicaid—thus reducing both state and federal support for Medicaid. For example, this legislation permits states to impose as much as a 10% co-pay on the cost of health care services for individuals with family income between 100% and 150% of the federal poverty level and up to 20% for individuals with family income above 150% of the federal poverty level (Congressional Budget Office, 2006, p. 40). The Congressional Budget Office estimates that, as a result of these Medicaid program cutbacks, 65,000 Americans will lose their Medicaid coverage.

Based on historical experience, it seems reasonable to predict that such co-pays will impose a strong incentive on the part of the poor to avoid even much needed health care, and further incentives on the part of health care providers to avoid making health care available to the poor. This is not an accidental by-product of the co-pays, but (as any credible health economist can explain) their intended effect.[26] It should be noted that the significant cuts in health care for the poor contained in the Deficit Reduction Act of 2005 also are made to support the agenda by the Bush administration and its allies to make the temporary tax cuts passed in the early years of the administration permanent. Although the billions cut from Medicaid may appear to make the billions granted to wealthy Americans in permanent tax cuts fiscally viable, there is significant dissent even from within Bush's own party on this point.[27] Whatever the outcome of this particular debate, there is a larger political agenda embedded in the Deficit Reduction Act of 2005 than the continuation of generous tax cuts to the wealthy at stake—the further shrinkage of

[25] Passed by the U.S. Senate, December 21, 2005 and approved by the House of Representatives by a narrow (216 to 214) vote on February 1, 2006, this bill was signed by President George W. Bush on February 8, 2006.

[26] The position taken in this text is that the argument that the poor will avoid only "unnecessary" health care when confronted by co-pays they cannot afford is both preposterous and disingenuous.

[27] It is clear, even to some members of Bush's own party, that the tax cuts proposed to be made permanent more than offset any presumed savings contained in the Deficit Reduction Act. For example, George Voinovich (R-Ohio) described the proposed extension of the tax cuts an "immoral" burden on future generations (Congressional Record: February 1, 2006: S402).

the role of the federal government in the financing of health care for the poor.

The Devolution of the Safety Net Infrastructure: The Case of Charity Hospital in New Orleans

In the immediate wake of Hurricane Katrina on September 2, 2005, President Bush assured Senator Trent Lott (R-Mississippi) that his mansion that had been destroyed by Katrina would be rebuilt.[28] In defense of what many saw as an elitist remark that ignored the plight of those thousands of poor who had lost either family members or what little they possessed to Katrina, President Bush's staunchest defenders were quick to point out that the President meant his comment as a metaphor for his commitment to rebuild and restore the homes and communities that were equally reduced to rubble by Katrina. In fact, probably no better test for the Bush administration's commitment to such a rebuilding exists than Charity Hospital, the safety net hospital that became for a time the focus of national scandal when its patients and staff were left un-evacuated and essentially abandoned for days without clean water, electricity, food, and even the most basic emergency medical supplies (Berggren, 2005).

Known locally as "Big Charity," Charity Hospital of New Orleans was the second oldest hospital in the United States, opening its doors in 1736 just weeks after the first patients were admitted to Bellevue Hospital in New York. At the time Katrina hit New Orleans in August of 2005, Charity Hospital occupied a building that was constructed in 1939 to accommodate 2,680 inpatients (Medical Center of Louisiana at New Orleans, 2003). Although Charity's aged facility had been reduced to 565 staffed beds in more recent years, it remained among the busiest safety net hospitals in the United States. For example, in 2003 Charity Hospital provided 146,178 annual inpatient days of care and accounted for nearly 3,000 births (National Association of Public Hospitals and Health Systems, 2005). Of equal importance and more typical to critical safety net providers of comparable size, Charity Hospital of New Orleans also served as a regional trauma center and teaching hospital. Finally, Charity Hospital was Louisiana's and New Orleans' principal provider of hospital care for the poor—deriving 85% of its revenues from Medicaid (National Association of Public Hospitals and Health Systems, 2005).[29]

---

[28] "Out of the rubble of Trent Lott's house—he lost his entire house—there's going to be a fantastic house. And I'm looking forward to sitting on the porch." (Milbank, 2005).
[29] Figures as reported for year 2003.

Although both local and national authorities were quick to concede the floodwaters unleashed by Katrina had made the already decrepit hospital building unsalvageable, is was also apparent that there was nothing to replace the role Charity Hospital has long served as the hospital of last and only resort for the city's poor (Gesensway, 1999). Months after Charity's demise, uncertainty reigns in the state of Louisiana over the ultimate feasibility of rebuilding the hospital and the source of financing (Moller, 2006). Given the devastating effects of the Katrina disaster on Louisiana's economy and the other demands for reinvestment the state faces, it is difficult to foresee any way that a modernized version of a public hospital with an equal level of commitment to care for the poor and uninsured of Louisiana will rise again—at least in the current national health care policy environment.

The case of Charity Hospital provides two lessons concerning the devolution of the health care safety net. The first is that Charity's decrepit condition preceding its final destruction reflected a longstanding failure to reinvest in the buildings and equipment needed to sustain an adequate safety net—either directly through state level capital construction funds or indirectly through Medicaid and Medicare payment mechanisms. Although discussions in recent years among local health care planners had identified the replacement of the 65-year-old Charity Hospital building and related infrastructure as critical need, the pre-Katrina cash-strapped State of Louisiana was in no position to allocate the funds necessary to either refurbish the aging institution or provide the resources to enable the Charity Hospital system to adapt to a changing health care market (Gesensway, 1999). The second lesson is that absent a major overhaul of the system of health care finance for the poor and those without access to health insurance, other safety net providers like Charity Hospital will ultimately collapse under the burden of uncompensated and undercompensated health care costs. For example, in a survey of its member institutions the National Association of Public Hospitals and Health Systems found that in the year 2003 the average operating margins among the core safety net hospitals sank to one-half of 1%—though a 2% operating margin is considered the minimum that is essential for the long-term survival of both private and public sector hospitals (National Association of Public Hospitals and Health Systems, 2005). Given the most recent moves by Congress to cut the further funds from the Medicaid program, it is difficult to see how the average operating margins of safety net hospitals for the years ahead will escape staying out of the red—thus inducing a crisis of insolvency nationwide within the next decade.

CONCLUDING COMMENTS—THE PARADOXICAL UNDERACHIEVEMENT OF THE U.S. HEALTH CARE SYSTEM

For decades the health care reform debate has been framed by the assumption that primary deficits in the U.S. health care system pertain to its failure to provide universal access to health care. However, the evidence continues to mount that the U.S. health care system, despite its being the most expensive in the world, fails to achieve the population health outcomes of nations that spend far less per capita on health care. While many of the factors that influence population health are only peripherally affected by the organization of the health care system, the prevalence of the diseases that contribute the most to disability and early death are also a function of the adequacy of the health care system. The United Kingdom, a nation with a rigid social class structure that spends over 50% less per capita than the United States on health care, has an adult population that is in remarkably superior health *at all levels of the social class gradient* (Banks, Marmot, Oldfield, & Smith, 2006). Rich, middle income, or poor, British adults in middle age have dramatically lower prevalence rates of diabetes, hypertension, heart disease, and cancer than U.S. citizens of the same socioeconomic status (Banks et al., 2006, p. 2039). Because these disadvantages in relative health affect affluent Americans as much as well Americans in poverty, it cannot be claimed that the primary deficits of the U.S. Health care system are attributable to the health insurance gap. What else could be wrong?

In truth, there is no clear answer or scientifically unequivocal explanation to this paradoxical underachievement of the U.S. health care system. By some accounts, the disconnect between the dollars and resources spent on health care in the United States and deficits in population health lies almost entirely outside of the health care system, through such mechanisms as poverty, racism, social isolation, and rising levels of income inequality (Phelan, Link, Diez-Roux, Kawachi, & Levin, 2004; Wilkinson, 1996). A second take, from a more Marxist perspective, is that the health care system paradox is nothing more and nothing less than a reflection of the system's success at achieving its latent function, the reinforcement of class structure and the expansion of opportunities for capital class exploitation. A third account suggests that the paradox arises from the U.S. health care system's orientation toward disease treatment and symptom management rather than the key factors that shape individual health behaviors and use of health services (Fuchs, 2004). Although there are strains of truth in each of these explanations (as well as a range of other accounts not mentioned), the common thread is that flaws in the organization of the health care system are complex, endemic, and deeply embedded in other aspects of social structure. In the chapters that follow, many of these interconnections will be illuminated—as well some of the key implications for health care system reform.

REFERENCES

AHA. (2005a, November 14). *Fast facts on U.S. hospitals from AHA Hospital Statistics.* Retrieved January 23, 2006, from http://www.aha.org/aha/resource_center/fastfacts/fast_facts_US_hospitals.html.

AHA. (2005b, November 14). *Fast facts on U.S. hospitals from AHA Hospital Statistics.* Retrieved February 2, 2006, from http://www.aha.org/aha/resource_center/fastfacts/fast_facts_US_hospitals.html#community.

Altman, S., Shactman, D., & Eilat, E. (2006). Could U.S. hospitals go the way of U.S. airlines? *Health Affairs, 25*(1), 11–21.

Andrulis, D. P., & Duchon, L. M. (2005). *Hospital care in the 100 largest cities and their suburbs, 1996–2002: Implications for the future of the hospital safety net in metropolitan America.* New York: SUNY Downstate Medical Center.

Ashton, C. M., Souchek, J., Petersen, N. J., Menke, T. J., Collins, T. C., Kizer, K. W., et al. (2003). Hospital use and survival among Veterans Affairs beneficiaries. *N Engl J Med, 349*(17), 1637–1646.

Banks, J., Marmot, M., Oldfield, Z., & Smith, J. P. (2006). Disease and Disadvantage in the United States and in England. *Journal of the American Medical Association, 295*(17), 2037–2045.

Berggren, R. (2005). Unexpected necessities—Inside Charity Hospital. *New England Journal of Medicine, 353*(15), 1550–1553.

Bodenheimer, T., & Grumbach, K. (2002). *Understanding health policy: A clinical approach* (3rd ed.). New York: Lange Medical Books/McGraw-Hill.

Brush, B. L., Sochalski, J., & Berger, A. M. (2004). Imported care: Recruiting foreign nurses to U.S. health care facilities. *Health Affairs, 23*(3), 78–87.

Buerhaus, P. I., Staiger, D. O., & Auerbach, D. I. (2000). Implications of an aging registered nurse workforce. *JAMA, 283*(22), 2948–2954.

Bureau of Labor Statistics. (2005). *Career guide to industries.* Washington, DC: U.S. Department of Labor.

Canadian Labour and Business Centre. (2003). *Physician workforce in Canada: Literature review and gap analysis.* Ottawa, Canada: Canadian Medical Forum.

Colombo, F., & Tapay, N. (2004). *OECD health working papers—Private health insurance in OECD countries: The benefits and costs for individuals and health systems* (No. 15). Paris, France: Organization for Economic Cooperation and Development.

Congressional Budget Office. (2006). *Congressional Budget Office Cost Estimate: S. 1932 Deficit Reduction Act of 2005.* Washington, DC: United States Congress.

Conrad, D., & Shortell, S. (1996). Integrated health systems: Promise and performance. *Frontiers of Health Services Management, 13*(1), 3–40.

Cooper, R. A., Getzen, T. E., McKee, H. J., & Laud, P. (2002). Economic and demographic trends signal an impending physician shortage. *Health Affairs, 21*(1), 140–154.

Council on Graduate Medical Education. (2005). *Physician workforce policy guidelines for the United States, 2000–2020.* Rockville, MD: Health Resources and Services Administration, Department of Health and Human Services.

Cuellar, A. E., & Gertler, P. J. (2003). Trends in hospital consolidation: The formation of local systems. *Health Affairs, 22*(6), 77–87.

Darcy, K., & Pope, J. (2006, January 9). FORCED TO CHANGE: Charity Hospital, an icon in trauma treatment and teaching, will never be the same after Katrina. *The Times-Picayune.*

Fuchs, V. R. (2004). Perspective: More variation in use of care, more flat-of-the-curve medicine. *Health Affairs,* 104.

GAO. (2005a). *Indian Health Service: Health care services are not always available to Native Americans* (No. GAO-05-789). Washington, DC: U.S. Government Accountability Office.

GAO. (2005b). *Testimony before the Committee on Ways and Means, U.S. House of Representatives—Nonprofit, for-profit, and government hospitals: Uncompensated care and other community benefits.* Washington, DC: General Accounting Office.

Gesensway, D. (1999). *How a legendary New Orleans hospital is struggling to finally change its ways.* Retrieved January, 2006, from http://www.acponline.org/journals/news/apr99/orleans.htm.

Grumbach, K. (2002). Perspective: The ramifications of specialty-dominated medicine. *Health Affairs, 21*(1), 155–157.

Hegner, R. (2001). *The health care safety net in a time of fiscal pressures.* Washington, DC: National Health Policy Forum.

Horowitz, J. (2005). Making profits and providing care: Comparing nonprofit, for-profit, and government hospitals. *Health Affairs, 24*(3), 790–801.

Hospital Corporation of America. (2004). *Hospital Corporation of America annual report to shareholders for 2004.* Nashville, TN.

HRSA. (2005a). *Bureau of Primary Care: Community Health Centers.* Retrieved July 1, 2005, from http://bphc.hrsa.gov/chc/.

HRSA. (2005b). *FY 2005 Budget in Brief—Health Resources and Services Administration.* Retrieved July 1, 2005, from http://www.hhs.gov/budget/05 budget.

Hughes, J. (2003). Can the Veterans Affairs health care system continue to care for the poor and vulnerable? *Journal of Ambulatory Care Management, 26*(4), 344–348.

IHS. (2005, February 7). *Indian Health Service Introduction.* Retrieved January 24, 2006, from http://www.ihs.gov/PublicInfo/PublicAffairs/Welcome_Info/IHSintro.asp.

IOM. (2000). *Institute of Medicine—America's health care safety net: Intact but endangered*. Washington, DC: National Academy Press.

Kaiser Commission on Medicaid and the Uninsured. (2005a). *Health insurance coverage in America: 2004 update*. Washington, DC: The Henry J. Kaiser Family Foundation.

Kaiser Commission on Medicaid and the Uninsured. (2005b). *Key facts on covering the uninsured—Growing need, strained resources*. Washington, DC: Henry J. Kaiser Family Foundation.

Kaiser Family Foundation. (2005). *Statehealthfacts.org*. Retrieved November 17, 2005, from http://www/statehealthfacts.kff.org.

Kaiser Family Foundation. (2006a). *Statehealthfacts: Distribution of nursing care facilities by ownership type*, 2003. Retrieved February 15, 2006, from http://statehealthfacts.org.

Kaiser Family Foundation. (2006b). *Statehealthfacts: Hospital admission per 1,000 persons 2003*. Retrieved February 2, 2006, from http://statehealthfacts.org.

Kaiser Family Foundation. (2006c). *Statehealthfacts: Hospitals by Ownership 2003*. Retrieved February 2, 2006, from http://statehealthfacts.org

Kaiser Family Foundation. (2006d). *Statehealthfacts: Registered Nurses per 10,000 population, 2002*. Retrieved February 15, 2006, from http://statehealthfacts.org.

Kane, R., Kane, R., & Ladd, R. (1998). *The heart of long term care*. New York: Oxford University press.

Medical Center of Louisiana at New Orleans. (2003, January 31, 2006). *The Beginnings of Charity Hospital*. Retrieved January 31, 2006, from http://www.mclno.org/.

Milbank, D. (2005, September 3). A day of contradictions. *The Washington Post*, p. A15.

Moller, J. (2006, June 23). Building costs could raise state debt: Hospital financing may collide with spending limits. *The Times-Picayune*.

National Association of public hospitals and health systems. (2005). *America's public hospitals and health care systems: Results of the Annual NAPH hospital characteristics survey*. Washington, DC: National Association of Public Hospitals and Health Systems.

National Center for Health Statistics. (2005). *Health, United States, 2005*. Hyattsville, MD: Centers for Disease Control and Prevention, U.S. Department of Health and Human Services.

OECD. (2005a). *OECD Health Data 2005: Life expectancy in years*. Retrieved February 18, 2006, from www.oecd.org/dataoecd/7/44/35530071.xls.

OECD. (2005b). *OECD Health Data 2005: MRI units per million population*. Retrieved February 16, 2006, from www.oecd.org/dataoecd/7/44/3553002.xls.

OECD. (2005c). *OECD Health Data 2005: Practicing physicians, density per 1,000 population, 1960 to 2003*. Retrieved February 18, 2006, from www.oecd.org/dataoecd/7/44/35529872.xls.

Phelan, J. C., Link, B. G., Diez-Roux, A., Kawachi, I., & Levin, B. (2004).

"Fundamental causes" of social inequalities in mortality: A test of the theory. *J Health Soc Behav*, 45(3), 265–285.

Rosenau, P. V. (2000). Managing medical technology: Lessons for the United States from Quebec and France. *International Journal of Health Services*, 30(3), 617–639.

Ross, S. J., Polsky, D., & Sochalski, J. (2005). Nursing shortages and international nurse migration. *International Nursing Review*, 52(4), 253–262.

Shi, L., & Singh, D. (2001). *Delivering health care in America* (2nd ed.). Gaithersburg, MD: Aspen Publishers.

Starfield, B., Shi, L., Grover, A., & Macinko, J. (2005). The effects of specialist supply on populations' health: Assessing the evidence. *Health Affairs*, W5-97.

Starr, P. (1982). *The social transformation of American medicine*. New York: Basic Books.

Stensland, J., & Milet, M. (2002). The variance of rural small-town hospitals' financial performance. *Policy Anal Brief W Series*, 5(3), 1–4.

Tenet Healthcare Corporation. (2006). *Corporate Website*. Retrieved February 9, 2006, from http://www.tenethealth.com/TenetHealth.

U.S. Census Bureau. (2004). *2002 economic census: Ambulatory health care services* (No. EC02-62I-01). Washington DC: U.S. Department of Commerce.

Waitzkin, H. (2005). Commentary—The history and contradictions of the health care safety net. *Health Services Research*, 40(3), 923–940.

West, D. (2005). *Wal-Mart and health care: Condition critical*. Seattle, WA: Center for a Changing Workforce.

Wilkinson, R. G. (1996). *Unhealthy societies: The afflictions of inequality*. London: Routledge.

CHAPTER FIVE

Long-Term Care of the Aged and Disabled

Long-term care involves the financing and delivery of an array of health and social services to the aged and disabled. In contrast to acute care, which is disease-based and curative in orientation, the orientation of long-term care is inherently holistic and function-based. The conventional definition of *long-term care,* provided by Kane, Kane, & Ladd's (1998) authoritative analysis of U.S. long-term care policy and services, is the "[h]ealth, personal care, and related social services provided over a sustained period of time to people who have lost or never developed certain measurable functional abilities" (p. 314). The scope of long-term care policies and services thus encompasses the aged, the developmentally disabled, the chronically ill, and persons disabled by trauma. Although there are many specific health care services and episodes of care that are typically defined and financed as a part of the acute care system, long-term care has a distinct identity in its own right (Kane, Kane, & Ladd, 1998). Ordinary acute care services are typically episodic in delivery, oriented toward specific gains in health, and are often experienced as a disruptive event in people's everyday lives. In contrast, the prolonged and holistic nature of long-term care leads to its becoming integral to people's lives (Kane, Kane, & Ladd, p. 4). Also in contrast to ordinary acute care, where there are formal boundaries between health care services, social services, and the supports provided through family, friendship networks, and the community, long-term care's boundaries are far more informal and permeable.

Although the public discourse pertaining to long-term care policy and services has generally been focused on the elderly, in reality the elderly account for between 50 and 60% of adults receiving long-term care services (Spector, Fleishman, Pezzin, & Spillman, 2000). The nonelderly long-term care users include the developmentally disabled, the mentally ill, persons with chemical dependencies, persons with chronic disabling illness (e.g., multiple sclerosis) and persons disabled through injury (Kane et al., 1998; Spector et al., 2000). Obtaining a precise estimate of the number of persons receiving long-term care services is relatively straightforward for those residing in institutional long-term care settings like nursing homes and long-term psychiatric hospitals, because counts of residents of these facilities are routinely reported to state and federal regulatory agencies. However, for the far majority of persons receiving community-based long-term care services, precise estimates are much more difficult to obtain. Through a methodology that combines household level survey data on the use of long-term care assistance and institutional data, the Agency for Health Policy and Research (AHPR) estimates that approximately 2.2 percent of adults between the ages of 18 and 64 (4 million) are long-term care recipients, while for those aged 65+, about 16.7 percent (6 million) are long-term care recipients (Spector et al., 2000; U.S. Census Bureau, 2005a).[1] It should be noted that while these estimates provide some idea of the number of long-term care users, like other health care utilization statistics they underestimate the number of persons actually in need of care.

THE LONG-TERM CARE SERVICES SYSTEM

The very broad definition of long-term care as encompassing "health, personal care, and related social services provided over a sustained period of time" (Kane, Kane, & Ladd, 1998, p. 314) suggests that it can be thought about in a number of ways. The approach taken by the AHPR distinguishes three general types of long-term care: formal care provided in the community setting, informal care provided in the community setting, and institutional care. Because formal care refers to care that is provided by paid persons as opposed to care that is provided by family, friends, and volunteers, institutional care is inherently formal (Spector et al., 2000). Although there is great local variation in the relative balance between the three general types of long-term care, the AHPR's (2000) *Characteristics of Long-term Care Users* reveals some interesting general trends:

---

[1] These estimates apply to the proportion of persons using long-term care services estimated by the Agency for Health Policy and Research to the most recent census projections. The Agency for Health Policy and Research estimates on long-term care use were derived from the 1994–95 National Health Interview Survey (NHIS-D) and the 1994 National Long-Term Care Survey (NLTCS).

- Only about 4% of the nonelderly recipients of long-term care (those aged 18–64) are institutionalized, while 27% of the elderly long-term care recipients (those aged 65+) receive their care in institutional settings.[2]
- For the nonelderly population of long-term care recipients living in the community, most (about 70%) rely exclusively on informal supports. For the elderly long-term care recipients living in the community, it is more common to rely on a mixture of formal and informal supports.
- About 30% of the informal caregivers of the elderly long-term are themselves elderly, and most (63.1%) are women. By far the most common category of informal caregivers are adult daughters (27%).[3]

Taken together, these trends portray a long-term care system that has a significant institutional bias with respect to the elderly, and a system of care that is also enormously dependent upon the social norms that define women as the prime caregivers of the elderly. Though the three general types of long-term care (informal community-based care, formal community-based care, and institutional care) are structurally distinct, they address the same array of long-term care needs—generally defined as forms of assistance with either ADLs (activities of daily living) or IADLs (instrumental activities of daily living). ADLs refer to tasks of everyday self-care that are basic or essential: getting in and out of bed, dressing, eating, toileting, and bathing. IADLs refer to the more complex tasks of everyday living that draw upon more highly developed capacities in cognition, communication, physical dexterity, and stamina: cooking, doing laundry, driving a car, paying bills, and buying groceries. In contrast to acute care, where the prevalent kinds of health services attend to sophisticated things untrained people are unable to do for themselves, in long-term care the prevalent kinds of service attend to ordinary things people have either lost or been unable to develop the capacity to do.

Community-Based Long-Term Care Services

Community-based long-term care services, as the name implies, provide services to the elderly and otherwise disabled who are able to live in the

[2] See Spector et al. (2000) Table 10. Characteristics of Long-Term Care (LTC) Users by Age and Setting, 1994 and 1996.

[3] See Spector et al. (2000) Table 9. Characteristics of Active Family Caregivers: Spouses and Children of Elderly Long-Term Care (LTC) Users, 1994.

community. Although the bases of many community-based long-term care services were developed as a specific alternative to institutional care or as a way to reduce the risk for institutionalization, much if not most of their value pertains to their ability to enhance the range of functional capacity and improve quality of life. While some forms of community-based long-term care are designed to be rehabilitative and others designed to maintain functioning, in reality there is a continuum of both design and true effect. Sometimes rehabilitative services do little more than maintain functioning and sometimes so-called custodial forms of long-term care that are guided by a strong philosophy of optimism and capacity maximization promote incremental recovery. Another significant contrast between acute care health services and long-term care services is that while the target of intervention in acute care is the so-called primary patient, long-term care services tend to be structured around the impaired person's caregiving network. For example, participation in an adult day care center generally benefits the functioning of the participating older adult and promotes the resilience of the elder's informal caregiver through the provision of emotional support and respite. The major components of community-based long-term care services typically include in-home services (skilled nursing, restorative therapies, personal care, companions, and chore services), residential care (adult foster homes, group homes, assisted living facilities), voluntary multiservice agencies, senior centers, adult day health centers, hospices, public social and health service agencies, and case management services from any number of sources.

In-Home Services

Although Medicare provides payment for a limited array of professional home care services that are specific to an episode of illness, the in-home services that more typically fall under the definition of long-term care involve long-term assistance with ADLs and IADLs. Because ongoing skilled nursing services are prohibitively expensive, individuals requiring that level of care for protracted periods tend to become institutionalized. For most persons in need of in-home long-term care services, the specific services needed typically entail personal care (assistance with getting in and out of bed, dressing, eating), companions (persons able to provide supervision and socialization), and chore services (housekeeping, laundry, shopping). These services are either paid for privately, through long-term care insurance, or funded by Medicaid. In-home services are the most likely services that would be provided by an able and willing family member, and they are also the services that are the most critical in terms of preventing institutionalization. For this reason, states are often strongly motivated to fund these services for the poor and more severely disabled, aside from the judicial imperatives to do so that extend from the Olmstead decision.[4]

Residential Care

Residential care encompasses a variety of living arrangements that have the common feature of providing group living in a community environment. Adult family homes (also referred to as adult foster homes) typically provide shelter, supervision, and assistance with ADLs and IADLs to the extent necessary, for from two to six residents. Adult Family Homes are licensed by states and provide residential care for the mentally ill, the developmentally disabled, and the elderly. While they have the advantage of providing a range of supports to their residents and in many states have prevented further expansions of the nursing home industry, the lack of professional staff and the low costs of entry into the market have also attracted a minority of unscrupulous operators. Group Homes are basically larger versions of Adult Family Homes, serving a larger number of residents. They are often operated by voluntary agencies. Unlike Adult Family Homes, they serve the mentally ill and developmentally disabled more than they do the elderly. Assisted Living Centers are large congregate care homes that are akin to retirement homes, except that they offer some limited in-house or contracted nursing and personal support services to their (typically elderly) residents. More than nursing homes and Adult Family Homes, they tend to attract middle-class and more affluent elderly and have a large presence of for-profit corporate ownership.

Multiservice Agencies

For many of the elderly and nonelderly disabled, their ability to retain optimal independence is contingent upon an array of social services that include information and referral, advocacy, skills training, counseling, transportation, and contracted case management services (which will be defined later). They are voluntary local agencies organized to serve specific populations of the disabled (e.g., the developmentally disabled, the severely visually impaired, the mentally ill, and the elderly) and are

---

[4] In 1999, the U.S. Supreme Court in a 6–3 decision interpreted the ADA as affirming the right of individuals with disabilities to live in their community and required states to place persons with mental disabilities in community settings rather than in institutions. States are required to make community-based long-term care available, where treatment professionals determine that community placement is appropriate, it is not opposed by the affected individual, and where such arrangements can reasonably be accommodated. See Olmstead V. L. C. (98-536) 527 U.S. 581 (1999).

funded by a mixture of public and local private funds. Many qualify for federal funding as designated Centers for Independent Living, a federally funded program established under the Rehabilitation Act of 1973 to serve broad classes of the disabled (Kane et al., 1998).

Senior Centers

Strictly speaking, as originally conceived, senior centers were not organized as long-term care service providers so much as they were social and recreational organizations for older adults. However, in recent decades they have evolved to places where older adults can obtain meals, be offered nutrition and health education services, and obtain a limited array of important social and health care services, such as flu shots, health screening, counseling, and assistance with health insurance (Shi & Singh, 2001). For many fragile elders, the local Senior Center plays a central role in their lives and offers the critical supports needed to sustain independent living.

Adult Day Centers

Like senior centers, Adult Day Centers (ADCs) are oriented toward seniors and provide an array of supportive services. Unlike senior centers, ADCs function as a carefully structured and protective environment for elderly adults with substantial cognitive and physical impairments. Adult Day Centers have been organized by voluntary community groups, as extensions of community hospital programs, and even by for-profit providers as an alternative to nursing home care. As noted by Shi and Singh (2001), ADCs often serve as a means of respite to caregivers of elders. Akin to conventional day care centers, ADC's generally operate during hours that permit other members of the elders family to work normal day jobs. Although ADCs vary in their relative emphasis on rehabilitation, health maintenance, and social–psychological support, in general they all provide a socio–medical milieu that permits very fragile elders to "age-in-place" as opposed to be segregated in institutions (Cutchin, 2003; Shi & Singh, 2001). While in many respects the long-term care support needs of modestly impaired residents of Assisted Living Centers and modestly impaired participants in ADCs are identical, there is a tendency for ADCs to serve lower income elders unable to afford the costs of living in an Assisted Living Center (Cutchin, 2003). These trends not only reflect the disadvantages of social class accrued over the life course, but also state and federal policies that have favored the for-profit nursing home industry as the long-term care solution for the aged poor. This issue will be revisited in the next section of this chapter.

Hospice Programs

Even though hospice care in the United States originated as an extension of the acute health care benefits of Medicare and private insurance, the history of the hospice concept and the nature of hospice care (as an integrated array of social and medical care services delivered over a sustained and often indefinite period) makes hospice care and hospice agencies an integral part of the long-term care system. The hospice concept originated in England with the pioneering work in the care of the dying by British physician Cecily Saunders. Although the beginnings of U.S. hospice movement can be traced to a visit Saunders made to Yale University in 1963, hospice care in the United States did not become a conventional approach for care of the dying until after Congress made hospice care a permanent feature of the Medicare benefit package and an optional component of state Medicaid programs in 1986 (NHPCO, 2006). Despite widespread support for hospice care among the public and across the health professions, in many communities the growth of hospice care has been constrained by curative biases within the local medical community and the political economy of private medical practice. The specific benefits of hospice vary by the form of insurance coverage, but in general hospice benefits follow the Medicare model, which includes physicians' services, and provides intermittent home nursing care, medical supplies, outpatient drugs, home health aide services, social work, professional therapies (physical, occupational, and speech), short-term inpatient care for respite/symptom management, and spiritual counseling. The caveats are that the hospice recipient must be diagnosed by a physician as terminally ill within a specified period (conventionally 6 months), and must voluntarily accept hospice care benefits as an alternative to standard benefits. By definition, the hospice benefits provided are for palliative care as opposed to curative care.[5]

Public Social and Health Service Agencies

As mentioned previously, the long-term care population is comprised of the aged, the developmentally disabled, and also poor persons who have become disabled by injury or chronic illness at some point in their lives. Obviously, all of these characteristics are nonexclusive and are frequently overlapping. For the mentally ill, the developmentally disabled, and the

---

[5] The receipt of hospice care does not preclude a recipient from pursuing cure, either through a decision to withdraw from hospice care or to pay for curative health care services out of pocket. For the far majority of hospice patients, they have made the transition from the pursuit of cure to an emphasis on optimal quality of remaining life. However, it is also true that hospice care is not inconsistent with the retention of some hope—a point that is frequently misunderstood by the general public and many health care professionals.

aged there are generally local (county and municipal) public agencies that both provide an array of publicly funded social and health services and at least help mediate the benefits of other public programs. The origins of these agencies are either major federal programs aligned with major deinstitutionalization initiatives at different points in history, or policy initiatives more generally designed to enhance the well-being and quality of life for a specific group. An example of the former is the *1963 Community Mental Health Centers Construction Act/Mental Retardation Facilities Construction Act (PL 88-164)* which funded the construction of comprehensive community centers for the community-based care of the developmentally disabled and the mentally ill. An example of the latter is the *1965 Older Americans Act (Pl 89-73)*, which established grants to states for community planning and services programs for older adults and ultimately a network of more than 600 local "Area Agencies on Aging" to both plan and contract services for older adults (Kane et al., 1998).[6] For nonelderly persons who are disabled through injury or illness, their entry into long-term care services is via the local branch of the state agency charged with attending to the needs of the so-called "worthy" poor, that is, those with a legitimized reason for not being employable. In contrast to the local public agencies with a mandate to advocate on behalf of a specific population (the developmentally disabled, the mentally ill, and the elderly), state agencies with a more general scope of responsibility for the poor are more known for creating bureaucratic barriers to program benefits and services. Thus persons who are disabled and in need of community-based long-term care services due to injury or chronic illness are more often seen through the lens of poverty and character deficits rather than through their status as a disabled person.

Case Management

Case management is at once a particular kind of service and a major structural component of community-based long-term care. Some also claim it as a distinct profession. Although case management is applied to a wide variety of client-centered activities, in general there are two general kinds of case management—both of which are relevant and essential to community-based long-term care. Managed care approaches to case management entail an organized approach to social and health care needs assessment, the acquisition of appropriate services through the most cost effective setting and providers, coordinating service delivery, and

---

[6] Later amendments to the Older Americans Act funded such key services to older adults as community nutrition programs, meals to the homebound, services targeted at low-income minority elders and to Native American elders, health promotion programs, and advocacy services.

monitoring the ongoing delivery and quality of services (Shi & Singh, 2001, p. 582; Kane, Kane, & Ladd, 1998, p. 46). Although the managed care model of case management can involve a health professional with a distinct set of individual ethical and legal obligations toward the client, case managers that work within the managed care model are often paraprofessionals with a bureaucratic orientation and agenda. In contrast, clinical case management is delivered by health care professionals (physicians, nurses, social workers) who are accountable to a distinct set of professionally prescribed ethical obligations that transcend organizational interests and requirements. Although most of the activities will look similar (assessment, planning, care coordination, and service monitoring), clinical case management also involves careful attention to the engagement of the client in the care planning process, consultation with the client's family and system of natural supports, collaboration with other involved clinical professionals, and crisis intervention (Kanter, 1989). In truth, well functioning community-based long-term systems rely on both models of case management, because managed care organizations and health care professionals bring different structural benefits to an integrated system of long-term care.

The Institutional Component of Long-Term Care: The American Nursing Home Industry

The institutional component of long-term care is comprised of long-term psychiatric hospitals, state institutions for the developmentally disabled, long-term rehabilitation facilities, prisons, and nursing homes.[7] The primary distinction between institutional long-term care and community-based long-term care involves institutional segregation from the nondisabled population and a related emphasis on protective confinement. Other common features include the "medicalization" of ordinary needs and services, extensive restrictions on personal autonomy, and the prevalence of a medical model pathology-based interpretation of disablement. It is for these reasons that over 50 years of long-term care policy have placed an emphasis on deinstitutionalization. As a general trend, the legislation and litigation that have defined the deinstitutionalization movement have been dramatically successful in reducing the populations of state institutions—a trend that has favored the developmentally disabled and the mentally ill far more than it has the aged. Care for the aged disabled still retains a strong institutional emphasis, for a variety of reasons that include changes in family structure and role expectations, labor force trends and policies,

---

[7] Prison populations include a large number of persons who are disabled by mental illness and diminished intellectual capacities. Critics of the deinstitutionalization movement often cite this fact.

a longstanding federal policy bias toward nursing home care, formidable challenges in creating an integrated network of community-based long-term care, the acute care orientation of health care financing, the historic medicalization of the aging process, and an entrenched for-profit nursing home industry.

Nursing Home Utilization

Only a very small proportion of the elderly reside in nursing homes at any one time (3.8% of those aged 65+). However, about 42% of adults over age 70 will have some exposure to nursing home care before death (Merlis, 1999). On a more positive note, only about one fifth of the elderly will have spells of nursing home care in excess of one year (Merlis, 1999). As Figure 5.1 shows, if entry into nursing home care for a relatively short period is considered (less than 1 year), there is a linear trend toward an increased risk of nursing home use as a person ages (see bar graph for nursing home stays of less than 1 year). That is, at age 70 roughly one-fifth of persons will enter a nursing home for no more than 1 year, while by age 85 the proportion entering short-term nursing home care will grow to roughly one third. Generally speaking, nursing home spells of less than 1 year are comprised of two populations, those that go into nursing home care to convalesce after a debilitating spell of illness or in order to recover from surgery and those for whom entrance into nursing home care presages death. Concerning the latter category, this is often an

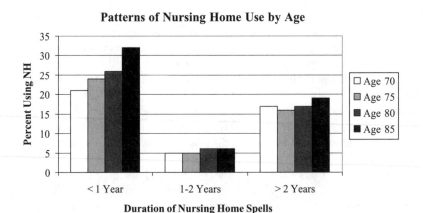

Figure 5.1 Risk of Nursing Home Use by Age and During of Spells. (Source: Calculated from projections by Merlis, *Financing Long Term Care in the Twenty-First Century: The Public and Private Roles.* New York: Institute for Policy Solutions, 1999, Table 3.)

inevitable event in the dying process. However, in many cases entry into nursing home care is a shock event that itself precipitates death.

The graphs in Figure 5.1 that correspond to longer spells of nursing home care show an amazing level of consistency across all ages shown. This suggests that where long-term residence in a nursing home is considered, past a certain point in life age by itself is a poor discriminator. The patterns shown in the latter two graphs reflect the population level effects of the complex interplay between levels of morbidity and impairments, and the network of formal and informal supports either available or not available to the fragile aged. In this regard, there has long been an extensive literature on the role of race, ethnicity, and cultural variation in nursing home utilization (Almgren, 1990). For example, African Americans are far less likely to end their days in a nursing home than either non-Hispanic Whites or Hispanics, even where the confounding effects of age, sex, income, education and cause of death are accounted for (Iwashyna & Chang, 2002).

The Structure of the Nursing Home Industry

As previously discussed (see chapter 4 on the Organization of Health Care), the most recently available economic census of the United States

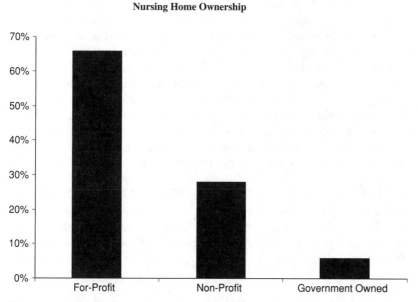

Figure 5.2 Distribution of Nursing Home Ownership. (Source: Data obtained from Kaiser Family Foundation. (2006). *Statehealthfacts: Distribution of Nursing Care Facilites by Ownership Type*, 2003: http://statehealthfacts.org.)

estimates that there are 16,479 nursing homes nationwide with a collective revenue of nearly $74 billion annually (U.S. Census Bureau, 2004). As Figure 5.2 shows, in contrast to the hospital industry, which is 80% either public or nonprofit, in the nursing home industry 66% are operated on a for-profit basis. Very large corporate nursing home chains account for a significant share of the industry (U.S. Census Bureau, 2005a).

Although the for-profit sector of the nursing home industry was dominated by independent owners through the late 1970s, by 1985 approximately 70% of for-profit homes had become a part of a nursing home chain (Almgren, 1990). However, like the hospital industry, there is great statewide variation in the extent to which the for-profit sector of the industry is dominant. For example, in Texas and Arkansas, 80% of all nursing homes are for-profit, while in states with a more established tradition of not-for-profit nursing home care, like Minnesota and the Dakotas, the for-profit sector of the industry holds a minority share of the market (Kaiser Family Foundation, 2006).

There are enduring policy questions in nursing home research pertaining to whether the form of ownership makes a difference in the quality of nursing home care, and whether different forms of ownership serve different segments of the population. With respect to the question on ownership and quality of care, the prevailing belief among the broad public and health care professionals is that nonprofit nursing homes are inherently of higher quality, because they have a fundamentally different reason for being in business and because they are mandated to reinvest their profits into their facilities and services. As intuitive as this might seem, the evidence is actually quite equivocal (Almgren, 1990; O'Brien, 1988; O'Brien, Saxberg, & Smith, 1983; Spector, Seldon, & Cohen, 1998). In large part this is because many studies fail to control for confounding effects or use measures of quality that pertain to clinical outcomes. However, a particularly rigorous study that employed a range of critical outcome measures (e.g. mortality, hospitalizations, and clinical conditions pertaining directly to quality of care) found no significant differences in clinical care outcomes—other than fewer hospitalizations among patients in nonprofit homes (Spector et al., 1998).[8]

With respect to the second question, whether different forms of nursing home ownership serve different segments of the population, it is indeed the case that the nonprofit sector of the nursing home caters to the more socially advantaged (Almgren, 1990; O'Brien, 1988; Spector et al., 1998). Both Almgren (1990) and O'Brien (1988) concur that nonprofit

[8] There was some limited evidence to suggest that nonprofit nursing homes also reduced adverse outcomes relative to for-profit homes. See Spector et al. (1998) pp. 649–650.

nursing homes, because they tend to have a higher level of public confidence, are better able to support selective admissions policies aimed at avoiding the medically indigent. Another dimension of segmentation in the nursing home industry, aside from the form of ownership, is the division between the relatively small number of nursing homes that carry a very high proportion of Medicaid patients, and those nursing homes that have a higher mix of private and publicly financed residents. According to Mor, Zinn, Angelleli, Teno, & Miller (2004) the former class of nursing homes comprise roughly 15 percent of the industry, tend to be disproportionately located in poor areas, and tend have a higher representation of African American residents. These nursing homes also have lower levels of staffing, a higher number of citations for deficiencies, and are more likely to be terminated from the Medicaid/Medicare program—thus in effect forcing their closure (Mor et al., 2004). While closure of these medicalized almshouses might be seen as a positive action, their disappearance will not affect the likelihood that impoverished frail elderly will then be able to access the higher quality tiers of the nursing home industry.

The Origins of the Nursing Home Industry

In contrast to other modern democracies, the United States has placed a particular emphasis on an institutional solution for the care of the aged (Kane et al., 1998). While there are many reasons cited for this, including the dominance of a highly individualistic perspective and an overzealous faith in market solutions to most problems, much of the reason has to do with the development of an entrenched proprietary (private for-profit) nursing home industry that has adapted well to the mixed private and public model of health care financing. The primary origins of the proprietary actually can be traced to the Social Security Act of 1935.

Care of the Aged Before 1935. A common myth about earlier generations of Americans is that they took care of their frail elderly, largely through the mechanisms of the multigenerational household and extensive kinship ties. While it is true that throughout most of U.S. history there were few homes for the aged and no nursing homes, in fact an early precursor to the modern nursing home was the almshouse.[9] Were it true that frail elders were at one time well attended by children and kin, it would be expected that the population of early 20th century almshouses would be dominantly comprised of children and working age adults. However,

---

[9] Almshouses, or poor houses as they were also called, were buildings appropriated and operated by local authorities to shelter and feed the destitute in the years preceding the Social Security Act of 1935.

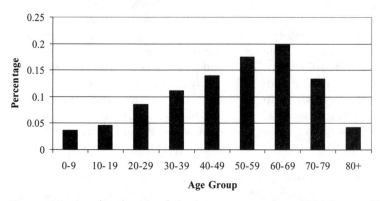

Age at Admission, Paupers in Almhouses 1904

Figure 5.3   Age distribution of almshouse entrants from 1904 Census. (Source: Adapted from Table XX, Census of 1904 Special Report, Paupers in Almshouses. U.S. Census Bureau, Washington D.C.)

as shown in Figure 5.3, that is hardly the case. Indeed the most common age category for those entering almshouses at the turn of the century were elderly between the ages of 60 and 69, which given the 49-year life expectancy of 1900 was very old age (Almgren, 1990). This was also the age category at which the elderly of the working class were likely to become unemployable due to diminished physical capacities. Given the lack of a national old-age pension program before 1935, the early 60s would be the peak age to be at risk for destitution for working class elders. The drop off of admissions to the almshouse after age 70 likely represents the reality that those who were both old and impoverished did not tend to survive to very old age. Although progressive era social reformers embarked on a national campaign to eliminate the almshouse as the method for providing for the poor, this movement favored women and children more than it did the elderly. As late as 1923 more than 70 percent of those that remained in diminishing number of almshouses were persons over age 65 (Vladeck, 1980).

The other precursor to the nursing home was the mental institution, typically a state asylum. In the early 1900s about 2% of all persons age 65+ were in some kind of institutional setting. Of these institutionalized elderly the almshouses accounted for about 57%, while the remaining 43% were confined to mental institutions (Almgren, 1990; Manard, Kart, & Gils, 1975). Although it is likely that cognitive deficits were the largest factor in determining whether an impoverished and abandoned elder ended up in a mental institution as opposed to an almshouse, the major drivers to institutionalization were age, poverty, the lack of informal social supports, and the lack of any federalized safety net for the aged poor.

The Social Security Act of 1935 and the Beginnings of the for-Profit Sector of Nursing Home Industry. There were two provisions of the Social Security Act of 1935 that in many respects were specifically intended to empty to the nation's poorhouses of their elderly. The first was the Old Age Assistance (OAA) program itself, which established the monthly Social Security pension check that remains an essential buffer between old age and poverty. The second provision precluded from eligibility the aged residents of public and private institutions that could be classified as custodial, correctional, or curative in nature (Thomas, 1969). Although the intent of the latter provision was in effect an attempt to deinstitutionalize the elderly, in a classic paradox of unintended policy consequences it became the founding cornerstone of the modern proprietary nursing home industry. The basis of the paradox involves a specific *disadvantage* this provision of the Social Security Act extended to the nonprofit sector of the nursing home industry, formally known as "Homes for the Aged."

Prior to the availability of the OAA pension program, churches, fraternal organizations, and immigrant self-help organizations throughout the country were erecting nonprofit "Homes for the Aged" as a benign and enlightened alternative to the almshouse. Though established from diverse sources, these nonprofit old-age homes established within a few decades the voluntary sector of the nursing home industry, which (as previously shown in Figure 5.2) composes 28% of the nursing home industry. Although a far superior alternative to the poorhouse and in many respects a model of care for the frail aged, the OAA pension program provisions aimed at eliminating the institutionalization of elderly in almshouses and mental institutions tarred these nonprofit homes with the same brush. Vladeck (1980) attributes this tragic error of public policy to the domination of new immigrant groups in sponsoring these voluntary homes for the aged rather than middle-class reformers. Whatever the underlying motivations, the effect of this policy ultimately provided the impetus for the establishment of the private sector of the nursing home industry.

Even the meager purchasing power granted by the OAA monthly pension enabled the aged without family resources to either live totally independently or to make their living arrangements in a boarding home. As a result, cities and towns throughout the United States had a burgeoning private boarding home industry that catered to the new social class of elderly pensioners. Most of these homes were large, old multistory family structures with several rooms available to accommodate boarders (Gruber, 1967). As would be expected, those elders that elected to live in a boarding home were more likely to have functional impairments. There is also evidence to suggest that some boarding homes provided nursing care to gain a competitive edge over others (Dunlop, 1979). While some proprietary nursing homes were founded as such, with the passage of time many of the larger homes that had their beginnings as room and board enterprises gradually transformed to nursing homes. Key to this process of transformation was several pieces of enabling federal legislation, beginning with amendments to the Social Security Act that followed the first National Conference on Aging in 1950[10] (Almgren, 1990).

By 1953, Congress passed various amendments to the Social Security Act that provided direct payments to providers of nursing home care, enabled residents of voluntary and public homes for the aged to receive OAA pensions, and required states to establish licensing and inspection programs for nursing homes as a condition for receiving federal matching funds for nursing home care. Collectively these provisions established the essential structural basis for federal financing and oversight of nursing home care in both the voluntary and proprietary sectors of the nursing home industry. Between 1954 and 1959, Congress followed up with a massive infusion of federal dollars into all three sectors of the growing nursing home industry (private, voluntary, and public) via funding programs for nursing home construction and upgrades. In 1954 the Hill–Burton Act was extended to provide construction and upgrade funds for the voluntary and public parts of the nursing home industry. Largely as a result of pressure from the newly formed proprietary nursing home lobby (The American Nursing Home Association), in 1956 and 1959 Congress amended both the Small Business Administration Loan Program and the Federal Housing Administration Mortgage Insurance Program to similarly support the proprietary sector of the nursing home industry (Dunlop, 1979; Pegals, 1981). Thus it can be said that by the end of the 1950s federal policy had been thoroughly committed to an institutionalized approach to long-term care—one that privileged the further growth of private sector institutions.

Medicaid/Medicare and the Establishment of the Modern Nursing Home Industry. While the 1950s had witnessed the entrenchment of institutional solutions to aging and long-term care policy issues, there remained critical gaps in financing, licensure, and quality assurance. In particular, there were no uniform standards in the definition of what constituted a nursing home or uniform standards pertaining to facility construction and operation. All began to change with the passage of the 1960 Kerr–Mills Medical Assistance to the Aged Program, which

---

[10] This became the precedent for later national conferences on aging that beginning in 1961 were designated as a "White House Conference on Aging."

committed the federal government to the funding of skilled nursing services for the medically indigent and introduced a categorical in-kind assistance program to the nursing home industry. This legislation presaged the Social Security Act Amendments of 1965, which through the financial clout of the Medicare and Medicaid program dollars enabled the federal government to impose uniform definitions of nursing home care, uniform standards for nursing home construction and operation, and uniform requirements for facility inspection. Later amendments (in 1967 and 1972) went even further in expanding nursing home care benefits as well as uniform standards of services, cost, and utilization review (Almgren, 1990). In sum effect, these policies increased the purchasing power of families who might be in the market for the nursing home placement of an elder, assuaged their concerns about nursing home quality, and reinforced the perception of a dichotomy of choice between family-based solutions to long-term care and institutional solutions.

The Growth in Nursing Home Utilization. Between 1960 and 1970, the nursing home utilization rate for the population aged 65+ increased by a phenomenal 74 percent (Dunlop, 1979). There is a general consensus that much of this increase is attributable to the massive infusion of public subsidies to the nursing home industry that characterized the long-term care policies of the 1960s (Dunlop, 1979; Kane et al., 1998; Manard et al., 1975; Morony & Kurtz, 1975; Vladeck, 1980). This argument is further reinforced by the fact that in the immediate nine-year period following the introduction of the Medicaid and Medicare subsidies, the annual rate of nursing home beds increased by an average 19% (Almgren, 1990). However, the enduring state-by-state variations in nursing home utilization suggest there are other factors at work. From the demand side of nursing home utilization, the factors that are most plausible include advancements in medical care that increased the survival rates of elderly in advanced stages of frailty (Chiswick, 1976; Crimmons, Saito, & Ingegneri, 1989), increased rates of internal migration with geographic separation of parents and children (Rabin & Stockton, 1987), an increase in the *dependency ratio*[11] arising from increased old-age survivor-ship (Chiswick, 1976), growth in the survival disparities between men and women in old age (Chiswick, 1976), a decrease in the number of multigenerational households (Almgren, 1990; Treas, 1977), and the growth in

[11] The old-age dependency ratio is defined as the number of persons aged 65+/number of persons aged 15–64, and refers to the number of persons at risk for old-age dependency relative to the number of persons available for caregiving or economic support. There are many ways to adjust the composition of this ratio to account for different subgroups of aged and subgroups of caregivers.

female labor force participation that characterized the 1960s (Almgren, 1990).

In particular, it is likely that the interaction between an increase in the dependency ratio (i.e. the population size of elderly relative to the population size of potential caregivers) and the increase in the number of women employed outside the home during the 1960–1970 period accounted for a large share of the increased demand for institutional care of the aged. During the period in question, it was well established that women acted as the primary caregivers of the elderly and that women (more than men) believe that dependent elderly should reside with their children (Seelbach & Sauer, 1977; Select Committee on Aging, 1987).[12] As the 1960s unfolded, both the increase in the average number of hours women worked outside the home and the growth of the elderly population collided in ways that, for many families, made nursing home care seem the only realistic alternative. While it may have seemed like prudent public policy to provide various forms of subsidies for families that would better enabled them to provide care for their elders, Congress favored subsidies to the nursing home industry instead as a part of a larger agenda to invest in the infrastructure of the health care system.

Policy Initiatives to Reduce Nursing Home Utilization. In all likelihood, there will never be a consensus on the relative merits of supply side factors versus demand side factors behind the dramatic 1960–1970 period growth in nursing home care. In an attempt to develop an effective policy response to demand side of nursing home utilization, during the 1970s and early 1980s there were several federally funded community-based care demonstration projects aimed at decreasing the necessity of nursing home placement. The common premise of these demonstration projects was that through public investments in the right mixture of community-based care services to elders and their informal care networks, a net savings in tax dollars could be realized through a decrease in the use of nursing home care. It was also hoped that the results from these projects would pave the way to the most cost-efficient benefit structures for the private long-term insurance market. In a widely disputed (but nonetheless influential) analysis of these demonstration projects published in *Health Services Research*, William Weissert[13] concluded that "Community care rarely reduces nursing home or hospital use; it provides only limited outcome benefits; and to this point, it has usually raised overall use of health services as well as

[12] As discussed earlier in this chapter, the caregiving of elders remains largely in the hands of women.
[13] At the time a Professor of Health Policy and Administration at the School of Public Health, University of North Carolina at Chapel Hill.

total expenditures" (Weissert, 1985, p.424). In fact, his study concluded that the sickest and most dependent patients may be more cheaply served in a nursing home. As Weissert saw it, the evidence from these projects suggested that the principal benefits to community-based care were not in net cost savings or the even marginal reductions in nursing home care, but in making life somewhat better for elderly and their caregivers (Weissert, 1985). Although it is convincingly argued that Weissert's findings failed to take into account the favorable effect of community-based care on nursing home care utilization over time (see Kane, Kane, & Ladd, 1998, p. 71), there is no question that Weissert's conclusions caused policy makers to take a more skeptical view of the potential of community-based care as a cost-effective substitute for nursing home care—thus turning policy attention back toward the supply side.

One very straightforward approach to reducing the growth in nursing home utilization is to simply reduce the growth in the supply of nursing home beds. One argument for this approach is transparent: by constraining the supply of nursing home beds over time the proportion of the population of elderly in institutional care will decline as the population of elderly increases. The other argument for constraints on the supply side of nursing home care is based on something commonly known in the health services research field as "Roemer's Law." In a nutshell, Roemer's Law holds that *supply tends to induce its own demand where a third party guarantees reimbursement of use* (Roemer, 1961).[14] In the context of institutional care like hospitals and nursing homes, this predicts that to the extent that public funds are available to subsidize the costs of care, a market dynamic of "build the beds and they will come" emerges. Applied more directly to the nursing home industry, Roemer's law suggests that to the extent that more nursing home beds are built and financial subsidies for nursing home care are made available, more of the elderly will become institutionalized.

In fact, beginning in the 1980s many states adopted very restrictive policies aimed at constraining the supply of nursing home beds, including outright moratoriums on new nursing home construction (Kane et al., 1998). The central mechanism for enabling states to do this was the so-called certificate-of-need legislation, which enables states to deny licensure and reimbursement to health care facilities that have not been granted a "certificate-of-need" through the state's health care planning agency.[15]

---

[14] Roemer's Law is named for Milton Roemer (d. 2001), formerly Professor of Health Services at UCLA. The arguments and findings of Milton Roemer were highly influential among legislators and health policy administrators.

[15] In 1972, the Social Security Act was amended to require states to review capital expenditures for health care facilities and equipment in excess of $100,000 as a condition of

Other supply-side state level initiatives involve the restriction of access to Medicaid subsidies for nursing home care through such mechanisms as a mandatory preadmission comprehensive functional assessment—an approach that is generally linked with assessment and referral to community-based care alternatives that in effect reduce the demand for nursing home care. Despite some level of skepticism among many policy makers concerning the ability of community-based long-term care services to be a cost-effective alternative to nursing home care, for a variety of reasons most states opted to invest in subsidies to community-based care in combination with efforts to restrict the growth of nursing home bed supply. Between 1992 and 1997, Medicaid waivers to allow subsidy of community-based long-term care services spending grew by almost 260% (The Urban Institute, 2001).

In the Balanced Budget Act 1997, Congress established the Medicare PACE Program (Program of All-Inclusive Care for the Elderly), which integrates Medicare and Medicaid financing in order to provide a comprehensive array of medical and community-based long-term care services to at-risk elderly. In order qualify for enrollment, the applicant must be over aged 55 and be certified by the cooperating state agency to be eligible for nursing home placement. The PACE program is modeled on the On Lok Social Health Maintenance Organization (S/HOM) demonstration project in San Francisco, California—broadly recognized as a highly successful HCFA demonstration project.[16]

As a result of these supply-side and demand-side efforts to constrain nursing home utilization, the proportion of nursing home beds to the population of persons over age 65 stabilized at about 5% nationwide for several years and more recently has declined to 4% (Kaiser Family Foundation, 2006; Kane et al., 1998; U.S. Census Bureau, 2005a). While this is an encouraging trend, national long-term care policy remains burdened by the unintended policy consequences of the past—and quite belated in its response to the formidable challenges of the immediate future.

---

receiving Medicare and Medicaid reimbursement for capital expenditures. Over time this federal legislation was very effective in enabling states to restrict the further expansion of nursing home bed capacity.

[16] A Social Health Maintenance Organization (S/HMO) is a comprehensive community-based care program that integrates medical care and social supports under a model of capitated financing. Typical S/HMO benefits include case management, personal in-home support services, adult day care, respite care (including short-term nursing home care), and coverage for pharmaceuticals. Although it was hoped that the S/HMO model would quickly evolve as a substitute for nursing home care, the mixed outcomes of the early S/HMO projects retarded the widespread adoption of the S/HMO approach to long-term care.

FINANCING LONG-TERM CARE

There are a set of givens to long-term care policy that should guide policy makers at all levels: (1) the population of the oldest old (those 85+) will have expanded nearly five fold between the census of 2000 and 2050 (U.S. Census Bureau, 2005b); (2) the newest generation of aged (like those of the past) favor "aging in place" to institutional care; (3) the newest generation of aged (like those of the past) are also ill-prepared to pay for the "aging in place" community support services that have proved an essential adjunct to informal supports from family and friends; (4) the next waves of aged have fewer children available as a resource for informal care than previous generations;[17] and (5) the country is already too deeply in debt to greatly expand public entitlements to long-term care services in absence of a radical restructuring of both the Medicare and Medicaid programs. As summarized by a recent Government Accountability Office's report on long-term care to Congress (GAO, 2005), the primary policy challenges facing both state legislatures and the Congress that pertain to the financing of long-term care include:

- Determining societal responsibilities.
- Considering the potential role of social insurance in financing.
- Encouraging personal preparedness.
- Recognizing the benefits, burdens, and costs of informal caregiving.
- Assessing the balance of state and federal responsibilities to ensure adequate and equitable satisfaction of needs.
- Adopting effective and efficient implementation and administration of reforms.
- Developing financially sustainable public commitments (GAO, 2005, p. 3).

Of all the above policy challenges, the most immediate concerns the financial sustainability of public commitments to long-term care.

Current Long-Term Care Expenditures and Future Projections

As estimated by the Government Accountability Office, in 2003 the national expenditures on all forms of long-term care for all age groups summed to roughly $183 billion, or about 13% of all national health

---

[17] While demographic projections are always disputable, those currently at the cusp of retirement are not bearing more children. It is also unlikely that there will be significant declines in old-age longevity (and ergo the population of aged) in isolation from a catastrophic public health event that will affect all age groups.

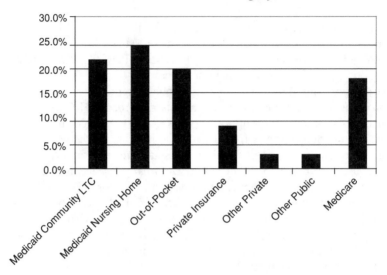

Figure 5.4   GAO Estimates of Long Term Care Funding Sources, 2003. (Source: Adapted from Figure 1: Funding Sources for Long-Term Care, 2003, in *Testimony Before the Subcommittee on Health, Committee on Energy and Commerce, House of Representatives: Long-Term Care Financing: Growing Demand and Cost of Services Are Straining Federal and State Budgets.* (April 27, 2005) GAO, Washington D.C.)

expenditures (GAO, 2005). As a relative share of the domestic economy (the GDP), long-term care expenditures accounted for about 2% in 2003. As is shown in Figure 5.4, the lion's share of long-term care expenditures are funded by public sources: Medicare accounts for 18% of expenditures while Medicaid accounts for 47%. Obviously, the magnitude of public expenditures on long-term care is problematic at a point when those most likely to use long-term care services (those over age 85) are about 4.5% of the population—what about when this population doubles, triples, and quadruples over the immediate next decades?

The prime driver of future long-term care expenditures, whether public or private, is not age per se but a complex interaction between the growth of the aged population, the prevalence of disability in the aged population, and the availability of informal supports. The magnitude of public expenditures is further affected by the distribution of income, wealth, and long-term care insurance coverage among the disabled aged—as well as federal and state policies that determine the eligibility criteria for public long-term care subsidies. All of these factors (plus several that have not been introduced) makes the forecasting of public expenditures for long-term care exceedingly uncertain. However, the

Urban Institute estimated that *under the current regime of public policy*, the overall spending on institutional and home care for the aged would increase from the 2000 level of $98 billion to $208 billion by 2025, and then $379.5 billion by the year 2050 (The Urban Institute, 2001).[18] Notably, the Urban Institute projects that while public expenditures through the Medicare and Medicaid programs will increase to unsustainable levels, spending on long-term care services from family resources will double by 2025 and more than triple by 2050. Such a growth in private expenditures for long-term care would make it exceedingly difficult for most families to invest in higher education for their children and grandchildren or afford to save for retirement and other contingencies, and certainly make home ownership even more difficult for working class families than it is today. Given these grim prospects, what are the alternatives?

DIRECTIONS FOR LONG-TERM FINANCING POLICY

As dismal as the future looks for the affordability of long-term care for most families, as it stands currently the financing long-term care is actually highly favorable to middle-class families. This is because the federal rules governing Medicaid subsidies for nursing home care that are intended to keep elderly out of poverty also enable reasonably savvy families to shield a large share of the assets of the older generation for intergenerational transfers—often without taxation. A likely secondary effect of this policy, aside from the direct effect in increasing the level of Medicaid expenditures for long-term care, is that it plausibly retarded the growth of the long-term care insurance market.

Private Long-Term Care Insurance

Decades ago it was established that catastrophic long-term care expenditures for nursing home care met the criteria for an insurable event under the prevailing assumptions of insurance markets. That is, nursing home care is a financially burdensome event with a known probability of risk, people are averse to nursing home care, and the probability of extended periods of nursing home care relative to its costs is sufficiently low. In the 1980s, a large share of policy planners and administrators believed that the development of a mature long-term care insurance market would

---

[18] The Urban Institutes projections assume annual reductions in mortality rates of 0.6% and reductions in disability among the old-age population, fixed age- and sex-specific utilization rates for institutional and community-based long-term care services, no changes in public policies, and a modest inflation rate for long-term care services of 1.2% (The Urban Institute, 2001, p. 38).

ultimately curtail the growth of public long-term care expenditures. For a variety of reasons, this has turned out not to be the case. Early generation long-term care policies were written in ways that excluded the highest risk conditions from coverage, many elderly believed that their Medicare and Medigap policy benefits would provide adequate coverage for nursing home care and other long-term care services, most elders and their families regard nursing home care as something they would never accept, and in particular, those who were most at risk for the need for nursing home care tended not to purchase long-term care insurance (Wilson & Weissert, 1989). Although long-term care insurance carriers have greatly improved their products[19] and their marketing strategies, at this point long-term care insurance still covers only small proportion of the more affluent elderly. Only about 10% of the population of elderly aged 75+ have private long-term care insurance, and the group that purchases long-term care insurance over represents those with the higher income and assets (Johnson & Uccello, 2005; The Urban Institute, 2001). Clearly, if private long-term care insurance is not the solution to the financing of long-term care, then what can be?

Social Insurance, Private Insurance, or Both?

There have been hundreds of articles over the past 2 decades written by very credible scholars from all points of view that propose solutions for financing long-term care. Although the arguments are often detailed and quite complex, there are four plausible policy directions:

1. Stay the current course, and watch the growth of Medicaid-funded long-term care grow to $87.8 billion annually by 2020 (per Congressional Budget Office estimates).[20]
2. Pursue an aggressive strategy of promoting, principally through tax subsidies, the long-term care insurance market.
3. Expand the social insurance approach of Social Security and Medicare to include long-term care services.
4. Employ a mixed strategy of (2) and (3), which would involve a more limited mandatory wage-based payroll contribution for community-based care and limited nursing home care, with tax-incentives to purchase commercial long-term care insurance via vouchers for higher level asset protection.

[19] Including expanded benefits that include an array of essential community-based long-term services.
[20] CBO. (1999). Projections of Expenditures for Long-Term Care Services for the Elderly. Washington DC: Congressional Budget Office. Table 2 Projection of National Long-Term Care Expenditures for the Elderly, Assuming No Increase in Long-Term Care Insurance.

At this point, several years after the Congressional Budget Office estimated the cost of the first alternative (CBO, 1999), the nation remains mired in the first strategy. The second strategy has not been pursued, though given the performance of the long-term care insurance market to date this seems like a dubious solution. The third strategy, expanding the social insurance model to include long-term care insurance, is popular among progressives, but less defensible as a major social investment than a social insurance fund for basic health care. The fourth strategy, a version of which was proposed by the 1990 Pepper Commission, appears to strike the best balance of reciprocity between generations. As proposed by the Pepper Commission, the social insurance fund would provide home and community-based care services to supplement informal family supports, and would cover the first 3 months of nursing home care. Longer nursing home stays would be partially funded with some assurance of minimum asset protection. Those elders and families wanting higher levels of asset protection would have the option of purchasing tax-subsidized private long-term care insurance (O'Shaughnessy, Lyke, & Storey, 2002).

Each of the last three strategies for the financing of long-term care must, in the final analysis, reconcile very different perspectives on individual responsibility and mutual obligations in order to become policy. The financing of long-term care, while it involves the pragmatics of economic principles and political bargaining, is ultimately embedded in a social justice discourse. The central question in that discourse involves the degree to which rights and obligations pertaining to general health care extend to the domain of long-term care, and the implications that follow for the structure of long-term care finance.

CONCLUDING COMMENTS—A SOCIAL JUSTICE PERSPECTIVE ON THE FINANCING OF LONG-TERM CARE

As discussed in other chapters (see in particular chapter 1 on theories of social justice and chapter 8 on health care system reform), it seems very clear that Rawls' theory of justice encompasses a positive right to health care. The primary basis for this conclusion is health care's social function as an essential determinant of fair equality of opportunity. However, among the several constraints to an *unlimited* positive right to health care are conflicts between young and old over limited resources (Daniels, 2002). In the last available formulation of his Theory of Justice (*Justice as Fairness: A Restatement*, 2001: Harvard University Press), Rawls acknowledged that special problems arose when considering more extreme health care needs, as in the case of the severely handicapped (and presumably those disabled by age as well). As Rawls saw it, the primary problem involved determining the limit of duties toward disabled citizens when the weight of such duties compete with other basic claims, as in the case of funds for long-term care versus funds for basic education (Rawls, 2001). As a reflection of the complexity of the problem, Rawls himself was uncertain as to whether his theory of justice could be extended to provide a satisfactory resolution to this fundamental conflict: "At some point, then, we must see whether justice as fairness can be extended to provide guidelines for these cases; and if not, whether it must be rejected rather than supplanted with some other conception." (Rawls, 2001, p. 176, n59). At the time Rawls wrote this, he was beyond a doubt well aware of the dilemmas facing the nation as a consequence of population aging—thus his reluctance to give a clear ruling on the issue must also give us pause.

However, there are three basic ideas from Rawls' theory (whether or not Rawls would agree with their application) that seem particularly relevant to the formulation of a just approach to the financing of long-term care. The first is the positive right to health care, the second is that there are limits to that right that involve competing commitments to the provision of other primary goods (like an adequate scheme of basic education), and the third is Rawls' emphasis on the principle of reciprocity as a cornerstone to his conception of justice (Rawls, 2001, p. 77). Reciprocity comes into play as one thinks about the obligations that flow between generations as pertains to Social Security: thus far each generation of workers funds a large share of the retirement for the next. Conversely, it seems incumbent on each generation not to place an undue burden on the opportunity structure of the next—thus limiting each generation's claim to the extent of public entitlements in old age. This of course would extend to publicly financed long-term care entitlements. Although this perspective is offered as a plausible application of Rawls' theory of justice, this is perspective is also a fairly common point of view.

Whatever the policy final direction, it is likely that the public discourse about intergenerational obligations will become more pronounced as the newest generation of retirees takes full advantage of the social insurance fund set aside by the generation of their grandparents, and encounters the blessings and burdens of old age.

REFERENCES

Almgren, G. (1990). *Artificial nutrition and hydration practices and the American nursing home: Currents of social change and adaptation by an industry in transition.* Unpublished doctoral dissertation, University of Washington, Seattle.

CBO. (1999). *Projections of Expenditures for Long-Term Care Services for the Elderly.* Washington DC: Congressional Budget Office.

Chiswick, B. (1976). The Demand for Nursing Home Care: An Analysis of Institutional and Noninstitutional Care. *Journal of Human Resources, 9,* 295–315.

Crimmons, E., Saito, Y., & Ingegneri, D. (1989). Changes in Life Expectancy and Disability-Free Life Expectancy in the United States. *Population and Development Review, 15*(2), 229–254.

Cutchin, M. P. (2003). The process of mediated aging-in-place: A theoretically and empirically based model. *Social Science & Medicine, 57*(6), 1077–1090.

Daniels, N. (2002). Justice, health and health care. In R. Rhodes, M. Battin & A. Silvers (Eds.), *Medicine and social justice.* New York: Oxford University Press.

Dunlop, B. (1979). *The growth of nursing home care.* Lexington, MA: Lexington Books.

GAO. (2005). *Testimony Before the Subcommittee on Health, Committee on Energy and Commerce, House of Representatives: Long-Term Care Financing: Growing Demand and Cost of Services Are Straining Federal and State Budgets.* Washington DC: United States Government Accountability Office.

Gruber, H. (1967). A History of Nursing Homes—A Review. In *The Extended Care Facility: A Handbook for the Medical Society.* Chicago: American Medical Association.

Iwashyna, T., & Chang, V. (2002). Racial and ethnic differences in place of death: United States, 1993. *Journal of the American Geriatric Society, 50*(6), 1113–1117.

Johnson, R. W., & Uccello, C. E. (2005). *Is Private Long-term Care Insurance the Answer?* (No. 29). Boston: Center for Retirement Research at Boston College.

Kaiser Family Foundation. (2006). *Statehealthfacts: Distribution of Nursing Care Facilities by Ownership Type, 2003.* Retrieved February 15, 2006, from http://statehealthfacts.org.

Kane, R., Kane, R., & Ladd, R. (1998). *The heart of long-term care.* New York: Oxford University Press.

Kanter, J. (1989). Clinical case management: Definition, principles, components. *Hospital and Community Psychiatry, 40*(4), 361–368.

Manard, B., Kart, C., & Gils, D. v. (1975). *Old age institutions.* Lexington, MA.: Lexington Books.

Merlis, M. (1999). *Financing Long-term Care in the Twenty-First Century: The Public and Private Roles.* New York: Institute for Policy Solutions.

Mor, V., Zinn, J., Angelleli, J., Teno, J., & Miller, S. (2004). Driven to Tiers: Socioeconomic and Racial Disparities in the Quality of Nursing Home Care. *The Milbank Quarterly, 82*(2), 227–256.

Morony, R., & Kurtz, N. (1975). The Evolution of Long-term Care Institutions. In S. Sherwood (Ed.), *Long-term Care: A Handbook for Researchers, Planners, and Providers.* New York: Spectrum Publications.

NHPCO. (2006). *History of Hospice Care.* Retrieved May 3, 2006, from http://www.nhpco.org/i4a/pages/index.cfm?pageid=3285.

O'Brien, J. (1988). *The three sector nursing home industry.* Unpublished doctoral dissertation, University of Washington, Seattle.

O'Brien, J., Saxberg, B., & Smith, H. (1983). For-profit nursing homes: Does it Matter? *The Gerontologist, 23,* 341–347.

O'Shaughnessy, C., Lyke, B., & Storey, J. (2002). *Long-term care: What direction for public policy?* Washington, DC: Congressional Research Service, Library of Congress.

Pegals, C. (1981). *Health care and the elderly.* Rockville, MD: Aspen Systems Corporation.

Rabin, D., & Stockton, D. (1987). *Longterm care for the elderly: A factbook.* New York: Oxford University Press.

Rawls, J. (2001). *Justice as fairness.* Cambridge, MA: Harvard University Press.

Roemer, M. I. (1961). Bed supply and hospital utilization: A natural experiment. *Hospitals, 35,* 36–42.

Seelbach, W., & Sauer, W. (1977). Filial responsibility expectations and morale among the aged. *The Gerontologist, 17*(6), 492–499.

Select Committee on Aging. (1987). *Exploding the myth: Caregiving in America.* Washington DC: U.S. Congress, House of Representatives.

Shi, L., & Singh, D. (2001). *Delivering Health Care in America: A Systems Approach.* Gaithersburg, MD: Aspen.

Spector, W. D., Fleishman, J. A., Pezzin, L. E., & Spillman, B. C. (2000). *The characteristics of long-term care users.* Rockville, MD: Agency for Health Care Policy and Research.

Spector, W. D., Seldon, T., & Cohen, J. (1998). The impact of ownership type on nursing home outcomes. *Health Econ.* 7: 639–653 (1998).

The Urban Institute. (2001). *Long-term care: Consumers, providers, and financing: A chart book.* Washington DC: The Urban Institute.

Thomas, W. (1969). *Nursing homes and public policy: Drift and decision in New York State.* Ithaca, NY: Cornell University Press.

Treas, J. (1977). Family support systems and the aged: Some social and demographic considerations. *The Gerontologist, 17,* 486–491.

U.S. Census Bureau. (2004). *2002 economic census: Nursing homes and residential care facilities* (No. EC02-62I-03). Washington, DC: U.S. Department of Commerce.

U.S. Census Bureau. (2005a). *Table 2: Annual estimates of the population by selected age groups and sex for the United States: April 1, 2000 to July 1, 2004 (NC-EST2004-02).* Washington, DC: U.S. Census Bureau.

U.S. Census Bureau. (2005b). *Table 2a: Projected population of the United States, by Age and Sex: 2000 to 2050.* Washington, DC: U.S. Census Bureau.

Vladeck, B. (1980). *Unloving care: The nursing home tragedy.* New York: Basic Books.

Weissert, W. (1985). Seven reasons why it is so difficult to make community-based long-term care cost-effective. *Health Services Research, 20*(4), 423–433.

Wilson, C., & Weissert, W. (1989). Private long-term care insurance: After coverage restrictions is there anything left? *Inquiry, 26*(4), 493–507.

CHAPTER SIX

Disparities in Health and Health Care

The central concern of this text encompasses the relationships between social inequality, health, and health care policy. This is the first of two chapters that examine the incidence and causes of disparities in health and in health care in the United States. Although both chapters have both descriptive and causal components, they differ in their emphasis. This chapter concerns itself primarily with the descriptive aspects of disparities in health and health care, while the next focuses on the causal aspects of these disparities.

CONCEPTUALIZING DISPARITIES IN HEALTH AND IN HEALTH CARE

The National Institutes of Health defines *disparities in health* as "differences in the incidence, prevalence, mortality, and burden of diseases and other adverse health conditions that exist among specific population groups in the United States" (NIH, 2001a). The U.S. Department of Health and Human Services (HHS) employs a more encompassing definition that includes both the *health* and *health care* dimensions of disparity (HHS, 2000; AHRQ, 2004). According to HHS, "All differences among populations in measures of *health* and *health care* are considered evidence of disparities..." (AHRQ, 2004, p. 7). The distinction between *disparities in health* and *disparities in health care* is a huge one, both conceptually and politically. Disparities in health concern differences between populations and population subgroups in the overall level of health and the distributions of disease and death, while disparities in health care encompass both the health outcomes of care and other dimensions of health care that include access, quality, and equity.

221

Although the above definitions of *disparities in health* are generally accepted, the position of HHS that "all differences among populations in measures of *health care* are considered evidence of disparities" is far more controversial. In its recent analysis of racial and ethnic disparities in health care (IOM, 2003), the IOM limited its definition of disparities in health care to differences in "the quality of healthcare that are not due to access-related factors or clinical needs, preferences, and appropriateness of intervention" (IOM, 2003, p. 32). A similarly limited conceptualization of disparities in health care was put forth in a recent article in *Annals of Internal Medicine,* in which disparities in health care are argued to be limited to differences in health care that (1) represent shortfalls in appropriate care that are both associated with adverse health consequences and (2) cannot be explained by differences in patient factors (such as needs and preferences) (Rathore & Krumholz, 2004).

As exemplified in the IOM definition of health care disparities, the choice of a narrow conceptualization of health care disparities has significant political implications.[1] While the U.S. Congress charged the IOM with the task of analyzing health care disparities, the mandate given IOM very deliberately excluded analysis of disparities in health care that arise from access factors. By shaping the discourse on health care disparities in this way, Congress avoids or at least significantly deflects discussions of disparities in health care access that provide political leverage for advocates of radical health care reform. On the other hand, the limited conceptualization of health care disparities conveyed in the *Annals of Internal Medicine* represents resistance in the medical profession to a definition of health care disparities that implies a general culpability on the part of physicians and other clinicians for any and all differences in health care that are correlated with race, ethnicity, sex, and other characteristics linked with social inequality.

In part, resistance within the medical profession to a more encompassing definition of disparities in health care is provoked by the implicit (and often explicit) tendency in much of the literature on health care disparities to cite any and all differences in health care as further evidence of the multiple biases in the diagnosis and treatment of various patients from disadvantaged groups. Although the medical profession is indeed deeply

---

[1] The Institute of Medicine (IOM) developed this narrow definition of health care disparities in response to the limited definition of disparities conveyed by the U.S. Congress in its original charge to the IOM to perform an analysis of health care disparities. Although the IOM acknowledges that the exclusion of access factors from the definition of health care disparities results in a definitional distinction that is "artificial" (IOM, 2003, p. 30), it is argued here that the IOM's narrow definition of health care also serves to downplay the role of access factors in production of health care disparities.

implicated in multiple aspects of disparities in health care, including the evolvement of a system of finance that keeps millions of U.S. residents from various disadvantaged groups out of the health care system altogether (Starr, 1982), it is important to concede four points in favor of the defenders of the medical profession:

1. Much of the literature on disparities in health care also confuses correlation with causality.
2. Disparities in health care can arise from patient need and preferences, the system, or the health care practitioner.
3. All of the health professions share culpability for disparities in health care.
4. Differences in health care by such factors as gender, race, or age are not in and of themselves either malevolent in intent or detrimental in outcome.[2]

However, there are two troubling aspects of a perspective on health care disparities that narrows the definition of health care disparities to factors exclude *access* and individual *needs and preferences* for health care.

Concerning access, it is well established that access to health care in the United States varies by income, race, gender, nativity. and a variety of other factors related to status, material resources, and social power. Further, it is also well established that groups that encounter barriers to health care access have poorer health (AHRQ, 2004). Thus, it is arbitrary if not disingenuous to limit the definition of disparities in health care only to differences in health care for those privileged to receive it. A similarly restricted definition of malnutrition would exclude differences in the nutritional status of individuals who, for any number of reasons, are kept from food. The effect of excluding issues of access as a key component of the definition of disparities in health care is a denial and negation of the culpability of all individuals and groups responsible for the delivery of care (hospital boards, hospital administrators, physicians, and allied health professionals) for any and all aspects of differences in health that arise from issues of access.

In this regard, the Institute of Medicine correctly concedes that multiple factors related to access cannot be kept distinct from other processes affecting the quality of health care provided (IOM, 2003, p. 31). For example, although a Medicaid voucher may provide the appearance of

---

[2] In fact, there are many differences in care by such factors as race, age, and gender that are based on optimal care, for example, racial differences in the prevalence of hereditary disease, age differences in metabolism, etc.

access to care, the stigma attached to being a Medicaid patient can bias the clinical assessment of health care needs as well as a patient's willingness to articulate preferences (Gurwitz et al., 2002; Obst, Nauenberg, & Buck, 2001).

Excluding *needs and preferences* from the calculus of health care disparities denies the very subtle ways in which individual preferences are shaped through the clinical encounter. There is a central paradox embedded in the clinical encounter that arises from a conflict between the criteria for achieving an unbiased expression of patient preference for care and the patient's dependence on the clinician for critical information. The achievement of unbiased patient preference requires that the patient possess the same information about risks and benefits of treatment as that possessed by the clinician. Although the ethical principles espoused in Western medicine obligate the physician to provide information about the risks and benefits of various treatment alternatives in an unbiased fashion, these conversations occur in a context of differences in race, socioeconomic class, ethnicity, gender, and age that profoundly influence perceptions of choice, best interests, and the norms of expressing preference. Put another way, the patient preferences are rarely antecedent to, or independent of, the sociology of the clinical encounter.[3]

The summary point of the preceding discussion of the definition of health care disparities is this: Although some differences in health care by such characteristics as race, ethnicity, and gender may be either benign or even beneficial, all differences in health care from any source qualify as disparities worthy of thoughtful investigation.

The Three Dimensions of Disparities Relevant to Health Care Policy

As shown in Figure 6.1, there are huge differences in the death rates of middle-age persons in the United States by race and Hispanic ethnicity. Among the groups compared, non-Hispanic blacks between the ages of 45 and 54 have the highest death rates, nearly twice that of non-Hispanic Whites and more than twice that of Hispanics. It is also clear that Native Americans between the ages of 45 and 54 have death rates that are significantly above those for both Hispanics and non-Hispanic Whites.

Differences in death rates for persons between the ages of 45 and 54 are particularly illuminating because they are premature deaths that

---

[3] A useful anecdotal example is a physician that elects to prescribe less expensive medications to Medicaid patients due to personal biases against public assistance recipients. It seems unlikely that the physician shares the full range of the pharmaceutical options with the Medicaid patients that are the targets of the physician's discrimination.

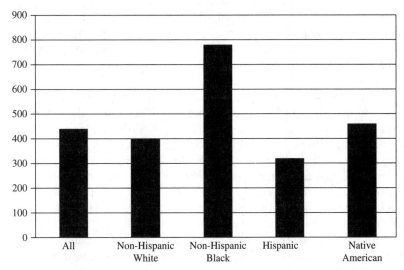

Figure 6.1 Deaths per 100,000 Persons Aged 45 to 54, U.S. 2003.
Source: Based on *Deaths: Preliminary data for 2003*, Table 6.1 National Center for Health Statistics (Hoyert, Kung, & Smith, 2005.)

reflect the cumulative and combined effects of disparities between population subgroups in three key dimensions of disparities in health: in the *burden of disease* carried by a subgroup, in the subgroup's relative *access to health care*, and in the *quality of health care* available to the subgroup. All three dimensions of disparity are of central concern to health care policy, however, the *burden of disease* is the most complex and influential dimension of disparity.

Conceptually, any population's (or population subgroup's) *burden of disease* refers to the prevalence and distribution of diseases, disabilities, and mortality that is carried by the population. Depending upon the application and central questions, *burden of disease* measures can be highly specific to one particular disease or cluster of related diseases, or can be global measures of population health that capture the overall impact of disease, disability, and death on a population.[4] The *burden of disease* that

---

[4] A innovative example of a global burden of disease measure is the Disability Adjusted Life Year(DALY), developed for the World Health Organization by the Harvard School of Public Health (Murray & Lopez, 1996). In essence, The DALY estimates the number of life years lost to premature death and years of healthy life lost due to disabling conditions. DALY estimates can be disease specific (e.g. years of healthy life lost due to breast cancer) or can be calculated to measure the summed impact of all diseases.

is carried by a population or population subgroup incorporates the susceptibilities and exposures to disease that arise from the interaction of biology and social environment as well as those differences in health that can be attributed to disparities in health care arising from such factors as ethnic and racial discrimination.

Unlike disparities in the *burden of disease*, which in part are produced by disparities in health care access and outcomes, disparities in *access to health care* and *quality of health care* do not in and of themselves reflect differences in health.[5] From the perspectives of health care policy and more broadly public health, this is a critical distinction. For example, the higher *burden of disease* that is reflected in the mortality rates of Native Americans and non-Hispanic Black Americans aged 45–54 relative to those of other racial/ethnic groups (per Figure 6.1) can likely be reduced by policy initiatives aimed at eliminating the disparities in health care access and quality experienced by both groups (AHRQ, 2004)—but only to a limited degree given sources of disease, death, and disability that lie outside of the health care system (e.g., economic displacement, disadvantages in education, and racial segregation). Although health and health care policy encompasses consideration of all factors that are relevant health disparities, specific policy questions and interventions must make clear the distinction between factors that are most closely linked to the organization and processes of the health care system and those factors that are tied to the larger structural context of disparities in health.

The Social Production of Disparities in Health

Disparities in health are associated with a variety of social characteristics, including age, race, ethnicity, gender, foreign birth, geographic location, and social class (education, occupation, and income) (AHRQ, 2004; Collins, Davis, Doty, & Ho, 2004; Denton & Walters, 1999; Finch, 2003). Although the next chapter will address the theories and evidence pertaining to the causal relationships between particular population characteristics and health, what follows is a brief overview of the ways in which population characteristics interact with the health care system to produce disparities in health.

---

[5] Even though disparities in access to health care and quality of health care do not "in and of themselves" reflect differences in health, they are correlated with them to the extent that there are patterns of disease that influence health care access and quality. An example of this is treatment of HIV, which remains encumbered with fear, stigma, and denial of appropriate care.

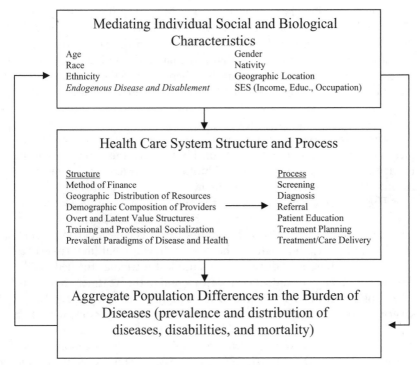

Figure 6.2   A Heuristic Model of Health Disparity Generation.

As shown in the heuristic model[6] depicted in Figure 6.2, health disparities (aggregate population differences in the burden of disease) are associated with social characteristics in two ways. The first, a direct causal pathway is depicted by the downward arrow at the right side of the model. The term *direct causal pathway* is used to convey the idea that there are particular social and biological characteristics of individuals (age, race, gender, etc.) that act as mediators for the determinants of disease prevalence in populations. As one example, race is less a direct determinant of disease than it is a social and biological characteristic that acts as mediator of various determinants of disease risk that have complex biological and social origins.[7] The same relationship holds for age, gender, ethnicity and

---

[6] The term "heuristic" is attached to the model as an acknowledgment of the model's simplification of extremely complex processes. In particular, the model shown omits the social and biological determinants that link the manifestations of disease to particular individual characteristics. These issues are taken up in the chapter that follows.

[7] For example, the prevalence of the gene that causes cystic fibrosis is higher among Whites than it is among other racial groups. This does not mean that race is a causal factor in

the other mediating characteristics shown in the top box of Figure 6.2. The middle pathway, shown in the downward arrows that connect the three boxes, conveys the idea that social characteristics also have an indirect effect on disease prevalence that is mediated through the health care system. For example, to the extent that there are racial characteristics of individuals that have detrimental effects on the availability and quality of health care, those same racial characteristics will lead to a higher burden of disease in the racial population.

The third arrow, pointing upward on the left side of the model, depicts a complex but important relationship between the differences in the burden of disease and the social and biological characteristics referred to as *endogenous disease and disablement.*

The term *endogenous* refers to the existence of a causal relationship that is internal to a model. As shown in Figure 6.2, an endogenous process takes place as particular diseases and disablements have a detrimental effect the availability and quality of health care in ways that (in turn) lead to an even higher burden of disease. For example, the stigma attached to HIV disease has in many instances been detrimental to the treatment of the disease, thus increasing the burden of disease both in terms of prevalence and severity in the populations at risk for HIV. In general, persons with high levels of chronic illness and disability confront various barriers to appropriate care related to stigma. Other examples of this endogenous causal process include STDs, asthma, cancer, epilepsy, tuberculosis, obesity, and psychiatric conditions generally (Becker, Janson-Bjerklie, Benner, Slobin, & Ferketich, 1993; Hayes, Vaughan, Medeiros, & Dubuque, 2002; Jacoby, Snape, & Baker, 2005; Joachim & Acorn, 2000; Michielutte & Diseker, 1982; Rogge, Greenwald, & Golden, 2004).

The relationship between diabetes and the Native American population illustrates the ways in which health disparities observed at the population level flow directly through individuals and are further generated through the health care system. Relative to persons racially identified as White, Native Americans are twice as likely to have diabetes listed as their cause of death (NCHS, 2005). Embedded in this statistic are differences between Whites and Native Americans in both the incidence and severity of diabetes. Although meeting the criteria for inclusion in the Native American racial category is a significant risk factor for diabetes, being classified as a Native American doesn't "cause" either the incidence or the severity of the disease. Rather, Native American origin is correlated

the risk of cystic fibrosis, but a risk factor associated with complex patterns of hereditary transmission.

with multiple causal determinants of diabetes, including but not limited to diet, obesity, lack of exercise, smoking, and genetic susceptibilities (Gohdes, 1995; NIH, 2001b). Although it is impossible to reconstruct the prevalence rates of diabetes among Native Americans preceding the conquest and displacement of indigenous peoples by Europeans, there is little doubt that the root causes of disproportionate prevalence of diabetes among Native Americans are embedded in the near eradication of indigenous culture that accompanied contact with Europeans. Specifically, a principal casualty of the socio-cultural genocide that accompanied the European conquest involved the elimination of ancient ways of food production, acquisition, and consumption that functioned together as crucial protective factors against diabetes. As a result of these aggregated individual level predisposing factors (and as shown in the right-hand arrow of Figure 6.2), there is a high and increasing prevalence of diabetes in the population of Native Americans that precedes exposure to the health care system.

As the U.S. health care system is structured, Native Americans confront a kind of double jeopardy: health care disparities that arise from race and health care disparities that arise from lower socioeconomic status. Although the Indian Health Service (IHS) has existed since 1955 to provide health care services to Native Americans, the IHS provides services to only about 60% of the Native Population (Acton et al., 2002). In large part, this is because a significant proportion of the Native American population is geographically isolated from IHS services. The 40% of the Native Americans that are not served by IHS must rely on a system of health care that disadvantages persons of lower socioeconomic status (SES) above and beyond issues of race. Notably, Native Americans lag in all three dimensions of SES: income, occupation, and education (U.S. Census, 2003). Aside from confronting barriers in *access* to health care, individuals of lower SES also receive lower *quality of care* in a variety of dimensions, including patient–provider communication, respectful treatment, timeliness of appointments, preventative treatment, and the provision of care that is appropriate to the condition (AHRQ, 2004). In the case of diabetic care, the clinical management of the disease that is critical to slowing its progression is shown to be significantly inferior for persons of lower SES (AHRQ, 2004). Although it is difficult to clearly disentangle the disparities that arise from socioeconomic disadvantage from those that arise from disadvantaged treatment on the basis of race, the evidence is irrefutable that Native Americans (1) continue to experience significant disparities in multiple dimensions of health care quality and access and (2) have a burden of diabetic disease that is disproportionately large and growing relative to other racial groups in the United States (Acton et al., 2002; AHRQ, 2004; Hoyert et al., 2005).[8]

These disparities in care and outcomes can be traced to specific structures and processes within the U.S. health care system (see the middle box of Figure 6.2). For example, the *method of finance* is clearly unfavorable to the working poor—a social class disproportionately representative of Native Americans (U.S. Census, 2003). As pointed out previously, the *geographic structure* of the health care system is very problematic to Native Americans in that a large proportion of Native Americans are spatially isolated from INS clinics. The *demographic composition of providers* is also very unfavorable to Native Americans. Of all racial groups in the United States, Native Americans are the least likely to encounter a provider of their own race (American Medical Association, 2005; U.S. Census, 2003). In fact, the lack of Native American providers in the health care system both reflects and perpetuates all of the structural origins of disparities in health care shown in Figure 6.2, including *detrimental overt and latent value structures,*[9] inadequate *training and professional socialization of non-Native American providers,* and *prevalent paradigms of disease and health* that conflict with indigenous conceptions of health, illness, and healing (AHRQ, 2004; Garroutte, Kunovich, Jacobsen, & Goldberg, 2004).

All of the processes of health care shown in Figure 6.2 (screening, diagnosis, referral, patient education, treatment planning, and treatment/care delivery) are determined by the structural components just discussed. Conceptually, it is useful to speculate on the extent to which any structural component depicted increases or decreases the likelihood that any particular process of health care will occur in a way that promotes health care disparities. For example, it is easy to see how a system of health care finance that makes it more likely that a health care provider will be reimbursed less for seeing a low-income patient than a middle-income patient impacts on the provider's willingness to invest equally in

[8] Between 1990 and 1998 there was a 71% increase in the reported incidence of diabetes in HIS service areas, and a 46% increase in adolescent diabetes. Although some of this increase likely reflects better reporting, there is also evidence to suggest that these estimates reflect a large true increase in disease prevalence (Acton et al., 2002).

[9] Overt value structures are those values that are espoused through formal statements, professional credos, rules of conduct, and laws, for example, statements pertaining to patient rights and provider responsibilities, laws pertaining to patient consent and confidentiality, and formal statements pertaining to issues like patient autonomy. Latent values are those that expressed through the de facto effects of policies and the attitudes and actions of health care providers. For example, most health care organizations now espouse the value of "culturally competent practice" while at the same time retaining institutionalized structures and processes that reinforce the dominant culture.

the clinical encounter with a low income patient—thus negatively affecting screening, diagnosis, patient education, and treatment planning and delivery. It is also readily apparent to see the ways in which dramatic differences between the race and class composition of providers and patients affect the trust and communication between patient and provider that influences all aspects of patient care. Given the interaction of health care financing and the class and race composition of health care providers, it is hardy surprising to find that low-income and minority patients perceive less respect on the part of providers, feel less listened to, and (in apparent consequence) receive generally poorer health care that contributes to a higher burden of disease (AHRQ, 2004; IOM, 2003).

MEASURING DISPARITIES IN HEALTH AND IN HEALTH CARE

As mentioned at the beginning of this chapter, measures of disparities involve three general categories of health and health care delivery: *burden of disease, access to health care*, and *quality of health care*. However, measures of disparity often overlap across categories. For example, the incidence rates of diseases that are sensitive to prevention (e.g. diabetes) act as measures of a population's *burden of disease* and reflect disparities in *health care access* and *health care quality* as well. In answer to this dilemma, both the Institute of Medicine (IOM) and the Agency for Healthcare Research and Quality (AHRQ) have engaged in a significant effort to identify measures of disparity that tend to be specific to key aspects of health care as it is organized and delivered in the United States. In contrast, the most innovative *burden of disease* measures have evolved from international health studies. The in-depth discussion of measures of disparity will begin there.

Measuring Disparities in Burden of Disease

Earlier in this chapter it was stated that any population's *burden of disease* refers to the prevalence and distribution of diseases, disabilities, and mortality that is carried by the population. So the first characteristic that typically determines one burden of disease measure from another is whether the measure concerns morbidity or mortality. *Morbidity* measures involve incidence rates of disease and/or disability in nonfatal or prefatal stages, while *mortality* measures refer to death rates. More recently, burden of disease measures have been developed that combine morbidity and mortality, such as the DALY (disability adjusted life year) measure discussed previously, and the   HALE (health adjusted life expectancy) measure. While the DALY estimates the number of life years lost to premature death and years of healthy life lost due to disabling conditions, HALE is interpreted as the number of years at birth a person can expect to live in full health (i.e. unencumbered by either ill-health or disability) (World Health Organization, 2001). The DALY has the advantage of being disease or disabling condition specific (Murray & Lopez, 1996), while the HALE is useful as a summary measure of population health. Another innovation in burden of disease measures, again developed at the international level, involves the estimation of disparities in population morbidity and mortality that are due to specific risk factors—such as exposure to environmental toxins and the prevalence of tobacco use (Ezzati, Lopez, Rodgers, Vander Hoorn, & Murray, 2002). The advantage of these types of burden of disease measures is that they are directly linked to important sources of health disparities and critical areas of risk that can be addressed by targeted health care policies.

Although burden of disease measures that have applied to the problem of health disparities in the domestic context have been limited to either disease specific measures or very general measures of population health like life expectancy at birth or infant mortality, there have been revealing exceptions. For example, a fairly recent study employed the disability adjusted life years (DALY) measure to examine the burden of disease disparities by race, ethnicity, and gender in Los Angeles County (Kominski et al., 2002). Aside from finding that African Americans were the most disadvantaged of all groups in terms of the overall burden of disease, it was found that employing the DALY measure established a different ranking of diseases in terms of overall population burden than the more typical approach based solely upon mortality rates.

Turning to the prevalent measures for burden of disease in the United States, the most dominant of the global measures of population burden of disease involve two closely related indices of population health, the infant mortality rate and life expectancy. Life expectancy refers to the average number of remaining years for a person at a given age, given the prevailing pattern of population mortality of the population. Although life expectancy at birth is the most frequently cited life expectancy statistic, tables of population life expectancy typically calculated in single-, 5-, and 10-year intervals that allow estimation of life expectancy at multiple ages for different populations. The National Center for Health Statistics regularly estimates and publishes updated life expectancies at the state and national levels by general categories of race, ethnicity, and gender, and there are multiple studies of life expectancies for very specific subpopulations published in the public health literature.[10] As a general measure of population mortality, life expectancy is invaluable as an overall measure of the relative health disadvantages confronting some groups. For most people, the observation that the life expectancy of African Americans is nearly 5 years less than the average for all Americans has more impact than citing the disparities in age-specific death rates that determine estimates of life expectancy (Hoyert et al., 2005). However, the biggest disadvantage of life expectancy as a general measure of health is that it can be badly distorted by high death rates in younger ages—particularly in infancy. Thus, while African American males have an average life expectancy at birth that is 8.5 years less than the average for the United States, a significant component of that disparity is attributable to infant death rates.[11]

Disparities in life expectancy that are attributable to particular causes of death can also be calculated by the use of multiple decrement life table methods and related life table methods.[12] Basically, such methods identify life years that are lost to a population due to particular diseases or social characteristics associated with premature mortality (Schryock & Siegal, 1976). The general burden of disease measures that are yielded by such methods are the summary "years of potential life lost" (YPLL) statistic, which refers to all deaths that occur prior to a selected benchmark of average life expectancy and YPLLs due to specific causes of death associated with premature mortality (e.g. lung cancer deaths caused from tobacco exposure). As an example, the Centers for Disease Control estimated YPLLs per 100,000 persons for each state by five leading causes of death.[13] One startling exemplar from among many dramatic contrasts in the CDC report are the 1.7 years of potential years of life lost from heart disease in Mississippi relative to each year of potential years of life lost from heart disease in Connecticut—likely reflecting the interaction of state differences in racial composition, poverty, and access to health care (Centers for Disease Control and Prevention, 2003).

---

[10] Life expectancies are generally calculated from vital records (birth and death records) and population counts, although there are also methods to calculate life expectancies from household level survey data.

[11] By age 65, the life expectancy gap between African American males and the general U.S. population is 3.5 years (Hoyert et al, 2005).

[12] It should be pointed out that multiple decrement life tables are only a crude approximation of differences in life expectancy that are due to the impact of particular causes of death, because individuals dying of natural causes often have other potentially fatal co-morbid conditions.

[13] These YPLLs were also adjusted for age.

Of the many *burden of disease* measures, the one that is most often used in referencing health disparities is cause-specific death rates. *Cause-specific death rates* are calculated from cause of death data extracted from death certificates by county and state public health authorities, with the "underlying cause of death" typically used as the statistically relevant cause of death. Although multiple disease processes often contribute to death events, the underlying cause of death represents the coroner's evaluation of the disease process that is the most determinant causal factor a person's death.[14] Thus, while a person might have advanced heart disease, diabetes, and lung cancer, heart disease is identified as the cause of death only if it is the factor most implicated in the series of physiological events which resulted in death. This is an important point, because it should now be clear that cause-specific death rates don't by themselves reflect the full burden of disease carried by individuals or populations. However, for a variety of reasons discussed in more detail below, it is a powerful and highly informative measure of both health disparities and the root causes of disparities. The cause-specific death rate is typically calculated as the number of deaths per 100,000 persons from a given cause in a given year or month. However, there are also methods to adjust for differences in population age distribution, which for disease processes like cancer are often necessary to capture the relevant sources of disparity.

There are several reasons why cause-specific death rates are favored as a burden of disease measure that is illustrative of health disparities. Among the most important is the fact that in most countries, and all parts of the United States, all deaths are registered along with the determinant causes of death. Also, diagnoses in death records are more complete and scrutinized than other health records. Although death records are not immune to error and even fraud, on the whole they are much more accurate than clinical encounter records and moreover, ultimately capture disease prevalence rates from persons who don't ordinarily utilize health care. Another important advantage of cause-specific death rates is that they both measure the most critical health disparities (as death is considered the most extreme form of health disparity) and often reflect underlying social causes.

To illustrate this key point, the cause-specific death rates shown on Table 6.1 provide a glimpse of the health care disparities between persons that are classified as Hispanic versus those classified as non-Hispanic

---

[14] Causes of death are based upon an internationally recognized method for classifying diseases and causes of death, currently the World Health Organization *International Statistical Classification of Diseases and Related Health Problems Manual—Revised Version 10* (commonly called the *ICD-10*). In the parlance of ICD-10, accidents and acts of violence are coded as externally caused diseases.

Table 6.1 Age-Adjusted Deatth Rates (per 100,000) for Selected Causes of Death by Hispanic Origin

	Hispanic or Latin	White, Not Hispanic	Difference	Ratio Hisp/ White N-H
All Causes	629.3	837.3	−208.2	0.8
Diseases of the Heart	180.5	239.2	−58.7	0.8
Ischemic Heart Disease	138.3	171.0	−32.7	0.8
Cerebrovascular Diseases	41.3	54.6	−13.3	0.8
Malignant Neoplasms	128.4	195.6	−67.2	0.7
Trachea, Broncus and Lung	23.7	57.5	−33.8	0.4
Colon, Rectum, and Anus	13.7	19.5	−5.8	0.7
Prostate	21.6	25.8	−4.2	0.8
Breast	15.5	25.6	−10.1	0.6
Chronic Lower Respiratory Disease	20.6	46.9	−26.3	0.4
Influenza and Pneumonia	19.2	22.6	−3.4	0.8
Chronic Liver Disease and Cirrhosis	15.4	9.0	**6.4**	**1.7**
Diabetes Mellitus	35.6	22.2	**13.4**	**1.6**
HIV Disease	5.8	2.1	**3.7**	**2.8**
Unintentional Injuries	30.7	38.0	−7.3	0.8
Motor Vehicle Accidents	15.2	16.0	−0.8	1
Suicide	5.7	12.9	−7.2	0.4
Homicide	7.3	2.8	**4.5**	**2.6**

Source: NCHS, Health, United States, 2004. Data from Table 29 Age Adjusted Death Rates for Selected Causes According to Sex, Race and Hisptanic Origin., United States, Selected Years 1950–2003. Hyattesville, Maryland.

Whites (NCHS, 2004b). Note that the death rates are adjusted for age, which is important given the younger age distribution of Hispanics.

For most leading causes of death, Hispanics have lower death rates than non-Hispanic Whites. This phenomenon is referred to generally as the "Hispanic Paradox," because the socioeconomic status of Hispanics relative to non-Hispanic Whites would predict a significant mortality disadvantage. Although there are competing causal explanations for the Hispanic Paradox, the most recent findings show that the Hispanic mortality advantage is driven by the prevalence of low adult mortality among the foreign born—which suggests that selective migration plays an important role in the Hispanic mortality advantage (Palloni & Aria, 2004). The basic idea of selective migration is that Hispanic immigrants to the United States tend to be drawn from the healthiest of adults (those able to both work and withstand the rigors of the migratory journey). There is also the possibility of a selective return migration effect that arises as

Hispanic immigrants who become too ill to work return to their country of origin before dying.[15]

As shown on Table 6.1, the Hispanics that are resident in the United States have a mortality disadvantage relative to non-Hispanic Whites in only 4 of the 13 leading cause of death categories: chronic liver disease and cirrhosis, diabetes, HIV, and homicide. What is significant in this pattern is that this particular cluster of diseases is consistent with a working age mortality pattern found among the most highly disadvantaged African Americans (Guest, Almgren, & Hussey, 1998; Palazzo, Guest, & Almgren, 2003). All four causes of death are associated with premature death during what should be the most productive years of adulthood, and arise from detrimental exposures (interpersonal violence) and risky health behaviors (alcoholism, I.V. drug abuse). These particular risks and exposures are associated with disadvantages in stable employment, and fit with the employment barriers that confront Hispanics immigrants—in particular undocumented workers.

Measuring Disparities in Access to Care

Access to health care is generally defined as the ability to engage in timely use of the health care services that achieve the optimal health outcomes (IOM, 1993). As noted by the *2004 National Health Care Disparities Report* (AHRQ, 2004), access to health care involves gaining entry, getting to the geographic and physical locations where the needed health care is delivered, and finding appropriate providers for the needed care. Obviously, access barriers can arise in any one or all of these three steps to gaining access. The approach to measuring access that was undertaken by the Agency for Healthcare Research and Quality (HHS) involves three general categories of access measures: structural measures, patient assessments of care, and measures of health care utilization (AHRQ, 2004, p. 59). Structural measures involve the presence or absence of resources that enable health care (e.g., health insurance, health care providers within geographic proximity). Patient assessments of care, while subjective, are critically important to the process of seeking and acquiring appropriate care. Measures of health care utilization provide a more objective appraisal of the adequacy of the connection between health risk and conditions and the health services accessed.

---

[15] The prominent alternative explanation of the "Hispanic Paradox" places emphasis on the cultural factors, in particular the protective factors of close family and community ties. Although this is a compelling thesis, the most recent rigorous analysis of this question (see Palloni & Aria, 2004) failed to find evidence that cultural factors, as opposed to selective factors, accounted for the Hispanic mortality advantage.

It should be noted that disparities in access to health care, and the measures that reflect them, revolve around issues of equity. Equity of access actually involves two conceptually distinct dimensions of equity, *need-based equity* and *similar treatment for similar cases* (Aday & Andersen, 1981). Equity based on need acknowledges that differences between groups in health care utilization or the allocation of health care resources do not in and of themselves suggest disparities in health care access. For example, fewer oncologists and fewer hospital beds dedicated to oncology care within some Hispanic communities might reflect the lower prevalence of cancer among the Hispanic population. On the other hand, to the extent that diabetes is more prevalent among Hispanics a *need-based* approach to equity would require a higher level of specialized services for the prevention and treatment of diabetes among Hispanics than other groups at lower risk. *Similar treatment for similar cases* refers to the notion that given the same identified health care need, access to appropriate care should not differ by such extraneous factors such as race, social class, gender, age, geographic location, or insurance status.

Although differences in health insurance coverage by income, race, and employment status are the most frequently cited measure of disparities in access to health care, another important measure is the extent to which there are differences in having a source of regular and ongoing health care. For example, people who must rely upon hospital emergency rooms and urgent care clinics for their health care needs are unlikely to either build a trusting relationship with a physician or receive essential preventative care.

Figure 6.3, provided by the *2004 National Health Care Disparities Report* (AHRQ, 2004), shows that in the period between 1999 and 2001, the trends in having a regular and ongoing source of care moved in opposite directions for other racial groups and African Americans, with a significant trend downward for African Americans. In stark contrast to African Americans, American Indians and Alaska Natives (shown as AI/AN) experienced dramatic gains in having a regular and ongoing source of care. These access trends reflect important aspects of health care policy, specifically the increased fiscal appropriations during this period for Indian Health Service programs (Indian Health Service, 2004) and the continued neglect of the employer-based health care insurance system and the urban health care infrastructure that places the health care of African Americans in increased jeopardy.[16]

---

[16] The interpretation of the upper graph in Figure 6.3 in this text is different from than that published in the 2004 National Healthcare Disparities Report, which states that American Indians and Alaska Natives did not improve relative to other racial groups. It appears the latter is in error.

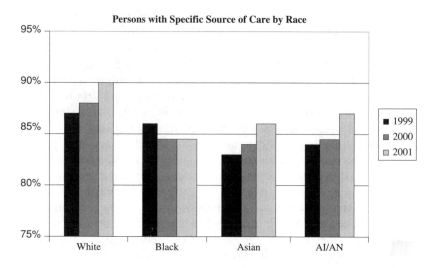

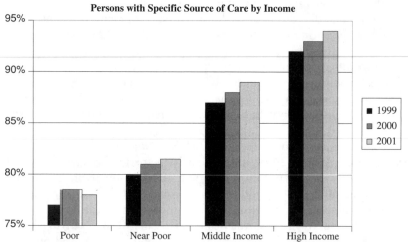

Figure 6.3   Persons with a Specific Source of Ongoing Care by Race and Income Leval.
Source: AHRQ. 2004 National Healthcare Disparities Report. Rockville, Md: U.S. Department of Health and Human Services. Figure 3.3.

The lower graph in Figure 6.3 also shows the dramatic differences in usual source of care by income, with the most disadvantaged group showing the least favorable trend over time. Given the higher burden of disease carried by the poor, from the standpoint of need-based equity of access, this is a particularly disturbing observation. As noted in the 2004 National Health Care Disparities Report, no racial or income group shown in Figure 6.3 achieved the Health People 2010 (HP 2010) goal of 96% of Americans having a specific source of ongoing care, although those with the highest income are very close to this goal. Despite the laudable intents of this HP 2010 goal, from the standpoint of a Rawlsian approach to social justice, closing the income gap in equity of access should be the clear policy priority.

Measures of Disparity in Health Care Quality

As can be surmised at this point, the measurement of disparities in health care access and quality is a highly complex enterprise. In fact, there are decades of research on the conceptualization and measurement of health care access and quality—with the escalating debate concerning disparities in health care even further raising the stakes. The approach undertaken by the Agency for Healthcare Research and Quality (AHRQ) represents the most current and encompassing approach to measuring disparities in health care quality and access (Kelley, Moy, & Dayton, 2005). Although a more complete overview of the AHRQ model of access and quality measurement is provided by Kelly et al. (2005), the graphic version of the AHRQ model shown in Figure 6.4 conveys the fundamentals.

First, it is shown that all aspects of health care access and quality serve four very general purposes: promoting health, recovering from illness, living with chronic disease and disability, and coping with the end of life. It is also shown quality of care is conceptualized as encompassing four specific aspects: effectiveness, safety, timeliness, and patient centeredness. The quality aspect that perhaps is the most abstract, patient centeredness, incorporates the notion that the care provided "is respectful of and responsive to individual patient preferences, needs, and values" (AHRQ, 2004, p. 21). Figure 6.4 also depicts the idea that access to care and quality of care are in part relative to the level of health care need, and that disparities in health care by race, ethnicity, and social class are observed in multiple aspects of health care access and quality.

An example application of the AHRQ framework for disparities in quality of health care, shown in Figure 6.5, concerns the racial disparities in the *patient safety* aspect of quality—specifically in the incidence of septicemia. Septicemia is a life-threatening infection of the bloodstream, and always a risk whenever surgery is performed. Protections against

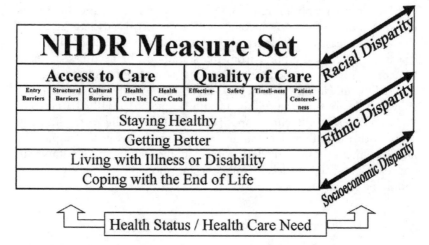

Figure 6.4   The Agency for Healthcare Research and Quality's Approach to the Conceptualization and Measurement of Disparities.
Source: Kelley, E.P., E.M.D. Moy, D.M.D. Stryer, H.M.D.M.P.H. Burstin, and C.M.D. Clancy. 2005. "The National Healthcare Quality and Disparities Reports: An Overview." *Medical care* 43(3):3–8. Figure 2.

septicemia include a sterile surgical field, sterilization of surgical instruments, the rituals of vigorous hand and arm scrubbing, "gowning-up" in the sterile vestments of surgery, and proper wound care following surgery. The risk of septicemia is minimized to the extent that hospitals and surgical staff are vigilant in all aspects of sterile procedure, and made substantial where there is inattention to patient safety at any point prior to, during, or after surgery.

As shown in Figure 6.5, the national rates of septicemia vary by race, with the rate of septicemia much higher among African Americans and Hispanic patients than Whites. Although the mechanisms of differential exposure to septicemia by race are not specified in the *2004 National Health Care Disparities Report*, the dramatic differences suggest that disparities in access to quality hospitals play a significant role and that race-based indifferences to issues of patient safety are implicated as well. Notably, the differences in the prevalence of septicemia cannot be explained by patient characteristics other than race, and thus stand as a significant indictment of the U.S. Health Care system. Sadly, other measures of regard for patient safety also reflect dramatic racial disparities, including accidental lung punctures, postsurgical pulmonary emboli, and hospital acquired infections (AHRQ, 2004).

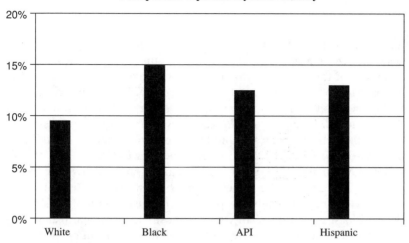

Figure 6.5 Incidence of Postoperative Septicemia by Race Per 1,000 Elective Surgery Discharge of More Than 3 Hospital Days, Year 2001 (Adjusted for Age, Gender, Comorbidities, and Diagnosis Related Group).
Source: AHRQ. 2004. "2004 National Healthcare Disparities Report." Rockville, Md: U.S. Department of Health and Human Services. Figure 2.10.

SOCIAL CHARACTERISTICS ASSOCIATED WITH DISPARITIES IN HEALTH AND HEALTH CARE

Disparities in health and in health care are structural in origin, meaning that they reflect the multiple forms of social hierarchy that are embedded in the organization of social relationships at all levels of society. According to "fundamental social cause" theory,[17] disparities in the burden of disease (and ergo in health care) arise wherever and whenever there are differences between groups in access to power, knowledge, and resources that are critical to health (Link & Phelan, 1995). In the United States, and to a greater or lesser extent elsewhere, differences in power, knowledge, and access to resources are associated with a broad variety of social characteristics, including age, race, SES (education, occupation, and income), gender, nativity (U.S. vs. foreign born), and also geography. As previously mentioned in this chapter, because disease and various forms of disablement are sources of disempowerment and deprivation, they further

---

[17] The theory of "fundamental social causes of disease" (Link & Phelan, 1995) will be covered extensively in the next chapter, which is devoted more specifically to social epidemiology.

accentuate health disparities that may have arisen from other determinant factors (e.g., poverty).

Given the breadth of social characteristics associated with disparities in health and in health care, the evidence concerning either is difficult to summarize in a way that is adequately comprehensive. However, the remainder of this chapter draws from the findings from three ambitious attempts to do so: *Living and Dying in the U.S.A.*, a sociological analysis of the adult mortality undertaken by Rogers, Hummer, and Nam (2000); the *2004 National Health Care Disparities Report*, published by the U.S. Department of Health and Human Services; and *Unequal Treatment: Confronting Racial and Ethnic Disparities in Health Care*, the Institute of Medicine's 2003 analysis of disparities in the delivery of health care. As rigorous and comprehensive as these studies are, even in total they provide only an incomplete portrayal of the disparities that arise in the wealthiest nation on earth with the most expensive and technologically advanced health care system. Occasionally data from other sources will be added to at least somewhat complete this tragic and ironic picture.

DISPARITIES IN HEALTH AND BURDEN OF DISEASE: GENERAL FINDINGS

Before examining the specific factors that are correlated with disparities in health, a few exemplars are provided to offer some sense of the magnitude of the disadvantages. First to be considered are racial and ethnic disparities in the "years of potential life lost" (YPLL) statistic described earlier in the chapter. Again, the YPLL statistic refers to either the life years lost in a population due to all deaths that occur prior to a selected benchmark of average life expectancy or life years lost due to specific causes of death associated with premature mortality. Figure 6.6 shows the recent time trends by race and by sex in the years of potential years of life lost (per 100,000 persons) from all causes of premature death combined.[18]

For example, the top graph shows that between 1990 and 2000, the years of potential life lost among African Americans dropped from just over 16,000 years per 100,000 persons to about 12,000. However, it is also clear that among the other racial and ethnic groups compared, the mortality disadvantage of African Americans remains both substantial and, in relative terms, largely unchanged. Aside from having the highest number of potential years of life lost of any racial group compared, there is

---

[18] Premature deaths are deaths that occur from diseases that can either be delayed until old age or death from external causes that are preventable (e.g., accidents, interpersonal violence).

Years of Life Lost (Age Adjusted) by Race

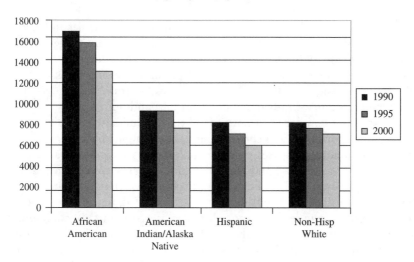

Years of Life Lost (Age Adjusted) by Sex

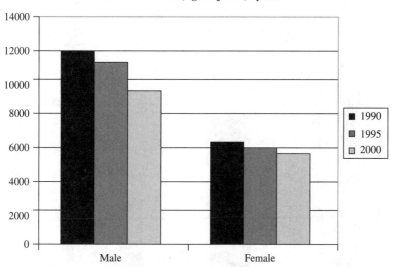

Figure 6.6   Years of life lost (YPLL) before age 75 per 100,000 persons for all causes of death, according to sex, race, and Hispanic origin. It should be noted that the death rates used to estimate the YPLL statistics are age adjusted.
Source: *Health, United States 2004*. NCHS Hyattesvilled, Maryland. Based on data from Table 30.

also an enormous gap in premature mortality between African Americans and all other groups.

The lower graph in Figure 6.6 also illuminates disparities in health by sex. Despite improvements in the years of potential years of life lost by males during the 1990s, the gender gap in preventable mortality remains highly unfavorable to males. The toll of premature mortality is particularly devastating for African American males, a group that suffers the combined mortality disadvantages of both race and sex.

A second exemplar of disparities in health illuminates the role of social class in mortality from chronic and noncommunicable diseases, and from communicable diseases. In Figure 6.7, recent trends in age-adjusted death rates from chronic and communicable diseases are contrasted by levels of education—a key dimension of social class that correlates with both occupational status and income. The first thing that is apparent is the huge contrast in levels of mortality from chronic and noncommunicable diseases (e.g. asthma, diabetes) by level of education. Secondly, it is apparent that the mortality advantages are significantly greater for those

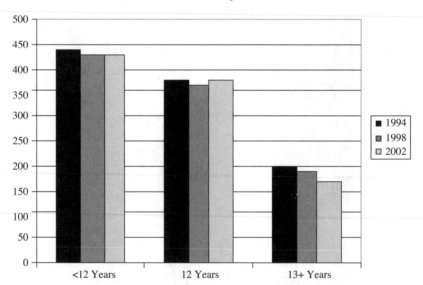

Age Adjusted Death Rates from Chronic and Non-Communicable Diseases by Education

Figure 6.7 Age adjusted death rates from chronic and non-communicable diseases for persons aged 25–64, by years of education.
Source: *Health, United States 2004*. N.C.H.S. Hyattesvilled, Maryland. Table 34. Age adjusted communicable disease death rates for adults aged 25–64 United States, selected years 1994–2002.

with at least 1 year of additional education beyond the standard 12-year education mark that generally signals high school completion. Thirdly, close examination of Figure 6.7 shows that the mortality advantage of those at the highest level of education has increased over the past several years.

However, it should be considered that the association between mortality from chronic and noncommunicable diseases and social class involves two causal directions. In essence, the burden of chronic disease reduces the likelihood that higher levels of educational attainment will be achieved[19] and conversely, the disadvantages associated with a limited education (e.g. poverty) contribute to the likelihood that chronic health conditions will emerge. Thus, disparities in mortality from chronic conditions are associated with social class, but the causal role of social class varies across individual cases.

In the case of mortality from communicable diseases (e.g. HIV), it is significantly less likely that lower levels of educational attainment are a result of ill health than is the case with chronic diseases. That is, communicable diseases are generally more likely to be acquired and progress to premature mortality as a function of disadvantaged socioeconomic status than to act as a determinant of socioeconomic disadvantage. While the opposite causal direction is quite plausible under a variety of circumstances, in general mortality from communicable diseases is more often an outcome of socioeconomic disadvantage. As shown in Figure 6.8, the mortality disadvantages of lower socioeconomic status (fewer years of education) are quite substantial where communicable diseases are the immediate cause of mortality. It is also apparent that despite significant improvements in the risk of death from communicable diseases during the mid-1990s (mostly attributable to decreased mortality from AIDS), the disparities by level of education remained little changed. For example, the lightest gray bar in Figure 6.8 shows that the most extreme education gap in age-adjusted mortality rates from communicable diseases remained at approximately 30 deaths/per 100,000 persons between 1994 and 2002— despite rather dramatic changes in the overall death rates.

Taken together, the exemplars shown in Figures 6.6, 6.7, and 6.8 illuminate two critical aspects of disparities in health. First, disparities by race and socioeconomic status are substantial. Second, despite general improvements in the overall level of health across all race and education groups shown, the relative mortality disadvantages associated with race and social class have remained largely unchanged. What can't be surmised

---

[19] For example, deaths from chronic and noncommunicable diseases disproportionately represent persons institutionalized due to severe cognitive deficits that preclude schooling.

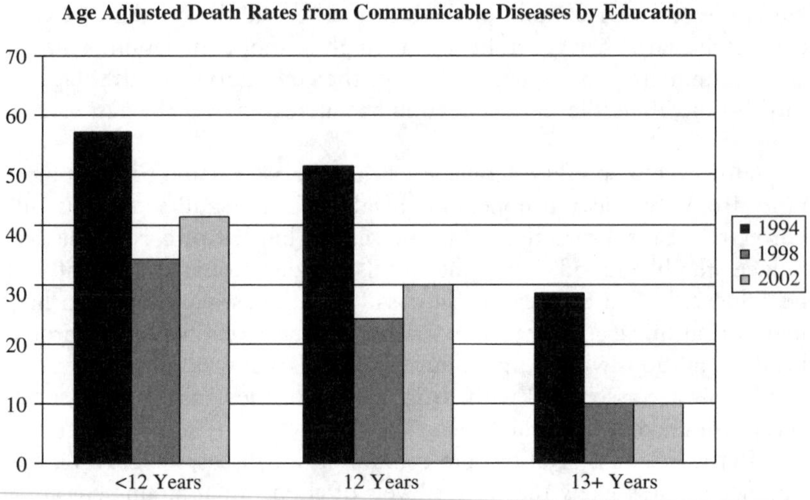

Age Adjusted Death Rates from Communicable Diseases by Education

Figure 6.8 Age adjusted death rates from communicable diseases for persons aged 25–64, by years of education.
Source: *Health, United States 2004*. N.C.H.S. Hyattesville, Maryland. Table 34. Age adjusted chronic and non-communicable disease death rates for adults aged 25–64 United States, selected years 1994–2002.

from these trends is the relative influence of race and social class on disparities in health. For that, we turn to the exhaustive analysis of disparities in adult mortality undertaken by Rogers, Hummer, and Nam in *Living and Dying in the USA* (2000).

Assessing the Relative Effects of Social Characteristics on Disparities in Health

Findings From Living and Dying in the USA

To the extent that socioeconomic status (SES) is associated with race, as is the case in the United States, determining the relative causal influence of either race or SES on disparities in health is not possible absent the ability to examine the lives of individuals with different racial and educational characteristics over time. The same is true for ethnicity, nativity (country of birth), marital status, sex, and a variety of other social characteristics that are associated with both health and SES.

Rogers, Hummer, and Nam (2000) tackled this problem by employing data prepared by the National Center for Health Statistics that linked survey information on individual social characteristics, health status, and health relevant behaviors to the death records of survey respondents who subsequently died. The linked survey and death records spanned a 9-year period (1986–1995) and involved a nationally representative sample—thus permitting generalization of multiple findings to the U.S. population as a whole.[20] Although the details of the study are quite complex, the statistical strategy employed Rogers, Hummer, and Nam produced findings that are straightforward to explain and interpret. In essence, the disparities in health that are attributable to different social characteristics are presented as "adjusted mortality differentials," that is, differences in the risk of death associated with a given social characteristic when all other factors are statistically controlled.

The graph shown in Figure 6.9 summarizes the findings from only one enlightening component of the exhaustive analysis of health disparities undertaken by Rogers, Hummer, and Nam.[21] Essentially, each social characteristic shown in Figure 6.9 is expressed as an adjusted mortality differential, meaning its effects on mortality are statistically adjusted for other potentially confounding factors—age, income, employment status, and marital status.[22] For racial/ethnic characteristics, all differences shown are relative to the mortality risks associated with the White Americans. Thus it can be seen that being of Asian-American descent reduces the likelihood of mortality something akin to 20% relative to White Americans when other relevant factors are taken into account. Conversely, there are distinct disadvantages in mortality risk attributable to those of African American or Puerto Rican descent relative to White Americans.

The mortality risks by lower levels of education are relative to the mortality levels of persons with 13+ years of education (shown in Figure 6.9 as the reference category). It is readily apparent that net of race, ethnicity, gender, and other social characteristics that the mortality disadvantages of fewer years of education are powerful. Specifically, persons having only 12 years of education (equivalent to a high school education) have about a 15% mortality risk disadvantage relative to those with greater than 13 years of education and persons of less than 12 years of education have about a 30% mortality risk disadvantage. Although

---

[20] There are caveats and important limitations that Rogers, Hummer, and Nam explain in detail. Interested readers are referred to Rogers, Hummer, and Nam (2000), pages 18–20.

[21] See the full analysis in Rogers, Hummer, & Nam (2000).

[22] The relative mortality risks shown in Figure 6.9 are derived from multivariate techniques that statistically control for the confounding effects of all other social characteristics shown in Figure 6.9 plus age, income, employment status, and marital status. Thus for example, the 28% mortality disadvantage associated with being of Puerto Rican descent (as opposed to being of White American descent) is net of or in addition to whatever mortality disadvantages are imposed by lower education levels, lower income, unfavorable marital status, age effects, and even being male.

Adjusted Mortality Differentials by Selected Social Characteristics

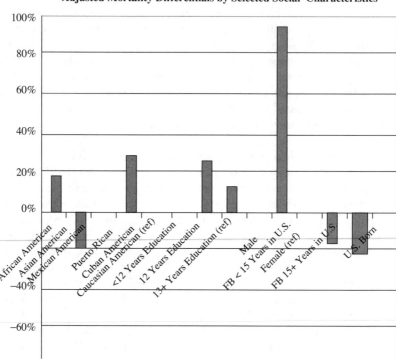

Figure 6.9 Mortality Differentials by Race, Educaion, Sex and Nativity, Adjusted for all Social Characteristics Shown plus Age, Income, Employment Status, and Marital Status. All references social characteristics (those used for relative comparison) show a 0% mortality differential.
Source: Rogers, R.G., R.A. Hummer, and C.B. Nam. 2000. *Living and dying in the USA: behavioral, health, and social differentials of adults mortality.* San Diego: Academic Press. Table 4.3.

the education and race/ethnicity effects on relative mortality risks are substantial, the most powerful social characteristic is gender. Relative to females (the reference or comparison category), males carry nearly twice the mortality risk of females when all other social characteristics are taken into account. The reason that males don't actually die at twice the rate of females is that (on an individual level) males are buffered by such protective factors as income, education, employment, relative age, and favorable marital status. Still, the mortality disadvantage in males is expressed in a variety of statistics, including a 5.4 year disadvantage in life expectancy at birth (NCHS, 2004a).

Interestingly though, being of foreign birth decreases mortality risk, again where differences in income, education, race/ethnicity, and other confounding social characteristics are taken into account. The most likely dynamic in the favorable mortality effects of foreign birth has to do with the selective migration process explained previously in this chapter (Palloni & Aria, 2004).

It is well beyond the scope of this text to summarize all of the findings from the exhaustive analysis of mortality disparities undertaken by Rogers, Hummer, and Nam. Indeed, the findings shown in Figure 6.9 that pertain to social characteristics associated with significant disparities in mortality are but a small but illuminating glimpse of their complete analysis. The other structural sources of disparities in mortality addressed in their investigation include the role of the occupational hierarchy,[23] disabilities, mental illness and addictions, and the mediating effects of specific health behaviors (e.g. exercise, smoking, and alcohol consumption). These issues are considered in more depth in chapter 7.

Social Characteristics Related to Disparities in Health Care

2004 National Healthcare Disparities Report: Background and Key Findings

The *2004 National Healthcare Disparities Report* (2004 NHDR) is actually the second of two studies authorized by the U.S. Congress and organized by the Agency for Healthcare Research and Quality.[24] Both these studies (the first was in 2003) are viewed as the foundation of an ongoing effort to describe and monitor disparities in health care delivery as they "relate to racial and socioeconomic factors in priority populations" (AHRQ, 2004, p. 7). The priority populations identified in the 2004 NHDR include racial and ethnic minorities, low-income persons, the elderly, residents of rural areas, women, children, and individuals with special health care needs (defined in the 2004 NHDR as including the disabled, persons in need of chronic care health services, and those in need of end-of-life care). As noted in the discussion of the measurement of disparities in health care earlier in this chapter, the 2004 NHDR measures disparities in two distinct domains: health care access and health care quality. The complete 2004 NHDR is a textbook and is packed with

---

[23] Notably, Rogers, Hummer. and Nam find that persons in the lowest status jobs experience a 25% excess risk of mortality, even when the effects of income and education are taken into account (Rogers, Hummer, & Nam, 2000, p. 155).

[24] The Agency for Healthcare Research and Quality is under the U.S. Department of Health and Human Services. The NHDR process was authorized by Congress under the Healthcare Research and Quality Act of 1999 (Public Law 106-129).

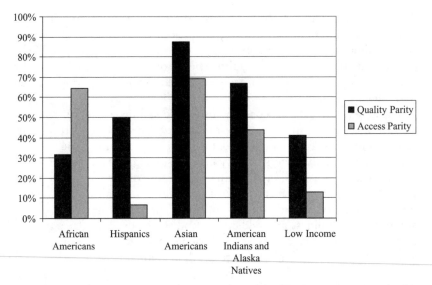

Figure 6.10 Relative parity in either quality of health care or access to health care by race, ethnicity, and income level.
Source: AHRQ. 2004. "2004 National Healthcare Disparities Report." Rockville, Md: U.S. Department of Health and Human Services. Based on data shown in Figures 4.1 to 4.5 and Figure 4.7.

tables and graphs of data pertaining to different aspects of disparities in health care—some of which have been highlighted previously. The focus here will be on the disparities that appear particularly relevant to different segments of the population.[25]

The first issue to be highlighted from the 2004 NHDR is quality and access to care by race, ethnicity, and income. As a way of illuminating the magnitude of the disparities reflected in the report, Figure 6.10 summarizes the findings from race, ethnicity, and income comparisons on an average of 28 measures of quality and 27 measures of access.[26] The strategy used to summarize the health care disparities is to show (for each racial, ethnic, or income group compared) the percentage of measures of either quality or access that show at least equity relative to a reference group receiving generally superior health care. In order to achieve 100% parity, the group identified would need to have every measure considered

[25] Readers are urged to review the full report, as well as the annual updates of the NHDR as they become available.
[26] The measures available from the data vary by the racial, ethnic, and income groups compared, from as few as 16 measures to as many as 38.

in equal or better health care than the reference group. For the racial and ethnic comparisons, the reference group is non-Hispanic Whites. For the income level comparison, persons at or below the federal poverty line are compared with those having an income of at least four times the federal poverty level.

As shown in Figure 6.10, with the exception of African Americans, there is more equity in measures of health care quality than in health care access—although the parity gaps in quality are large across race, ethnicity, and income. Asian Americans fare better than other racial groups, but even Asian Americans fall well short of complete parity in either health care quality or health care access. Low-income Americans (those at or below the federal poverty line) appear to be the most disadvantaged if access and quality are considered together, followed by Hispanics, then African Americans, and then those in the American Indian/Alaska Native category. If parity of access is considered apart from equity in health care quality, then the most disadvantaged group is Hispanics. If parity in quality of health care is considered apart from parity in access, then clearly African Americans are the most disadvantaged.

The second issue from the 2004 NHDR to be highlighted is the dramatic difference in the quality of care for heart disease. The 2004 NHDR examined a number of disparities in key areas pertaining to women's health, but no findings were more dramatic or consequential than those pertaining to gender differences in care for heart disease. As noted in the 2004 NHDR and elsewhere, although heart disease is the leading cause of death for women as well as men, women are significantly less likely to be offered adequate preventative care and cardiac rehabilitative care—thus contributing to the finding that women are more likely to die from a second heart attack than are men (AHRQ, 2004). As shown in Figure 6.11, women hospitalized for cardiac arrest are significantly less likely than men to receive beta-blocking medication (a therapeutic measure that reduces the likelihood of further heart damage) than men.

Equally disturbing is the observation that African American and Hispanic women are even less likely to receive postmyocardial infarction beta-blockers. In the case of Hispanic women, the disadvantages of race and gender are particularly egregious. The fact that the population studied is generally Medicare eligible suggests that the disparities observed are not due to income differences, but rather are due to biases based on gender, ethnicity, and race.

Findings From the Institute of Medicine

The Institute of Medicine (IOM) is a branch of the National Academy of Sciences established to seek and secure analysis of critical health policy

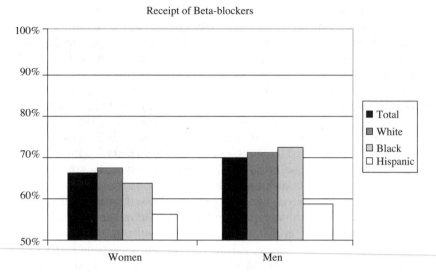

Figure 6.11 Elderly Medicare beneficiaries hospitalized for acute myocardial infarction who received beta-blockers (right) within 24 hours of admission by gender and race/ethnicity, 2000–2001.
Source: AHRQ. 2004. "2004 National Healthcare Disparities Report." Rockville, Md: U.S. Department of Health and Human Services. Figure 4.13.

issues from the most eminent members of the relevant professions—which in the case of the IOM is dominantly the medical profession. Although the American Medical Association can be described as the most influential voice of the medical profession's political interests, the IOM can be described as the medical profession's most authoritative voice in matters of scientifically informed health care practice and policy. At the early part of this chapter it was mentioned that the IOM restricted its definition of health care to differences in health care that did not involve issues of access, patient needs, and patient preferences (IOM, 2003, p32). As a result the IOM's *Unequal Treatment*[27] report (IOM-UTR) largely restricts its focus on disparities that arise within the health care system's structural context of clinical practice and sources of disparity that arise from patient–provider level discrimination. Also, the IOM-UTR is principally concerned with racial and ethnic discrimination (and even then largely restricted to

[27] Institute of Medicine, Committee on Understanding and Eliminating Racial and Ethnic Disparities in Health Care. 2003. *Unequal Treatment: Confronting Racial and Ethnic Disparities in Health Care.* Washington DC: National Academy Press.

comparisons between African Americans, Hispanics and Whites) as opposed to discrimination based upon age, income, gender, and other social characteristics. Despite these multiple shortcomings, the IOM-UTR makes some illuminating contributions in both establishing the historical context of disparities in health care and in highlighting the complexity of the processes that produce disparities in health care.

According to the IOM-UTR's conceptual framework, the sources of disparity in health care occur at three different levels: at the health care system level, at the patient level, and at the practitioner level (IOM, 2003, p. 126). As noted by the IOM-UTR, it is the clinical encounter[28] during the process of care that links sources of disparity with the various manifestations of unequal treatment. Although the cultural ideal of the clinical encounter is a face-to-face interaction between patient and provider that is founded upon mutual trust, honesty, empathy, objectivity, scientific knowledge, and deep concern for the patient's preferences and best interests, a variety of factors make this ideal exceedingly difficult to accomplish. In the reality of American health care, the clinical encounter typically involves three actors: the clinician (e.g., physician, nurse practitioner, or physical therapist), the physically absent but omnipresent utilization manager, and the patient. All three actors have the capacity to exercise discretion in what is shared and offered, and all three actors bring their own very subjective orientation to the "facts," purposes, and priorities of the encounter. Moreover, all three actors are encumbered by uncertainty and specific disadvantages with respect to critical information. Thus, the clinical encounter is not governed by objectivity, science, and clarity of purpose—but rather by a fog of uncertainty and discretion. To paraphrase the IOM-UTR on this point, despite benign intent "discretion and ambiguity create the conditions within which race and ethnicity may become salient and operative in ways that are more likely to produce disparities in health care" (IOM, 2003, p. 128).

As noted in the IOM-UTR, there are a number of ways in which each actor in the clinical encounter introduces the potential for disparities in care—absent the distrust, malicious intent, or overt negligence that is often assumed to be the basis of disparities in health care. For example, there is a substantial body of evidence from the literature in the behavior and social sciences establishing that patients vary greatly in their perception of symptoms, reporting of pain, in their conceptual frameworks of health

---

[28] As it is used here, the term clinical encounter is meant to refer to the typically face-to-face dialog between patient and health care provider that is focused upon the process of diagnosis and treatment.

and illness, and in health-seeking behavior—and that some of this variation correlates with race and ethnicity.[29] Differences between the patient and clinician by race, ethnicity, and social class only serve to compound the difficulties in clinical perception and interpretation. The sources of uncertainty that encumber the clinician include the often limited diagnostic information available from objective diagnostic tests, the often equivocal evidence concerning the relative efficacy of different therapeutic alternatives, and the often very limited knowledge or shared experience with the patient's world—thus leaving a large place for the clinician's subjective appraisal of the patient's needs and best interests. This of course is fertile ground for the introduction of stereotypes and biases into the process of health care (IOM, 2003).

Although the IOM-UTR takes the position that there is "no direct evidence that racism, bias, or prejudice among health care professionals affects the quality of care for minority patients" (IOM 2003, p. 176), this conclusion turns on a very narrow definition of direct evidence, that is, a perfectly controlled experiment. Instead, the IOM-UTR adopts the position that "indirect evidence from several lines of research" supports the statement that "[b]ias, stereotyping, prejudice, and clinical uncertainty on the part of healthcare providers may contribute to racial and ethnic disparities in healthcare" (IOM 2003, p. 178). In view of the multiple studies cited and summarized by the IOM-UTR demonstrating various examples of race-based discrimination in diagnosis and treatment, the logic of this conclusion appears tortured at best. A small partial sampling of the *indirect evidence* cited in the IOM-UTR includes studies that show:

- The lower probability of cardiac catheterization referral for African-American women relative to White men and women (Schulman et al., 1999).[30]
- The tendency of a White male physician to treat severe pain more aggressively for White patients than for African American patients suffering from identical symptoms (Weisse, Sorum, Sanders, & Syat, 2001).
- The propensity of White medical students (relative to minority medical students) to assess angina symptoms more seriously in White males that African American females (Rathore et al., 2000).

[29] This is a good instance to remember the oft-ignored adage that "correlation is not causality."
[30] This paper has attracted significant criticism on the basis of methods and findings, however the central findings that race and gender affected referral to catheterization are well defended by the evidence.

- The likelihood that African American patients are assessed more negatively on a variety of personal and clinical traits than White patients despite controls for socioeconomic status, personality attributes, and severity of illness (Van-Ryn & Burke, 2000).
- Lower incidence of cardiac bypass surgery and higher 5-year mortality for African American heart disease patients relative to Whites despite similar clinical characteristics (Peterson et al., 1997).

In fact, of the 13 studies on racial disparities in clinical care and outcomes selected by the IOM-UTR, all of which had appropriate controls for potentially confounding clinical characteristics, 11 (85%) found distinct patterns of racial disparities in care that could not be explained by patient characteristics other than race (IOM, 2003, pp. 380–383).

Whether one regards the IOM-UTR as a whitewash of the racism that pervades American health care or as a rigorous and dispassionate analysis of the possibility of racial and ethnic disparities in treatment, the report stands as a highly inclusive compendium and critique of the evidence on racial and ethnic disparities in health care. In addition, the IOM-UTR does an outstanding job of linking insights from behavioral science about the processes of stereotyping and discrimination to the deeply interpersonal processes of help-seeking and patient care. Interestingly, as cautious as the IOM-UTR language is regarding empirical support for the conclusions that personal biases and prejudices undermine the quality of health care for racial and ethnic minorities, the theoretical case that the IOM-UTR provides appears to make such a conclusion inevitable.[31]

CONCLUDING COMMENTS—THE DEEP ROOTS OF DISPARITIES IN HEALTH CARE

In contrast to the equivocal posture of the IOM-UTR, the position taken here is that the combined evidence from Rogers, Hummer, and Nam's *Living and Dying in the U.S.A.*, the *2004 National Health Care Disparities Report*, and the multiple studies cited in the IOM-UTR leads to one undeniable conclusion—disparities in U.S. health care system exist on the basis of a wide variety of social characteristics associated with other forms of social oppression and disadvantage. Differences in health care quality and outcomes are correlated with particular social characteristics because of human differences in beliefs and perceptions, because some

---

[31] See the discussion in chapter 4 of the IOM-UTR, pages 169–174.

organizations and individuals are biased and prejudiced, and because health care is embedded in a societal context that values and privileges some groups over others. Although disparities based on race are the most controversial and emotionally charged, all social forms of health care disparities are pervasive and pernicious, and involve both structural and individual level processes.

Pertaining to racism specifically, it can be argued that the IOM-UTR's reluctance to make a stronger statement on the effects of racism on quality of care based on the very evidence it cites itself perpetuates a key process in the production of health care disparities—institutional racism. Institutional racism, defined generally as institutional-level structures and processes that sustain the mechanisms of racial oppression with or without individual-level awareness or malicious intent, thrives where plausible denial of racism is permitted to exist. In this instance, the IOM-UTR's failure to offer a more definitive conclusion that bias, stereotyping, and prejudice all contribute to racial and ethnic disparities in health care (despite the evidence the report itself cites) lends the health care practitioners and organizations that perpetuate race-based disparities in health care the plausible deniability essential to resist change. Among the more deeply rooted and most difficult to eradicate sources of disparities in health care is the denial of institutional and individual agency in the processes that produce differences in care by race, ethnicity, and income.

In the next chapter, these issues are explored in more depth. In addition, that chapter considers theories that explain why disparities in health persist even where equity in health care is achieved.

REFERENCES

Acton, K. J., Rios Burrows, N., Moore, K., Querec, L., Geiss, L. S., & Engelgau, M. M. (2002). Trends in diabetes prevalence among American Indian and Alaska Native children, adolescents, and young adults. *American Journal of Public Health, 92*(9), 1485–1490.

Aday, L. A., & Andersen, R. (1981). Equity of access to medical care. *Medical Care, 19*(12), 4–27.

AHRQ. (2004). *2004 National healthcare disparities report* (No. AHRQ 05-0014). Rockville, MD: U.S. Department of Health and Human Services.

American Medical Association. (2005). *Total physicians by race/ethnicity—2003.* Retrieved March 21, 2005, from http://www.ama-assn.org/ama/pub/category/12930.html.

Becker, G., Janson-Bjerklie, S., Benner, P., Slobin, K., & Ferketich, S. (1993). The dilemma of seeking urgent care: Asthma episodes and emergency service use. *Social Science and Medicine, 37*(3), 305–313.

Centers for Disease Control and Prevention. (2003). *2003 state health profiles.* Atlanta, GA: U.S. Department of Health and Human Services.

Collins, S. R., Davis, K., Doty, M. M., & Ho, A. (2004). *Wages, health benefits, and worker's health.* New York: The Commonwealth Fund.

Denton, M., & Walters, V. (1999). Gender differences in structural and behavioral determinants of health: An analysis of the social production of health. *Social Science & Medicine, 48*(9), 1221–1222.

Ezzati, M., Lopez, A. D., Rodgers, A., Vander Hoorn, S., & Murray, C. J. (2002). Selected major risk factors and global and regional burden of disease. *The Lancet, 360*(9343), 1347–1360.

Finch, B. K. (2003). Early origins of the gradient: The relationship between socioeconomic status and infant mortality in the United States. *Demography, 40*(4), 675–699.

Garroutte, E. M., Kunovich, R. M., Jacobsen, C., & Goldberg, J. (2004). Patient satisfaction and ethnic identity among American Indian older adults. *Social Science & Medicine, 59*(11), 2233–2244.

Gohdes, D. (1995). *Diabetes in North American Indians and Alaska Natives* (NIH Publication No. 95-1468). Bethesda, MD: National Institute of Diabetes and Digestive and Kidney Diseases, National Institutes of Health.

Guest, A., Almgren, G., & Hussey, J. (1998). The ecology of race and socioeconomic distress: Infant and working-age mortality in Chicago. *Demography, 35*(1), 23–35.

Gurwitz, J. H., Goldberg, R. J., Malmgren, J. A., Barron, H. V., Tiefenbrunn, A. J., Frederick, P. D., et al. (2002). Hospital transfer of patients with acute myocardial infarction: The effects of age, race, and insurance type. *American Journal of Medicine, 112*(7), 528–534.

Hayes, R. A., Vaughan, C., Medeiros, T., & Dubuque, E. (2002). Stigma directed toward chronic illness is resistant to change through education and exposure. *Psychology Reports, 90*(3 Pt 2), 1161–1173.

HHS. (2000). *Healthy people 2010.* Washington, DC: U.S. Department of Health and Human Services.

Hoyert, D., Kung, H., & Smith, B. (2005). *Deaths: Preliminary data for 2003.* Hyattsville, MD: National Center for Health Statistics.

Indian Health Service. (2004, November 18). *Fiscal year 2001 appropriations.* Retrieved April 13, 2005, from http://www.ihs.gov/AdminMngrResources/Budget/Final_Appropriations.asp.

IOM. (1993). *Access to health care in America.* Washington, DC: National Academy Press.

IOM (Ed.). (2003). *Unequal treatment: Confronting racial and ethnic disparities in health care.* Washington, DC: National Academy Press.

Jacoby, A., Snape, D., & Baker, G. A. (2005). Epilepsy and social identity: The stigma of a chronic neurological disorder. *Lancet Neurology, 4*(3), 171–178.

Joachim, G., & Acorn, S. (2000). Stigma of visible and invisible chronic conditions. *Journal of Advanced Nursing, 32*(1), 243–248.

Kelley, E. P., Moy, E. M. D., & Dayton, E. M. A. (2005). Health care quality and disparities: Lessons from the first national reports. [Miscellaneous]. *Medical Care, 43*(3), 3–8.

Kominski, G., Simon, P., Ho, A., Luck, J., Lim, Y., & Fielding, J. (2002). Assessing the burden of disease and injury in Los Angeles County using disability-adjusted life years. *Public Health Reports, 117*(2), 185–191.

Link, B. G., & Phelan, J. (1995). Social conditions as fundamental causes of disease. *Journal of Health and Social Behavior*, Special Issue, 80–94.

Michielutte, R., & Diseker, R. A. (1982). Children's perceptions of cancer in comparison to other chronic illnesses. *Journal of Chronic Disease, 35*(11), 843–852.

Murray, C., & Lopez, A. (Eds.). (1996). *The global burden of disease: A comprehensive assessment of mortality and disability from diseases, injuries and risk factors in 1990 and projected to 2020.* (Vol. 1). Cambridge, MA.: Harvard School of Public Health on behalf of the World Health Organization and the World Bank.

NCHS. (2004a). Estimated life expectancy at birth in years, by race and sex: Death-registration States, 1900–28, and United States, 1929–2002. *National Vital Statistics Reports, 53*(6), Table 12.

NCHS. (2004b). *Health United States, 2004.* Hyattsville, MD: National Center for Health Statistics.

NCHS. (2005). Deaths and percentage of total deaths for the 10 leading causes of death, by race: United States, 2002. *National Vital Statistics Report, 53*(17).

NIH. (2001a). *Addressing health disparities: The NIH program of action.* Retrieved March 15, 2005, 2005, from http://healthdisparities.nih.gov/whatare.html.

NIH. (2001b, August 2001). *Diabetes in American Indians and Alaska Natives.* Retrieved March 16, 2005, from http://diabetes.niddk.nih.gov/dm/pubs/americanindian/index.htm.

Obst, T. E., Nauenberg, E., & Buck, G. M. (2001). Maternal health insurance coverage as a determinant of obstetrical anesthesia care. *Journal of Health Care for the Poor Underserved, 12*(2), 177–191.

Palazzo, L., Guest, A., & Almgren, G. (2003). Economic distress and cause-of-death patterns for Black and non-Black men in Chicago: Reconsidering the relevance of classic epidemiological transition theory. *Social Biology, 50*(1/2), 102–127.

Palloni, A., & Aria, C. (2004). Paradox lost: Explaining the Hispanic adult mortality advantage. *Demography, 41*(3), 385–415.

Peterson, E., Shaw, L., DeLong, E., Pryor, D., Califf, R., & Mark, D. (1997). Racial variation in the use of coronary-revascularization procedures: Are the differences real? Do they matter? *New England Journal of Medicine, 336*, 480–486.

Rathore, S., Lenert, L., Weinfurt, K., Tinoco, A., Taleghani, C., Harless, W., et al. (2000). The effects of patient sex and race on medical students' ratings of quality of life. *American Journal of Medicine, 108*(7), 561–566.

Rathore, S. S., & Krumholz, H. M. (2004). Differences, disparities, and biases:

Clarifying racial variations in health care use. *Annals of Internal Medicine, 141*(8), 635–638.

Rogers, R. G., Hummer, R. A., & Nam, C. B. (2000). *Living and dying in the USA: Behavioral, health, and social differentials of adult mortality.* San Diego, CA: Academic Press.

Rogge, M. M., Greenwald, M., & Golden, A. (2004). Obesity, stigma, and civilized oppression. *Advanced Nursing Science, 27*(4), 301–315.

Schryock, H., & Siegal, J. (1976). *The methods and materials of demography.* San Diego, CA: Academic Press.

Schulman, K., Berlin, J., Harless, W., Kerner, J., Sistrunk, S., Gersh, B., et al. (1999). The effect of race and sex on physicians' recommendations for cardiac catheterization. *New England Journal of Medicine, 340*(8), 618–626.

Starr, P. (1982). *The social transformation of American medicine.* New York: Basic Books.

U.S. Census. (2003). *2000 census of population and housing, characteristics of American Indians and Alaska Natives by tribe and language: 2000* (No. PHC-5). Washington, DC: U.S. Census Bureau.

Van-Ryn, M., & Burke, J. (2000). The effect of patient race and socio-economic status on physician's perceptions of patients. *Social Science & Medicine, 50,* 813–828.

Weisse, C., Sorum, P., Sanders, K., & Syat, B. (2001). Do gender and race affect decisions about pain management? *Journal of General Internal Medicine, 16*(4), 211–217.

World Health Organization. (2001). *World Health report 2001, statistical annex.* Retrieved March 28, 2005, from http://www.who.int/trade/glossary/story036/en/.

CHAPTER SEVEN

Social Epidemiology: Unraveling the Social Determinants of Disparities in Health

The term *social epidemiology* first appeared in the scientific literature in 1950, in the title of an article in the *American Sociological Review* that addressed the linkage between infant mortality and racial segregation[1] (Krieger, 2001c). The author later became the editor of the *American Journal of Public Health*, which in a serendipitous way underscores the interdisciplinary pedigree of social epidemiology in the more firmly established disciplines of sociology and public health (Krieger, 2001c).

Although inquiries into the social conditions that give rise to disease date back many centuries, arguably the French sociologist and philosopher Emile Durkheim is as much the founder of social epidemiology as he is of sociology. Rather than investigating suicide from the standpoint of an individual act with an internally embedded chain of causality, Durkheim approached the incidence of suicide as a social fact (sociological phenomenon) with a structural explanation (Kawachi, 2002, p. 1740). In fact, Durkheim's work on suicide captured the central defining feature of the discipline of social epidemiology: inquiries that focus upon structural explanations for the level and distribution of morbidity and mortality in human populations (Kawachi, 2002). Unlike traditional epidemiology, which incorporates social context as a background to its investigations into biological processes, social epidemiology "is distinguished by its

[1] Yankauer, A. The relationship of fetal and infant mortality to residential segregation: An inquiry into social epidemiology. *ASR* 1950:15(6)644–48.

insistence upon explicitly investigating the social determinants of population distributions of health, disease, and wellbeing ..." (Krieger, 2002 p. 7).

THE DISCIPLINE OF SOCIAL EPIDEMIOLOGY

Despite the legitimacy of its early origins, social epidemiology's recognition as a distinct discipline with its own place in the scientific community has been very recent and even then somewhat tenuous. In fact, the first textbook that employed "social epidemiology" in its title did not emerge until 2000[2] (Krieger, 2001c). Many reasons account for this. Chief among them is the fact that several well-established disciplines have significant bodies of research that in one way or another address linkages between social structure and population health outcomes, including among them medical sociology, social demography, anthropology, medical geography, political science, and public health. A second and related reason is the slow development, until the last decade, of any significant disciplinary infrastructure in social epidemiology: such as doctoral training programs, dedicated journals, and well funded research centers. The glacial emergence of a disciplinary infrastructure in social epidemiology is largely a consequence of social epidemiology's inherent character as a multidisciplinary enterprise and the tendency of scientific and academic recognition and reward structures to be very discipline-specific and conservative. A third reason for social epidemiology's tenuous hold as a unique discipline has to do with an arguably weak and underdeveloped theoretical structure in social epidemiology—a point taken up by critics within the discipline who identify themselves as social epidemiologists as well as those who consider social epidemiology to be little more than a pretentious fad (Kaplan, 2004; Kasl & Jones, 2002; Macdonald, 2001; Zielhuis & Kiemeney, 2001). Fourthly (but not exhaustively), social epidemiology is an inherently radical discipline. The central theme and line of inquiry of social epidemiology is, after all, the notion that inequalities in the distribution of disease in a population are a function of social inequalities.

Although it can be acknowledged that medical science and traditional epidemiology espouse as their ultimate purpose improvement of the human condition through knowledge of disease processes and treatment, neither is linked to an explicit agenda to identify and change the

[2] Berkman, I., & Kawachi I. (Eds.). *Social Epidemiology*. Oxford: Oxford University Press, 2000.

structural arrangements implicated in the prevalence and distribution of human diseases. As mentioned previously, Krieger defines social epidemiology as a scientific discipline that is "distinguished by its insistence upon explicitly investigating the social determinants of population distributions of health, disease, and wellbeing" (Krieger, 2002, p. 7). In the scientific community, where dispassionate objectivity and repudiation of a political agenda are central to the ethos, a field of inquiry that is predicated upon the assumption and illumination of detrimental social conditions is an anathema. Moreover, many of the central constructs employed by social epidemiologists in their theories and measures (e.g., discrimination, racism, sexism, social inequality) are derived directly from the discourse of the political left. Finally, social epidemiologists in general make little effort to distance their discipline from a view of a healthy society as one that is materially and socially egalitarian and driven by a deep respect for fundamental human rights (Burris, 2002). The prediction that arises from these observations is that, despite whatever significant advancements are made in the theories and methods of social epidemiology, to the extent that the theories and findings of social epidemiologists fundamentally challenge embedded hierarchies of power and privilege, the discipline will remain clouded in questions about its legitimacy.

The Theories and Methods of Social Epidemiology

The historical evolvement and current state of theory in social epidemiology have been well summarized in a series of articles written by social epidemiologist Nancy Krieger (Krieger, 1994, 1999, 2000, 2001a, 2001b, 20001c, 2002; Krieger & Davey Smith, 2004; Krieger & Smith, 2000). As noted by Krieger, the theoretical landscape of social epidemiology is dominated by three major frameworks that are listed in their order of emergence: psychosocial theories, political economy/social production of disease theories, and theories that derive from the ecological perspective (Krieger, 2001c).

The Psychosocial Theoretical Framework

The earliest to emerge, this model operates within the host-pathogen-environment paradigm and focuses upon the selective susceptibilities to disease that are created by the psychosocial context. Although structural constructs such as dominance hierarchies, material deprivation, victimization, and social isolation are identified as the fundamental social determinants, the chronic stress produced by these determinants and effect of chronic stress on the individual's biological defenses is viewed as the intervening mechanism of host–pathogen susceptibility (Krieger, 2001c, p. 669).

The mediating effects of stress are central to the arguments employed by Richard Wilkinson to bring social epidemiology to the forefront of the contemporary public health discourse (Wilkinson, 1996). In Wilkinson's highly influential book, *Unhealthy Societies: The Afflictions of Inequality,* chronic stress is emphasized as a critical intermediate mechanism through which societies embedded with status hierarchies both perpetuate the socio-economic status (SES) gradient and suppress population life expectancy—despite significant advances in health care infrastructure and per capita income. Although the hierarchy-stress-susceptibility link was not original to Wilkinson,[3] his extension of this paradigm as part of the explanation for emergence of a social inequality–mortality gradient at the societal level afforded the hypothesis renewed attention.

In Wilkinson's theoretical narratives (Wilkinson, 1996, 1999), the lower levels of social cohesion, trust, and social support that are prevalent in hierarchical societies promote both material deprivation and a pathogenic quality of social relationships that have direct effects on an individual's defenses against a wide array of diseases. In making his causal arguments, Wilkinson cites the linkage between social relationships and neuroendocrine system function at the individual level that were identified 20 years earlier by epidemiologist John Cassel (1976). Wilkinson also extends the identification of intermediate mechanisms to such factors as depression and interpersonal violence.

Political Economy/Social Production of Disease Theoretical Framework

This theoretical framework encompasses theories that derive from the classic political economy formulation of Adam Smith and the 19th-century Marxist critique of industrial capitalism (Swingwood, 2000). Central to this perspective is the assumption that the root causes of health inequalities are embedded in the economic and political structures and processes that promote and perpetuate economic and social privilege (Krieger, 2001c, p. 670). The main foci of this theoretical framework are the various structural determinants of health that are linked to disparities in social and economic power, such as poverty, detrimental working conditions, and spatial isolation from health care.

An important variant of this perspective places emphasis on disease as an outcome of a production function that serves the interest of the

---

[3] As noted by Krieger (2001c), John Cassel introduced the idea that both hierarchical social relationships and marginalized status are implicated in the impairment of individual level biological defense mechanisms (Cassel, 1976).

dominant social classes (Diamond, 1992). One can think about the production function of disease occurring in a number of ways: the direct exposure of disadvantaged populations to pathogens in a way that benefits the dominant class, the selective privileging of some threats to health and well-being over others, and in the social construction of disease and therapeutics.

The most obvious example of the first, exposure to pathogens, is easily and tragically exemplified in the class and race-targeted promotion of smoking in order to benefit investors in the tobacco industry (Balbach, Gasior, & Barbeau, 2003; Barbeau, Wolin, Naumova, & Balbach, 2005). An example of the selective privileging of some threats to health over others is observed in the juxtaposition of the influenza vaccine shortage of 2005 with the intense television advertising campaigns touting competing patent remedies for erectile dysfunction. Concerning the social construction of disease and therapeutics, there is extensive literature on historic linkages between the financial interests of the medical profession and the development of standards of practice related to the diagnosis and treatment of a variety of conditions (Starr, 1982), such as the ongoing controversy over the medical necessity of hysterectomies (Broder, Kanouse, Mittman, & Bernstein, 2000; Haas, Acker, Donahue, & Katz, 1993; West & Dranov, 1994; Dicker et al., 1982; Travis, 1985).

In a classic example of a social epidemiology investigation framed by a political economy perspective, Roderick Wallace linked patterns of homicide, suicide, drug abuse, low birth weight, and deaths from AIDS in the Bronx section of New York City to the class- and race-based withdrawal of basic municipal services—including fire protection (Wallace, 1990). Rather than attributing the high death rates of the African American and Hispanic inhabitants of the Bronx to the internal characteristics and social pathologies of their neighborhoods, Wallace's study showed how deliberate and targeted policies of "planned shrinkage" propelled these neighborhoods into chaos. In the political economy perspective of Wallace, the high death rates among Bronx inhabitants were less an outcome of poverty and political neglect than they were of a calculated policy of race and class-based neighborhood abandonment by the economic and political elites of the city.

It can be claimed without much controversy that the *Political Economy/Social Production of Disease* framework has dominated the empiricism of social epidemiology. A case can also be made that this theoretical dominance has been promoted by methodological innovations over the past several years, greatly aided by innovations in computer technology that can more precisely estimate the relative contributions of individual characteristics from contextual effects on health outcomes. Sometimes referred to generally as mixed, hierarchical, or multilevel modeling techniques, these approaches allow researchers to deal with the statistical anomalies that occur when observations at the individual level (e.g., health outcomes or specific behaviors) are nested within larger social units such as families, neighborhoods, or large communities. The ability to more precisely sort out the unique contributions of social context from individual characteristics has thus enabled social epidemiologists to better model and validate the theoretically suggested causal linkages between structural determinants at the societal level, the effects of proximate social context, and intervening mechanisms of disease at the individual level. Although in one way this synergy of theory and method represents a significant advance in science, in another way it has embedded social epidemiology further in a linear model of causality that fails to account for the complex, dynamic, and mutually generative interactions between social structure and biology that occurs at all levels.

The Ecosocial Theoretical Framework

As explained by Krieger (1994, 1999, 2001c), the ecosocial framework applies to a class of theories that move the ecological perspective from a general metaphor to a wide array of testable propositions based on a model of human health that situates "humans as one notable species among many co-habiting, evolving on, and altering our dynamic planet" (Krieger 2001c, p. 671). This is a significant advancement over the linear, albeit hierarchical model of social epidemiology that is the basis of the *political economy/social production of disease* model.

Briefly described, the ecosocial framework greatly enriches the theoretical basis of social epidemiology in several respects. First, it incorporates and contextualizes the basic principles and processes of the social production of the disease model within the framework of an ecological analysis (Krieger, 2001c). Thus it is a theoretical framework that is inherently concerned with the ways in which structural relationships are implicated in, and accountable for, the creation and perpetuation of inequalities in health. Second, the ecosocial framework is not driven by or confined within linear models and methods. Instead, the ecosocial perspective merges social and biological analyses in a way that examines their dynamic interplay at multiple levels as opposed to an analysis that is a linear and hierarchical approximation of reality. Third, the ecosocial perspective invites and embraces an array of theories that operate within and across different ecological levels that, in synthesis, promote an enhanced understanding of the complex and simultaneous processes through which particular social constructs and processes become biologically incorporated and expressed in disease (Krieger, 2002).

Ecosocial theory is built around four central concepts: *embodiment, pathways of embodiment, cumulative interplay between exposure, susceptibility, and resistance*, and *accountability and agency* (Krieger, 2001c). *Embodiment* refers to the means by which human beings "literally incorporate, biologically; the material and social world, from conception to death." *Pathways to embodiment* (the means of incorporation) are structured simultaneously by societal arrangements, the limits of possibilities of the biology that is shaped by evolution, and individual biological and social history. *Cumulative interplay between exposure, susceptibility, and resistance* is expressed in pathways to embodiment, with each of these factors and their respective distributions conceptualized at multiple ecological levels and in multiple domains, and manifested in processes at multiple *scales*[4] of time and space. *Accountability and agency* occurs in relation to social units at various levels of structure: institutions, households, and individuals—but also extending to the agents and agencies of science that privilege some theories and ignore others in the production of explanations for social inequalities in health (Krieger, 2001c, p. 672). In essence, these four central constructs function as heuristic lenses through which social epidemiologists can unveil and illuminate the patterns of health and disease that are a function of the complex interrelationships between the biological and social aspects of causality.

As Krieger suggests, the ecosocial perspective, aside from being derived from evolutionary theory, is akin to it as a general perspective for inquiry (Krieger, 2001c, p. 671). In the way that evolutionary theory provides the biological sciences with general guidance toward specific propositions, the ecosocial theoretical framework guides inquiry in social epidemiology toward "specificity within complexity." One way to conceptualize this notion is to examine the myriad ways in which race is *embodied* in the relative mortality levels of Native Americans living on the Pine Ridge Reservation.

Table 7.1 shows the relative age-adjusted death rates, reproductive health statistics, and the poverty rate for the Lakota (Sioux) Tribe inhabitants of Shannon County, South Dakota—located in the heart of the Pine Ridge Indian Reservation. Notably, the 52.3% poverty rate among the Lakota of Pine Ridge is over four times that of the national average. The Lakota die at over twice the rate of other residents of the United States, and for several causes (heart failure, accidents, respiratory diseases, diabetes, and kidney failure) their death rates are more than quadruple those prevalent for the United States as a whole.

---

[4] Krieger defines scales as "quantifiable dimensions" of spatial and temporal phenomenon, for example, kilometers and nanoseconds (2001, p. 372).

Table 7.1   Health Indicator Profile of Pine Ridge Tribal Reservation (Shannon County, SD) Relative to Entire United States

Mortality	United States	Shannon County, SD	Ratio
ALL CAUSES	847.3	1883.9	2.22
Heart Disease	241.7	379	1.57
Acute Myocardial Infarction	62.3	54.2	0.87
Heart Failure	19.6	84.1	4.29
Atherosclerotic Cardiovascular Disease	23.6	LNE	
Malignant Neoplasms (cancer)	193.2	291.9	1.51
Cerebrovascular Disease	56.4	103.9	1.84
Accidents	37	182.2	4.92
Motor Vehicle Accidents	15.7	133.7	8.52
Chronic Lower Respiratory Diseases	4.3	58.1	13.51
Influenza & Pneumonia	22.8	70.5	3.09
Diabetes Mellitus	25.4	158	6.22
Alzheimer's Disease	20.4	LNE	
Nephritis, Nephrotic Syndrome, & Nephrosis	14.2	69.2	4.87
Intentional Self-Harm (suicide)	11	21.5	1.95
Infant Mortality	7	13	1.86
Natality			
Percent Low Birth Weight Infants	7.8%	7.1%	0.91
Percent of Mothers Receiving Care in First Trimester	83.7%	63.1%	0.75
Percent of Mothers Who Use Tobacco While Pregnant	11.4%	19.3%	1.69
Percent of Mothers Who Consumed Alcohol While Pregnant	0.8%	7.3%	9.13
Teenage Pregnancy Rate	53.5	71.2	1.33
Population Under 100% of Poverty	12.4%	52.3%	4.22
Percent Native American	0.9%	95.1%	105.67

Source: South Dakota Department of Public Health, 2003 South Dakota Vital Statistics Report: Health Profiles by County.
Death rates are age adjusted deaths per 100,000, with the exception of the infant mortality rate. The teen age pregnancy rate is reported at events per 1,000 women aged 15-17. Cells labeled LNE refer to a number of events too low for statistical estimation.

The role of alcohol as one pathogen among many is not only evident in the death rates from motor vehicle accidents, diabetes, and nephritis (kidney failure), but in the prevalence of alcohol use during pregnancy as well—over nine times that of the national average. Also implicated in these death rates are the endemic exposures and susceptibilities to infectious diseases over the life course of the Pine Ridge Lakota.

The *pathways to embodiment* that are created and sustained by racial oppression include a tribal history and contemporary replication of racial isolation and deprivation; social policies that continue to promote endemic poverty and expropriation of resources by nonnatives; and the embedded exposures and susceptibilities to early death that are manifest in the harsh natural environment, dilapidated housing, diet, and even in the water.[5] *Accountability and agency* are seen not only in the U.S. government's historically genocidal policies toward Native Americans, but in the willful ignorance of the American mainstream—both in the historic and contemporary sense. Although the Pine Ridge Lakota were briefly in the national spotlight in the 2004 elections as potentially the only pocket of Democratic votes that could keep Senate minority leader Thomas Daschle from being swept from office, there was far more media attention to the political tactics aimed at the Lakota voters than on their dire living conditions and short life spans.

The "Fundamental Social Causes" Hypothesis

Although the ecosocial perspective represents the most elaborate and encompassing framework with which to advance the field of social epidemiology, at this stage of its development the most influential general theory in social epidemiology is the "fundamental social causes hypothesis" (Link & Phelan, 1995). Arising from the *political economy/social production of disease* perspective, this hypothesis resolves two enduring paradoxes of population health:

1. The growth of disparities in mortality and longevity by such factors as race, gender, and social class that follow significant advancements in the knowledge base, methods, and technologies of health care.
2. The tendency of intergroup disparities in mortality to persist even though the specific disease mechanisms linked to disparities in mortality change significantly over time.

---

[5] Aside from contamination of the ground water from nonnative sources of agricultural pesticides and residues from mining operations, over a third of homes on the reservations lack running water and sewage systems (Schwartz, 2002).

A decade ago sociologists Bruce Link and Jo Phelan advanced the theory that disparities in mortality endure over time because the "fundamental social causes" of health disparities arise from pernicious social inequalities rather than the intervening disease mechanisms that happen to link social inequalities to health disparities at any given point in time (Link & Phelan, 1995). Although this proposition may seem intuitive to many, it has not guided the thinking of the majority of the work in either investigating the causes of health disparities or ameliorating them through policy initiatives. Rather, the focus of attention of social epidemiology has been on the prevailing and transitory intervening mechanisms of group mortality differences (i.e., diseases, risk, and protective factors) that are operative at the historical moment (Phelan, Link, Diez-Roux, Kawachi, & Levin, 2004).

The result of this skewed attention toward intervening variables is a phenomenon somewhat akin to an epidemiological shell game. At the first stage of the game, science uncovers a salient linkage between a social factor such as race and selective mechanisms of disease, differential risk, and specific health behaviors or health care access issues that are causally implicated in mortality disparities. At the next stage, policy interventions take place that reduce the incidence of risk and disease for the disadvantaged group and it is widely assumed that health disparities associated with race will in turn be reduced. However, since disease ecology is a dynamic process that in large part is shaped by fundamental underlying social inequalities, racial disparities in mortality reemerge in the form of other diseases with different clusters of risk and protective factors that advantage one racial group over the other. This is the third stage of the epidemiological shell game and the point to begin anew.

The mortality patterns that reflect this process are clearly visible as the most recent 50-year trend in both overall disparities in life expectancy by race and age adjusted death rate are examined. As Figure 7.1 shows, although dramatic improvements in life expectancy for both Whites and African Americans occurred over this period, a significant disparity in the life expectancy of African Americans relative to Whites persisted (NCHS, 2004). At the conclusion of a 50-year period marked by dramatic improvements in standards of living, expansion of civil rights, and monumental advances in medical technology and health care system infrastructure a racial gap in life expectancy of 5.7 years remained. The persistence of disparities by race is the first mortality pattern that conforms to the epidemiological shell game.

The second conforming trend, as shown on Table 7.2, is the shift of the intervening disease mechanisms of mortality disparity from one set of mechanisms to another despite the persistence of the overall disparity

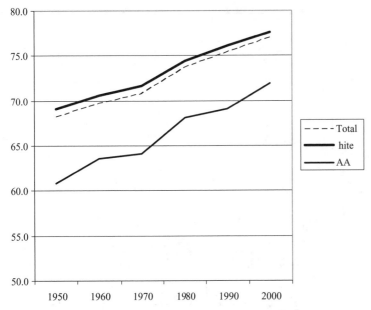

Figure 7.1 Population Life Expectancy Trends 1950–2000: Total, White and African American. (Source: *Health, United States 2004.* Table 27. Life expectancy at birth, at 65 years of age, and at 75 years of age, according to race and sex: United States, selected years 1900–2002. Hyattsville, MD: National Center for Health Statistics.)

itself[6] (NCHS, 2002). First, it should be noted that between 1950 and 2000[7] the mortality ratios from age-adjusted deaths by "all causes combined" actually became less favorable to African Americans in 2000 than in 1950 (see the tops of both the fourth column and the final column of Table 7.2). However, in the 50 years between 1950 and 2000, the principal intervening mechanisms of mortality (cause-specific death rates) changed from cerebrovascular diseases, infectious diseases, and homicides to heart disease, cancers (malignant neoplasms), and diabetes. This can be seen by comparing the columns showing the racial differences in death rates for the 1950 period and 2000 period (the three disease categories with the largest differences shown in bold type). It is worth noting

[6] Because U.S. life expectancy among Whites exceeds that among African Americans by several years, it is critical to adjust death rates by differences in population age distribution when comparing mortality patterns.

[7] Age-adjusted death rates for 1999 are used as estimates for the 2000 period and are sufficient for the particular comparisons made here.

Table 7.2 Age-Adjusted Death Rates (per 100,000) for Selected Causes of Death, According to Race 1950, 1980 and 2000

	1950 White	Period AA	Dif	Ratio	1980 White	Period AA	Dif	Ratio	2000 White	Period AA	Dif	Ratio
All causes	1410.8	1722.1	311.3	1.2	1012.7	1314.8	302.1	1.3	860.7	1147.1	286.4	1.3
Natural causes	—	—	—	—	945.0	1206.0	261.0	1.3	807.1	1075.7	268.6	1.3
Diseases of heart	584.8	586.7	1.9	1.0	409.4	455.3	**45.9**	1.1	263.4	336.7	**73.3**	1.3
Ischemic heart disease	—	—	—	—	347.6	334.5	−13.1	1.0	194.5	226.4	31.9	1.2
Cerebrovascular diseases	175.5	233.6	**58.1**	1.3	93.2	129.1	35.9	1.4	59.8	82.4	22.6	1.4
Malignant neoplasms	194.6	176.4	−18.2	0.9	204.2	256.4	**52.2**	1.3	199.8	254.4	**54.6**	1.3
Trachea, bronchus, and lung	15.2	11.1	−4.1	0.7	49.2	59.7	10.5	1.2	56.0	65.2	9.2	1.2
Colon, rectum, and anus	28.4	30.9	2.5	1.1	27.4	28.3	0.9	1.0	20.6	28.6	8.0	1.4
Prostate	32.4	25.3	−7.1	0.8	30.5	61.1	30.6	2.0	28.4	66.5	38.1	2.3
Breast	6.8	6.2	−0.6	0.9	32.1	31.7	−0.4	1.0	26.4	35.6	9.2	1.3
Chronic lower respiratory diseases	—	—	—	—	29.3	19.2	−10.1	0.7	47.5	33.7	−13.8	0.7
Influenza and pneumonia	44.8	76.7	**31.9**	1.7	30.9	34.4	3.5	1.1	23.4	25.6	2.2	1.1
Chronic liver disease and cirrhosis	11.5	9.0	−2.5	0.8	13.9	25.0	11.1	1.8	9.7	10.2	0.5	1.1
Diabetes mellitus	22.9	23.5	0.6	1.0	16.7	32.7	16.0	2.0	22.8	50.1	**27.3**	2.2
HIV disease	—	—	—	—	—	—	—	—	3.0	24.2	**21.2**	**8.1**
External causes	—	—	—	—	67.7	108.8	**41.1**	1.6	53.6	71.4	17.8	1.3
Unintentional injuries	77.0	79.9	2.9	1.0	45.3	57.6	12.3	1.3	35.7	40.9	5.2	1.1
Motor vehicle-related injuries	24.4	26.0	1.6	1.1	22.6	20.2	−2.4	0.9	15.6	16.2	0.6	1.0
Suicide	13.9	4.5	−9.4	0.3	13.0	6.5	−6.5	0.5	11.5	5.7	−5.8	0.5
Homicide	2.6	28.3	**25.7**	**10.9**	6.7	39.0	32.3	**5.8**	3.8	20.6	16.8	**5.4**

Source: NCHS. *Health, United States 2002*, Data from Table 30 Age Adjusted Death Rates for Selected Causes According to Sex, Race and Hispanic Origin, United States, Selected Years 1950–1999 Hyattsville, Maryland.

that by the end of this 50-year period the African American mortality disadvantage seems to have shifted toward a cluster of diseases that are highly influenced by early detection, treatment, and close management. In the discussion of fundamental social cause theory that follows, it will be shown that the shift from one set of intervening disease mechanisms of disparity to another is not random, but instead reflective of the advantaged group's differential access to critical adaptive social resources. This point can be extended to the mortality patterns for homicide and HIV, which also show a remarkable disadvantage for African Americans (see the bold typed AA/White mortality ratios for each).

The specific propositions of fundamental social causes theory have been advanced by Link and Phelan in a series of collaborative articles published over the past decade (Link & Phelan, 1995, 1996, 2002; Phelan et al., 2004). Their central ideas are summarized in five main points:[8]

1. *The focus of epidemiology, both in research and public dissemination of findings, has largely been centered on the proximate risk factors and specific causes of disease and related disparities in health outcomes reduced to the individual level. The emphasis on individual agency over structural context, because it resonates with the individualistic orientation of Western culture, has contributed to a bias in contemporary epidemiology toward individually based risk and protective factors to the neglect of the fundamental causes of disparities in health—the pervasive causal influence of social inequalities* (Link & Phelan, 1995, pp. 80–81).

2. *Although policy and program measures aimed at the intervening mechanisms of disease that link disparities in health outcomes to fundamental social causes might ameliorate health disparities in the short run, fundamental social causes will over time exert their effects in other intervening mechanisms* (Phelan et al., 2004, p. 280).

3. *The enduring nature of fundamental causes of disease, in essence the capacity to create and sustain disparities in health outcomes despite changes in the prevailing intervening mechanisms of disease, arises from structural disparities in access to resources that are critical to the avoidance of disease risk; and where disease occurs, minimization of its detrimental consequences. Resources that are critical to the avoidance of disease, and attenuation of its detriments to individual health, involve and include such social*

[8] Italicized type is employed to identify ideas that are closely paraphrased from the source articles.

assets as "money, knowledge, power, prestige and social connect-edness" (Link and Phelan, 1995, p. 87).

4. *Ultimately, sustained reductions or eradications of disparities in health outcomes cannot be achieved through exclusive focus on the ever changing mechanisms of disease and risk to the detriment of the attention given to the social structures and processes that determine access to critical adaptive resources: e.g. money, knowledge, power, prestige, and various aspects of social capital.* (Link and Phelan, 1995, p. 89; Link and Phelan, 1996, p. 472).

5. *The common features of the fundamental social causes within population disparities in mortality are that they (1) influence multiple disease outcomes, (2) affect disease outcomes through multiple disease factors, (3) reproduce their effects on mortality over time via the replacement of intervening disease and risk factor mechanisms, and (4) "involve access to resources that can be used to avoid risks or to minimize the consequences of disease when it occurs"* (Phelan et al., 2004, p. 268; Link and Phelan, 1995, p. 87).

Evidence for the "Fundamental Social Causes" Hypothesis

At this point in its development, the field of social epidemiology is dominated by studies that have focused on the identification of the prevailing intervening mechanisms that link disparities in mortality to various dimensions of social inequality (e.g. gender, race, ethnicity, social class). However, the limited number of studies that have sought to rigorously examine evidence for fundamental cause processes provides compelling support for the theory. For example, one test of the fundamental cause hypothesis would be to examine whether higher socioeconomic status confers mortality advantages through differential access to knowledge about health behaviors that would avoid and ameliorate the effects of "preventable" causes of death over the life course as opposed to "nonpreventable" causes of death that are by their nature not amenable to individual advantages in knowledge, money, power, prestige, or social capital.

Presumably, if SES confers significant advantages to the individual in knowledge and other resources critical to the reduction of the risk of death from any number of preventable causes, death rates from preventable causes of death should reflect a significantly stronger SES advantage than death rates from "nonpreventable" causes of death. If on the other hand, the SES effect on death rates is generally similar across both preventable and nonpreventable causes of death, this would undermine a key proposition of fundamental cause theory, namely that SES confers advantage in critical knowledge and other social assets tied to disease prevention.

To test the validity of this proposition, Phelan et al. (2004) employed data from the National Longitudinal Mortality Study to discern whether national population mortality patterns in fact conformed with theoretical expectations. Briefly described, they examined both the income and education dimensions of SES on the cause and age-specific death rates of a sample of 368,585 individuals representing a cross section of the U.S. adult population (those over age 25). Their central question was whether the magnitudes of the SES effects on death rates from preventable diseases were significantly larger for preventable causes than nonpreventable causes of death (Frisbie, Song, Powers, & Street, 2004). Although the details of the Phelan et al. analysis are far more complex than are reported here, the mortality trajectories by education for persons aged 25 to 44 shown by Figure 7.2 serve as a good example of their general findings.

Figure 7.2 depicts a series of survival trajectories observed over a 9.5-year (114 month) period for adults aged 25 to 44. As can be seen on the graph, the survival curves for individuals with different levels of education depict a very modest education effect for causes of death that have low probability of prevention, while for the highly preventable causes of death the survival curves differ dramatically by levels of education. Since education functions as an important component and measure of SES, the patterns observed fully conform to the theoretical proposition that SES confers significant advantages in access to knowledge and other resources that are tied to an individual's capacity to reduce the probability of preventable death. Notably, the Phelan et al. study found that SES effects on preventable causes of death are far less dramatic in old age, perhaps reflecting the cumulative effects of frailty on the effectiveness of interventions (Phelan et al. 2004, p. 278).

A second recent study that provides compelling support for the fundamental social causes hypothesis (Frisbie et al., 2004), examined the patterns of disparities in infant mortality by race. Race, like SES, is argued to fit the criteria as a "fundamental social cause" of disparities in health because its effects are at once pervasive and enduring despite significant changes in the prevailing regimes of morbidity and mortality. Although it is well established that disparities in infant mortality between Whites and African Americans have increased over the past 2 decades despite significant reductions in the overall rates of infant mortality for both groups, there is little scientific consensus on the chief reasons. Employing the fundamental social causes hypothesis as their framework (Link & Phelan, 1995, 1996, 2002), Frisbie et al. speculated that the growth in infant mortality disparities by race over the past 2 decades reflects the tendency of more advantaged groups to have earlier access to new

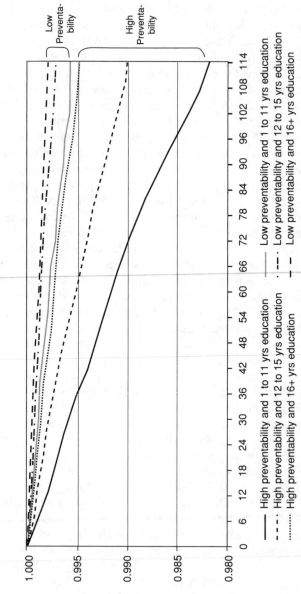

Figure 7.2 Cumulative Survival by Education and Preventability of Death Ages 25–44 at Baseline.
Source: Phelan, Link, Diez-Roux, Kawachi, and Levin. "Fundamental Causes" of Social Inequalities in Mortality:
A Test of the Theory. *Journal of Health and Social Behavior*, September 2004:45 (3), Figure 1.

innovations in health care, due to their differential access to the critical resources of knowledge, money, power, prestige, and interpersonal connections identified by Link and Phelan (1995, p.87).

As a test of their proposition, Frisbie and his colleagues examined the national data on infant death rates from respiratory distress syndrome (RDS) over two periods that represented different conditions in the availability of an important innovation in the treatment of RDS. During the first period (1989–1990), when the new RDS treatment was not available, African American infants were slightly less likely to die from RDS than White infants once disparities in prenatal care and other important factors relevant to infant survival were accounted for. During the second period (1995–1998), when the new innovation for treatment of RDS was made available, the relative risks of dying from RDS became higher for African American infants—as well as the risk of dying from all other causes (Frisbie et al., 2004, p. 789). These findings conform to the central tenet of fundamental social causes theory that racism, as one among several fundamental forms of social inequality, affords some racial groups more access to innovations in health care technology than others due to their privileged access to knowledge and the resources critical to their capacity to utilize it.

INCOME INEQUALITY AS A SOCIAL DETERMINANT OF HEALTH

Thus far the disparities in health that are the central concern of social epidemiology have been those that occur within populations, such as the socioeconomic class gradient in life expectancy. As discussed in the prior chapter, there is a powerful linear relationship between socioeconomic status and health that persists to varying degrees throughout the life course on a variety of dimensions of health and across all three dimensions of social class (income, occupation, and education). In an intriguing and related development over the last 2 decades, a second line of research has emerged which seeks to explain the relationship between income inequality and various indices of health at the population level. In part, the surge of interest in the role income inequality plays on health may have been fueled by rising levels of income inequality observed among wealthy nations in the wake of economic globalization (Alderson & Nielsen, 2002).[9]

[9] Alderson and Nielsen's analysis of the 16 OECD countries during the 1967–1992 period shows that 10 (63%) of these OECD member states experienced rising levels of income inequality during these years. Significantly, 1992 signaled the take-off point in the literature devoted to the population health effects of income inequality.

The earliest published study finding a relationship between population mortality and population income distribution appeared in 1979 (Rodgers, 1979), and by the mid-1990s a significant body of research had emerged from multiple sources of international data that implicated income inequality as a determinant of population mortality (Wilkinson, 1995). Although British social epidemiologist Richard Wilkinson was the chief proponent (and defendant) of the hypothesis that income inequality at the population level exerts a powerful effect on population mortality that is not explained by such factors as the absolute level of poverty, per capita income, population literacy, or the accessibility to health services, the "income inequality–population health hypothesis" garnered broad empirical support from other investigators. Remarkably, findings consistent with the "income inequality–population health hypothesis" also appeared to extend to populations at multiple ecological levels (e.g. states, communities), and not just national populations (Kaplan, Lynch, Cohen, & Balfour, 1996; Kawachi & Kennedy, 1997; Wilkinson, 1996).

As Figure 7.3 shows, there is a modest linear relationship ($r = .54$, $p < .05$) between the age-adjusted death rate in the 50 U.S. states and a

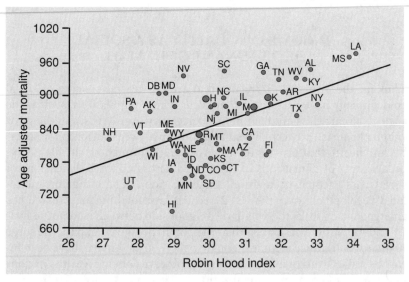

Figure 7.3 Mortality by Income Inequality (Robin Hood Index), U.S States in 1990.

Source: Kaplan GA, P. E., Lynch JW, Cohen RD, and Balfour JL. (1996). Inequality in income and mortality in the United States: analysis of mortality and potential pathways. *British Medical Journal*, 312(7037), 999–1003. Figure 1.

general measure of income inequality, termed the "Robin Hood Index."[10] It should be noted that the relationship shown in Figure 7.3 was little modified by adjustments for the overall poverty rate, median income, and race (Kaplan et al., 1996). Although the Robin Hood Index has strong merits as an indicator of income inequality, the relationship depicted in Figure 7.3 has been shown to be quite consistent across several other conventional measures in income inequality (Kawachi & Kennedy, 1997). Findings of this sort, replicated many times by various investigators, provoked two closely linked debates in the nascent discourse of social epidemiology, one theoretical and the other methodological.

The methodological debate considers whether in fact these findings reflect biased or flawed data and analyses, while the theoretical debate considers the causal linkages between income inequality and health. The first to be discussed will be the theoretical debate.

Theoretical Debates Concerning Income Inequality Effects

Setting aside the methodological questions for the time being, why *should* higher levels of population income inequality be associated with lower levels of population health? While at the individual level there are multiple well-established causal connections between relative deprivation and poor health (e.g., nutrition, exposure to occupational hazards, access to health care), at the population level the causal connections are far more contested. The theoretical and empirical debates aimed at illuminating the relationship between income inequality and population health have been dominated by two perspectives: a psychosocial perspective and one that takes a materialist political economy approach. While income inequality can influence health through material conditions, the quality of social participation, and the capacity to exercise choice (Marmot, 2002), the psychosocial perspective places far more emphasis on the importance of the latter two factors.

As mentioned previously in this chapter, the main proponent of the psychosocial perspective has been Richard Wilkinson (Wilkinson, 1992, 1995, 1996, 1999; Wilkinson, Kawachi, & Kennedy, 1998). The central thrust of this perspective is that extremes of income inequality are both associated with and implicated causally in the qualities of the social environment encountered by individuals at all strata of society. Accordingly,

[10] The Robin Hood Index, briefly stated, "approximates the share of total income that has to be taken from those above the mean and transferred to those below the mean to achieve equality in the distribution of incomes" (Kaplan et al., 1996, p. 2). The higher the index value, the higher the level of income inequality.

societies with high levels of income inequality are characterized by lower levels of "social cohesion," endemic distrust, and the pervasive social anxieties attendant with hierarchical relationships and low social status. The pathogenic mechanisms of the psychosocial environment identified by Wilkinson (and others) center around the quality of interpersonal relations and include such factors as depression, low attachment in early childhood, interpersonal violence, and (per the earlier work of John Cassel) disease susceptibilities linked to psychosocial social stress. On the other hand, according to this perspective, societies with low levels of income inequality have qualities of social cohesion, egalitarian relationships, and mutual trust that "are essential in ameliorating the effects of stress and poor living conditions" (Wilkinson, Kawachi & Kennedy 1998, p. 35).

For the better part of the last decade, the psychosocial perspective on the income inequality–population health link occupied center stage in the theoretical discourse of social epidemiology. In large extent, this can be attributed to a prevailing ideology within the field of social epidemiology that postulates the inherently detrimental nature of inequality in all of its forms—including social class. However, the popularity of the psychosocial perspective on income inequality–population health was also elevated considerably by its synthesis with social capital theory in sociology (Kawachi, Kennedy, Lochner, & Prothrow-Stith, 1997; Lomas, 1998; Wilkinson et al., 1998). While at the individual level, social capital refers to the quality and extent of a person's interpersonal networks, at the societal level social capital is defined as features of social organization that promote collective action toward mutual benefit, such as civic engagement, norms of reciprocity and high levels interpersonal trust, and norms of mutual aid and reciprocity (Kawachi et al., 1997; Lochner, Kawachi, & Kennedy, 1999).

Aside from the intuitive appeal of the connections between income inequality, social capital, and health, by the late 1990s a growing body of empirical support for these linkages had emerged in the public health literature. A seminal article in this line of research was a Harvard School of Public Health study that tested the evidence of linkages between income inequality, social capital, and population mortality (Kawachi et al., 1997). Using state-level data on income distribution and key dimensions of social capital and mortality, Ichiro Kawachi and his collaborators showed that states with higher levels of income inequality showed lower levels of social capital in three key areas: group membership, social trust, and perceptions of the helpfulness of others.[11] Consistent with theoretical expectations,

---

[11] These dimensions of social capital were measured on the bases of selected responses to the General Social Science Survey (the GSS), averaged over the 5-year period between

higher levels of population mortality (adjusted for age) were in turn linked to lower levels of social capital. Also consistent with theoretical expectations, their findings showed that the mortality effects of income inequality were largely mediated by the dimensions of social capital evaluated—in particular, beliefs about trust and fairness.

In contrast to psychosocial explanations of the link between income inequality and health, the materialist/political economy perspective concerns itself with the overall structural context that determines the distribution of power, status, and material resources (Navarro & Shi, 2001; Lynch et al., 2004; Lynch et al., 2001; Lynch, Smith, Kaplan, & House, 2000; Muntaner, 1999, 2001; Muntaner, Lynch, & Smith, 2001; Muntaner et al., 2002). Thus, the materialist/political economy perspective encompasses race, gender, social class, cultural norms, history, and political traditions. This makes the perspective an inherently far more complex one than the psychosocial perspective, which places its explanatory emphasis on a few key constructs—most notably social status and social capital. The basic narrative of the materialist/political economy perspective is that linkages between income inequality and overall levels of population arise from their shared association with "a combination of negative exposures and lack of resources held by individuals, along with systematic underinvestment across a wide range of human, physical, health, and social infrastructure" (Lynch et al., 2000, p. 1202).[12]

Because income inequalities and population health are both manifestations of material conditions, they are often associated. However, in the materialist/political economy explanation, there is no one common process that links income inequalities to population health across all populations—but many that are determined by the history, culture, and political economy that is specific to each population. A critical policy implication of this proposition is that income inequality and population health are not always associated, that is, structural arrangements that benefit health can occur that are independent of the income distribution (Lynch et al., 2000; Lynch et al., 2004).

1986 and 1999. The GSS is a national probability sample survey of adults on an array of social attitudes, beliefs, and behaviors that is conducted annually by the National Opinion Research Center at the University of Chicago. Although the investigators suggest that the selected GSS questions they employed measure four dimensions of social capital, two of the survey items employed appear to represent the same underlying dimension (see Kawachi et al., 1997, p. 1492).

[12] Lynch et al. use the term "neo-material" for this perspective rather than the "materialist/political economy" label applied here. The latter is preferred here because the principal origin of the perspective resides in political economy theory.

There is an important strain in the materialist/political economy perspective that places emphasis on social class over other structural determinants (Muntaner, 1999; Muntaner et al., 2002; Navarro & Shi, 2001). The basic argument of the class structure proponents is that vigorous labor movements and other aspects of working class power are associated with higher levels of income inequality, greater political representation for women, a more generous welfare state, and higher levels of population health. Although the social class perspective is not new, it was reinvigorated as a critique of the psychosocial perspective's neglect of the role of social class in health and the power of social class relations within societies to shape differences in population health outcomes. The central thrust of the social class critique of the psychosocial perspective is that the concept of social class and its effects encompass both the material and status inequalities that operate as key structural determinants of health, and that the social capital and "social cohesion" effects on population health touted by the psychosocial perspective are actually consequent to the structural effects of class. Accordingly, the road to increased population health lies in political change and not through strategies to enhance the quality of interpersonal relationships (Muntaner, 1999).

Methodological Debates Concerning Income Inequality Effects

Ten years after the *British Medical Journal's* publication of Richard Wilkinson's seminal paper showing a dramatic negative correlation between income inequality and life expectancy among wealthy nations (Wilkinson, 1992), an editorial in the very same journal conceded that the empirical support for the income inequality–population health hypothesis was rapidly waning—at least in cross-national population comparisons (Mackenbach, 2002). While income inequality effects at the population level appear evident within the United States (in comparisons among states) (Lynch et al., 2004), there is an emerging consensus among social epidemiologists today that (1) the correlations observed in earlier studies between income inequality and life expectancy at the international level were largely an outcome of significant flaws in data and methods and (2) the effects of income inequality on population health are far more complex and contextual than simple and generalized (Lynch et al, 2004, p. 81). The methodological critiques of the income inequality–population health hypothesis fall into two areas, the first concerned with the measurement of key constructs, and the second concerned with statistical modeling and sample selection effects.

Within the key constructs critique, most of the criticism pertains to the psychosocial perspective on the health effects of income inequality—specifically the constructs of social capital and social cohesion. As the critics note, social capital theory was developed in sociology at the level of the individual—not as a construct of societies or populations. As a result, within the psychosocial perspective there is theoretical ambiguity concerning the meanings of social capital and social cohesion that extends to a lack of specificity and consistency in measurement (Lomas, 1998). This problem is then compounded by the ad hoc measurement of these concepts via conveniently available population surveys (Forbes & Wainwright, 2001). The effect of all this is to cast serious doubt on whether particular statistical relationships used to support causal arguments have a clear theoretical interpretation.

The primary measurement critique specific to the materialist political economy perspective pertains to the measurement of income inequality. Although the relationship between income inequalities and population health has proved robust across a variety of measures in the context of the United States (Kawachi & Kennedy, 1997), the relationship at the cross-national level has been shown to be quite sensitive to the measure of income inequality employed (Judge, 1995). A second measurement problem that cuts across theoretical perspectives involves the measures of population health that are chosen. In essence, the critique here is that the some of the most influential studies used to argue a relationship between income inequality and population health relied upon a small set of very general indicators, such as average life expectancy, infant mortality, and homicide (Lynch et al., 2004).

At the heart of the sample selection critique of the income inequality–population health literature is the appearance of a statistical correlation that can arise when a small sample of cases is used, as was the case in the most famous of the early international studies used to argue the income inequality–population health hypothesis.[13] A second and related problem is that, under such circumstances, a few atypical cases can drive the results and lead to an erroneous conclusion. In fact, recent studies that were able to capture data on a larger number of countries have shown this to be the case (Judge, 1995; J. Lynch et al., 2001). The concluding critique in one that involves both issues of sample selection and statistical design is the spurious correlation between income inequality and health at the aggregate (population) level that arises where the effects of individual income on health are smaller as income rises (Gravelle, 1998). Since the diminishing returns of income on health correspond to the general pattern, this statistical artifact poses a significant problem to the evaluation of the income inequality–population health hypothesis. Although the use of

---

[13] This was Richard Wilkinson's (1992) *British Medical Journal* article that employed data from nine industrialized democracies to show a strong negative correlation between income inequality and life expectancy.

multilevel (population and individual) data and methods can mitigate this problem, this approach has largely been ignored in favor of population-level only studies (Lynch et al., 2004).

Does Income Inequality Directly Affect Population Health?

Debates about the relative importance of the psychosocial effects as opposed to the material effects of income inequality of health are predicated on the assumption that income inequality is a pervasive determinant of population health. So, theoretical pathways aside, we are left with the central question of whether or not income inequality affects health. On the basis of a comprehensive review involving the 98 studies published on this question between 1979 and 2004, John Lynch and his collaborators draw the conclusion that, *as a general phenomenon* among wealthy nations, *income inequality itself is not associated with population health differences* (Lynch et al., 2004, p. 81). However, their conclusion comes with several important caveats.[14]

First and most important, the lack of a consistent association between income inequality and population health at the international level does not preclude the effect of a relationship between income inequality and health *within* countries—in fact, such seems to be the case in the United States where there appears to be persistent state-level income inequality effects on health despite controls for a variety of confounding factors. As Lynch suggests, the income inequality effects on health may be more pronounced in national contexts (like the United States) where extremes of income inequality are juxtaposed with less evenly distributed social investments in goods and services that are relevant to health, such as high-quality public education and health care (Lynch et al., 2001).

Another important caveat is that income inequality, as a characteristic of a social system, can in many ways shape the life chances of individuals in ways that are not readily observable at the individual level (Lynch et al., 2004, p. 82). The fact that such "system effects" of income inequality are not as obvious and universal at the international level as once assumed does not mean that they are not important or in fact quite powerful—rather, it suggests that they are complex and highly contextualized by

---

[14] Lynch et al.'s conclusion that the income inequality effects in population health are not generalized among wealthy nations is largely based upon (1) the lack of evidence of a direct effect in more recent studies that use more complete data, (2) negative findings in the few international studies that employ multilevel methods to control for individual effects, and (3) inconsistent evidence within country studies that employ the appropriate multilevel methods.

the nation's specific cultural, historical, and political factors that affect health.[15]

Finally, Lynch and his collaborators earnestly point out that income inequality statistics at the population level reflect aggregate income disadvantages for individuals that are linked to poor health—thus implying the same fundamental public policy interventions—specifically, those policy interventions aimed at raising the income levels of the most disadvantaged (Lynch, 2004, p. 83).

Prospects for the Advancement of Social Epidemiology as a Discipline

Although the claims and controversies pertaining to the health effects of income inequality were heavily featured in social epidemiology's emergence as a distinct discipline over the last decade, income inequality is but one potential structural determinant of health among many. In fact, the rejection or revisions of popular theory on empirical grounds are the hallmark of a maturing discipline. The richness and scientific relevance that is inherent in the discipline of social epidemiology is not tied to the fate of any one meta-theory, but in what the discipline brings to the epistemologies of causality. In this regard the future of social epidemiology is very promising.

Perhaps social epidemiology's prospects as a discipline have been best articulated through an essay by Nancy Krieger published in the *International Journal of Epidemiology*, ironically in response to an editorial questioning the legitimacy of social epidemiology as a field of scientific endeavor (Zielhuis & Kiemeney, 2001).[16] As argued by Krieger, any complete explanation of disease, whether at the individual level or the population level, must take account of the fact that humans exist as both social and biological beings (Krieger, 2001a). Thus "epidemiologically adequate explanations of current and changing distributions of population disease [must] entail simultaneous social and biological explanations" (Krieger, 2001a, p. 44). By implication, there is an inherent merit to a discipline

---

[15] This more nuanced and contextualized view of the income inequality effects on health is quite consistent with the "fundamental social causes of disease" theory reviewed at an earlier point in the chapter. In essence, this theory suggests that the intervening mechanisms of disease through which income inequality influences health are likely to vary by historical period and social context—thus leading to inconsistency of results in cross-national comparisons of income inequality.

[16] Zielhuis and Kiemeney's essay seeks to keep epidemiology in the realm of the biological, and rejects the notion that investigators trained in social science can make meaningful contributions to epidemiology in absence of formal training in the biological sciences. Krieger's essay in response is one of several compelling rebuttals to this point of view.

that affords a niche for theoretical and methodological syntheses between the social and biological sciences.

However, because the disciplinary paradigm of social epidemiology encompasses at once the social and biological, it is exceedingly complex as well. Social epidemiologist George Kaplan illustrates this point by reference to his own work, specifically the Kaplan and Lynch model of the social epidemiology of cardiovascular disease depicted in Figure 7.4. (Kaplan & Lynch, 1999). As noted by Kaplan, the array of factors at multiple levels that are considered in Figure 7.4 is far more broad and complex than the models typically employed in other branches of science. While the model shown offers a general sense of the intricate web of causality that links structural determinants of health to specific mechanisms, it is still a gross oversimplification of the causal processes implied by a social and biological paradigm of disease.

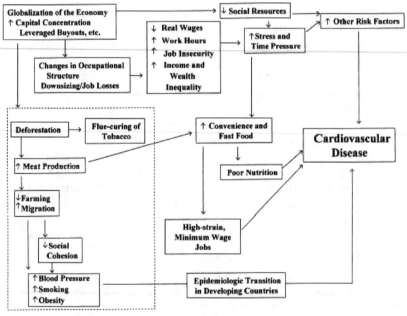

Figure 7.4   The Kaplan and Lynch Model of the Social Epidemiology of Cardio-vascular Disease. (Source: Reprinted from Kaplan, G. A. (2004). What's wrong with social epidemiology, and how can we make it better? *Epidemiology Review,* 26, 124–135. Originally published in Kaplan, G.A. and Lynch, G.W. (1999). Socioeconomic Considerations in the Primordial Prevention of Cardiovascular Disease. *Preventative Medicine,* 29, S30–S35.)

In order for social epidemiology to advance as a discipline and prove useful as a tool of medicine and social policy, complex multilevel modes like that shown in Figure 7.4 need to be validated and refined through empirical investigation. However, this imposes formidable challenges that have been well summarized by Kaplan in a general critique of the discipline (Kaplan, 2004). These challenges include surmounting obstacles in the acquisition of theory relevant data at multiple levels (e.g. physiological and health behavior data at the individual level, household characteristics and neighborhood level data relevant to psychosocial support networks, data pertaining to occupational status and work environment, data on the local health care infrastructure, and macro level data pertaining to such factors as job outsourcing, gaining disciplinary consensus on the meaning and measurement of key constructs (e.g. social cohesion), contending with the statistical complexities involved in estimating relative effects of variables at different ecological levels, contending issues of temporal effects and reciprocal causality, and overcoming the tendency to substitute general constructs (such as social class, gender, and race) for specific causal factors that are confounded with measures of the general construct. Although these challenges are not unique to social epidemiology, they are perhaps more prevalent given the complex nature of the theoretical paradigms in social epidemiology.

CONCLUDING COMMENTS—SOCIAL EPIDEMIOLOGY AS A TOOL OF SOCIAL POLICY

This chapter began with Nancy Krieger's observation that social epidemiology "is distinguished [from other sciences and branches of epidemiology] by its insistence upon explicitly investigating the social determinants of population distributions of health, disease, and wellbeing ..." (Krieger, 2002, p. 7). As much as this distinct purpose lends relevancy to the discipline, it also imposes a paradox in managing the boundaries between scientific inquiry, theory building, and political ideology. This paradox arises because (1) the social determinants of health tend to be structural in origin, and (2) such structural determinants of health are intertwined with hierarchies of power and privilege. Further (to reinforce a point made in the opening paragraphs of the chapter), to the extent that the theories and findings of social epidemiologists fundamentally challenge embedded hierarchies of power and privilege, the discipline will remain clouded in questions about its legitimacy. There is one sense in which social epidemiology should embrace and celebrate challenges to its legitimacy, and another sense in which social epidemiology should be worried.

Challenges to legitimacy that arise because the scientific inquiries of social epidemiologists either uncover or highlight social arrangements that are detrimental to health should be regarded as an affirmation that the social epidemiology is fulfilling a critical social purpose. Indeed, it seems that the more credible the theory and evidence that links power and privilege to detrimental social arrangements, the louder will be the outcry from the affected interests.[17] Ultimately though, such outraged protests about scientific legitimacy often portend the introduction of scientifically informed social policies.

On the other hand, to the extent that social epidemiologists fall into the trap of confounding the advancement of egalitarian political ideology with the advancement of epidemiological theory, other challenges to legitimacy arise that ultimately undermine the credibility of social epidemiology as a scientific discipline. This seems to have occurred in the popular consumption of theories that identified income inequality as a general determinant of population health, rather than as a more complex dimension of inequality with highly contextualized effects. While the proposition that income inequality functions as a readily observable *general determinant* of population health appears to be on the ever thinner ground, this is very different from the conclusion that income inequality fails to have significant and direct detrimental effects on population health under a variety of specific circumstances. In order to illuminate these more nuanced and policy relevant linkages between income inequality and population health, the discipline of social epidemiology will need to continue its very promising recent advances in theoretical specificity and methodological rigor.

REFERENCES

Alderson, A., & Nielsen, N. (2002). Globalization and the great U-Turn: Income inequality trends in 16 OECD countries. *American Journal of Sociology, 107*(5), 1244–1257.

Balbach, E. D., Gasior, R. J., & Barbeau, E. M. (2003). R.J. Reynolds' targeting of African Americans: 1988–2000. *American Journal of Public Health, 93*(5), 822–827.

Barbeau, E. M., Wolin, K. Y., Naumova, E. N., & Balbach, E. (2005). Tobacco advertising in communities: Associations with race and class. *Preventative Medicine, 40*(1), 16–22.

[17] The most notorious example is the U.S. tobacco industry and its decades-long disinformation campaign against cancer research. Of course, there are also the ongoing struggles between environmental science and the industrial sources of an array of environmental toxins.

Broder, M. S., Kanouse, D. E., Mittman, B. S., & Bernstein, S. J. (2000). The appropriateness of recommendations for hysterectomy. *Obstetrics & Gynecology, 95*(2), 199–205.

Burris, S. (2002). Introduction: Merging law, human rights, and social epidemiology. *Journal of Law and Medical Ethics, 30*(4), 498–509.

Cassel, J. (1976). The contribution of the social environment to host resistance: The fourth Wade Hampton Frost lecture. *American Journal of Epidemiology, 104*(2), 107–123.

Diamond, T. (1992). *Making gray gold: Narratives of nursing home care.* Chicago, IL: University of Chicago Press.

Dicker, R. C., Scally, M. J., Greenspan, J. R., Layde, P. M., Ory, H. W., Maze, J. M., et al. (1982). Hysterectomy among women of reproductive age. Trends in the United States, 1970–1978. *Journal of the American Medical Association, 248*(3), 323–327.

Forbes, A., & Wainwright, S. P. (2001). On the methodological, theoretical and philosophical context of health inequalities research: A critique. *Social Science & Medicine, 53*(6), 801–816.

Frisbie, W. P., Song, S. E., Powers, D. A., & Street, J. A. (2004). The increasing racial disparity in infant mortality: Respiratory distress syndrome and other causes. *Demography, 41*(4), 773–800.

Gravelle, H. (1998). How much of the relation between population mortality and unequal distribution of income is a statistical artefact? *British Medical Journal, 316*(7128), 382–385.

Haas, S., Acker, D., Donahue, C., & Katz, M. E. (1993). Variation in hysterectomy rates across small geographic areas of Massachusetts. *American Journal of Obstetrics and Gynecology, 169*(1), 150–154.

Judge, K. (1995). Income distribution and life expectancy: A critical appraisal. *British Medical Journal, 311*(7015), 1282–1285.

Kaplan, G. A. (2004). What's wrong with social epidemiology, and how can we make it better? *Epidemiology Review, 26,* 124–135.

Kaplan, G. A., & Lynch, J. W. (1999). Socioeconomic considerations in the primordial prevention of cardiovascular disease. *Preventive Medicine, 29*(6), S30–S35.

Kaplan, G. A., Lynch, J. W., Cohen, R. D., & Balfour, J. (1996). Inequality in income and mortality in the United States: Analysis of mortality and potential pathways. *British Medical Journal, 312*(7037), 999–1003.

Kasl, S. V., & Jones, B. A. (2002). Social epidemiology: Towards a better understanding of the field. *International Journal of Epidemiology, 31*(6), 1094–1097.

Kawachi, I. (2002). Social epidemiology. *Social Science and Medicine, 54*(12), 1739–1741.

Kawachi, I., & Kennedy, B. P. (1997). The relationship of income inequality to mortality: Does the choice of indicator matter? *Social Science and Medicine, 45*(7), 1121–1127.

Kawachi, I., Kennedy, B. P., Lochner, K., & Prothrow-Stith, D. (1997). Social capital, income inequality, and mortality. *American Journal of Public Health, 87*(9), 1491–1498.

Krieger, N. (1994). Epidemiology and the web of causation: Has anyone seen the spider? *Social Science and Medicine, 39*, 887–903.

Krieger, N. (1999). Sticky webs, hungry spiders, buzzing flies, and fractal metaphors: On the misleading juxtaposition of "risk factor" versus "social" epidemiology. *Journal of Epidemiology and Community Health, 53*(11), 678–680.

Krieger, N. (2000). Epidemiology and social sciences: Towards a critical reengagement in the 21st century. *Epidemiology Review, 22*(1), 155–163.

Krieger, N. (2001a). Commentary: Society, biology and the logic of social epidemiology. *International Journal of Epidemiology, 30*(1), 44–46.

Krieger, N. (2001b). Historical roots of social epidemiology: Socioeconomic gradients in health and contextual analysis. *International Journal of Epidemiology, 30*(4), 899–900.

Krieger, N. (2001c). Theories for social epidemiology in the 21st century: An ecosocial perspective. *International Journal of Epidemiology, 30*(4), 668–677.

Krieger, N. (2002). A glossary for social epidemiology. *Epidemiology Bulletin, 23*(1), 7–11.

Krieger, N., & Davey Smith, G. (2004). "Bodies count," and body counts: Social epidemiology and embodying inequality. *Epidemiology Review, 26*, 92–103.

Krieger, N., & Smith, G. D. (2000). Re: "Seeking causal explanations in social epidemiology." *American Journal of Epidemiology, 151*(8), 831–833.

Link, B. G., & Phelan, J. (1995). Social conditions as fundamental causes of disease. *Journal of Health and Social Behavior,* Spec No, 80–94.

Link, B. G., & Phelan, J. (1996). Understanding sociodemographic differences in health—The role of fundamental causes. *American Journal of Public Health, 86*(4), 471–473.

Link, B. G., & Phelan, J. C. (2002). McKeown and the idea that social conditions are fundamental causes of disease. *American Journal of Public Health, 92*(5), 730–732.

Lochner, K., Kawachi, I., & Kennedy, B. P. (1999). Social capital: A guide to its measurement. *Health & Place, 5*(4), 259–270.

Lomas, J. (1998). Social capital and health: Implications for public health and epidemiology. *Social Science and Medicine, 47*(9), 1181–1188.

Lynch, J., Smith, G. D., Harper, S., Hillemeie, M., Ross, N., Kaplan, G., et al. (2004). Is income inequality a determinant of population health? Part 1. A systematic review. *Milbank Quarterly, 82*(1), 5–99.

Lynch, J., Smith, G. D., Hillemeier, M., Shaw, M., Raghunathan, T., & Kaplan, G. (2001). Income inequality, the psychosocial environment, and health: Comparisons of wealthy nations. *Lancet, 358*(9277), 194–200.

Lynch, J. W., Smith, G. D., Kaplan, G. A., & House, J. S. (2000). Income inequality and mortality: Importance to health of individual income, psychosocial environment, or material conditions. *British Medical Journal, 320*(7243), 1200–1204.

Macdonald, K. (2001). Commentary: Social epidemiology. A way? *International Journal of Epidemiology, 30*(1), 46–47.

Mackenbach, J. P. (2002). Income inequality and population health. *British Medical Journal, 324*(7328), 1–2.

Marmot, M. (2002). The influence of income on health: Views of an epidemiologist. *Health Affairs, 21*(2), 31–46.

Muntaner, C. (1999). Invited commentary: Social mechanisms, race, and social epidemiology. *American Journal of Epidemiology, 150*(2), 121–126; discussion 127–128.

Muntaner, C. (2001). Social epidemiology: No way back. A response to Zielhuis and Kiemeney. *International Journal of Epidemiology, 30*(3), 625–626.

Muntaner, C., & Lynch, J. (1999). Income inequality, social cohesion, and class relations: A critique of Wilkinson's neo-Durkheimian research program. *International Journal of Health Services, 29*(1), 525–543.

Muntaner, C., Lynch, J., & Smith, G. D. (2001). Social capital, disorganized communities, and the third way: understanding the retreat from structural inequalities in epidemiology and public health. *International Journal of Health Services, 31*(2), 213–237.

Muntaner, C., Lynch, J. W., Hillemeie, M., Lee, J. H., David, R., Benach, J., et al. (2002). Economic inequality, working-class power, social capital, and cause-specific mortality in wealthy countries. *International Journal of Health Services, 32*(3), 423–432.

Navarro, V., & Shi, L. (2001). The political context of social inequalities and health. *Social Science & Medicine, 52*(3), 481–491.

NCHS. (2002). *Health, United States 2002, Data from Table 30 Age adjusted death rates for selected causes according to sex, race and hispanic origin, United States, selected years 1950–1999.* Hyattsville, MD: Author.

NCHS. (2004). *Health, United States 2004. Table 27. Life expectancy at birth, at 65 years of age, and at 75 years of age, according to race and sex: United States, selected years 1900–2002.* Hyattsville, MD: Author.

Phelan, J. C., Link, B. G., Diez-Roux, A., Kawachi, I., & Levin, B. (2004). "Fundamental causes" of social inequalities in mortality: A test of the theory. *Journal of Health and Social Behavior, 45*(3), 265–285.

Rodgers, G. (1979). Income and inequality as determinants of mortality: An international cross-section analysis. *Population Studies, 33,* 343–351.

Schwartz, S. (2002). *"Hidden away, in the land of plenty .... 2002 current statistics concerning the Pine Ridge Oglala Lakota (Sioux) Reservation."* Retrieved February 20, 2005, from http://www.wambliho.homestead.com.

Starr, P. (1982). *The social transformation of American medicine.* New York: Basic Books.

Swingwood, A. (2000). *A short history of social thought* (3rd ed.). New York: St. Martin's Press.

Travis, C. (1985). Medical decision making and elective surgery: The case of hysterectomy. *Risk Analysis, 5*(3), 241–251.

Wallace, R. (1990). Urban desertification, public health and public order: "Planned shrinkage," violent death, substance abuse and AIDS in the Bronx. *Social Science and Medicine, 31*(7), 801–813.

West, S., & Dranov, P. (1994). *The hysterectomy hoax* (3rd ed.). New York: Doubleday.

Wilkinson, R. G. (1992). Income distribution and life expectancy. *British Medical Journal (Clinical Research Ed.)*, *304*(6820), 165–168.

Wilkinson, R. G. (1995). Commentary: A reply to Ken Judge: Mistaken criticisms ignore overwhelming evidence. *British Medical Journal*, *311*(7015), 1285–1287.

Wilkinson, R. G. (1996). *Unhealthy societies: The afflictions of inequality*. London: Routledge.

Wilkinson, R. G. (1999). Health, hierarchy, and social anxiety. *Annals of the New York Academy of Sciences*, *896*(1), 48–63.

Wilkinson, R. G., Kawachi, I., & Kennedy, B. (1998). Mortality, the social environment, crime and violence. In M. Bartley, D. Blane, & G. Davey-Smith (Eds.), *The sociology of health inequalities* (pp. 19–38). Oxford, UK: Oxford Sociology of Health and Illness Monograph.

Zielhuis, G. A., & Kiemeney, L. A. (2001). Social epidemiology? No way. *International Journal of Epidemiology*, *30*(1), 43–44; discussion 51.

CHAPTER EIGHT

Competing Agendas for Health Care System Reform: A Social Justice Critique

The task taken up by this last chapter entails a review of the dominant and stable array of policy agendas arising from different interests and segments of the body politic. A pragmatic understanding of the policy priorities and arguments of the health care system's key stakeholders must be taken into account in any effort toward health care reform, whether incremental or fundamental. Although the "competitive agenda" approach will have a prominent place in the analysis provided, the chapter will conclude with a social justice analysis and critique of a general set of health care system reform typologies.

THE SOCIAL AND POLITICAL CONTEXT OF HEALTH CARE REFORM

Virtually every presidential administration since Lyndon Johnson's has needed to confront "the crisis in American health care" however it has been defined. Conservative politicians have tended to frame the crisis in terms of an unsustainable level of growth in federal health care spending and the disastrous consequences on the national economy that follow. In contrast, liberal politicians have typically framed the crisis in health care by the well-documented failures of the health care system to ensure the availability of essential health care for millions of Americans. Both positions are fundamentally correct. As discussed at length in an early chapter (chapter 3, Health Care Finance), 4 decades of mostly continuous health care inflation have been paralleled by the growth of federal expenditures for health care—principally via the Medicare and Medicaid programs. Conservatives rightly point out that over this same 40-year period there have been multiple expansions in the entitlements of both programs as well. On the other hand, just as liberals claim, the American health care system remains replete with disparities in access to health care across multiple categories of race, ethnicity, and social class.

Presidential administrations have tended to follow suit by defining the nature of the health care crisis largely in terms of one of these two perspectives—but not always in ways that are consistent with political party affiliation. The presidential administrations that have framed the health care crisis primarily as one of rising costs include Nixon (1969–1974), Carter (1977–1981), and Reagan (1981–1989). Each of these administrations introduced cost containment reforms with varying degrees of success that range from negligible to modest. In contrast, the Clinton administration (1993–2001) is the only presidency in recent history that defined the crisis in health care principally in terms of the lack of universal health insurance coverage. Two other administrations, those of George H. W. Bush (1989–1993) and George W. Bush (2001–present), have framed the crisis in health care in fairly narrow terms and thus have pursued very targeted reforms.[1]

Most significantly, no president in recent history has sought to actually radically reform the health care system in ways that would pursue both the curbing of health care inflation and assure universal access to health care. Even Clinton deferred from pursuing a health care reform agenda that would overtly challenge the key vested interests within the health care industry opposed to more than incremental reform—including the large share of physicians committed to the lucrative rewards of medical free enterprise, the for-profit and voluntary sectors of the hospital industry, the health care insurance industry, the pharmaceutical industry, and a significant share of the organized labor movement.[2]

[1] The George H. W. Bush administration (1989–1992) minimized the scope of the crisis in health care and disavowed any electoral mandate for health care reform (Roper, 1989). The George W. Bush administration has framed the crisis in health care in terms of the "affordability" of health care for ordinary Americans, and has pursued a reform platform that emphasizes tort reforms intended to reduce the burden of medical malpractice costs and the addition of Medicare prescription drug coverage for older Americans. The significant health care cost control measures implemented by the George W. Bush administration, primarily affecting the poor, were labeled as "deficit reduction" legislation.

[2] This strategy also failed, in large part because the complexity of the Clinton health care plan left many Americans confused and vulnerable to a well-financed campaign of oppositional rhetoric.

Public Preferences for Health Care Reform

Despite the fact that personal health care expenditures and the affordability of health care have been an ongoing concern of Americans for most of the last century,[3] public opinion on the nature and extent of the crisis in health care has varied dramatically from one national election to the next. In part, this is due to immediate economic and political issues that either illuminate or overshadow the problems embedded in the health care system. As a case in point, the 2004 presidential election witnessed the overshadowing of health care issues by the war in Iraq and related national security concerns—despite the resurgence of health care inflation and an increase in the number of both employed and unemployed Americans without health insurance (Kaiser Commission on Medicaid and the Uninsured, 2006).[4]

Public opinion on the nature and extent of the crisis in health care, as well as the most viable options for reform, has also been influenced by the political framing of the health care issue by politicians and the interests they represent.[5] Briefly described, *political framing* is a rhetorical tactic that reduces highly complex issues to simple ideas, assumptions, and contrasts that are put forth in highly biased terms. Sometimes referred to as "defining the terms of the debate," political framing tactics thrive where there is a convergence between public issue complexity, voter ambivalence about policy trade-offs, and strong vested interests in policy alternatives.

During the debate over the health care reform measures proposed by the Clinton administration, the crisis in health care and related reform proposals was politically framed as a tradeoff between extending health care coverage to a small minority of uninsured Americans and the surrendering of individual free choice in health care for all Americans. This was a very effective use of this tactic that clearly contributed to the decay of

---

[3] In a nationally representative survey conducted by the Kaiser Family Foundation in October of 2005, 72% worry about the rising costs of health care insurance and just over 60% worry about not being able to afford needed health care services (Kaiser Family Foundation, 2005).

[4] Although public polls that preceded the 2004 presidential election showed agreement among Democratic and Republican voters that something should be done about the problem of people without health insurance, at the time of the election only 17% of Republicans and 43% of Democrats indicated that this issue would be extremely important to determining their vote (Robert J. Blendon, Brodie, Altman, Benson, & Hamel, 2005).

[5] Political framing is defined as a rhetorical tactic through which political elites reduce and define a complex public issue into a limited set of assumptions and considerations that will influence how the public thinks about the issue (Koch, 1998). This is a very different and far more subtle form of persuasion than simply offering a political argument.

public support for the Clinton plan, despite the plan's objective to extend health care insurance coverage to all American households.

Although these factors have contributed to a high level of inconsistency in public opinion pertaining to the adequacy of the health care system and health care reform, over time there has been tremendous stability in public opinion pertaining to the role of the government in assuring access to health care. Since 1972, the General Social Survey has regularly asked a nationally representative sample of adults the same question pertaining to the role of the government (as opposed to the individual) in assuring affordable access to health care. Interestingly, the proportion of those surveyed during each decade since 1972 who believed the federal government should have little to no role in helping individuals to pay for doctors and hospitals has never exceeded 20%.[6] In contrast, most of those surveyed feel the government should either assume a large role in helping persons to pay for health care (48%) or at least assume a significant share of the responsibility (30–32%) (National Opinion Research Center, 2006).

Consistent with the General Social Survey findings, a series of public opinion polls conducted by the Kaiser Family Foundation and the Pew Research Center during the past decade also show that most Americans favor a strong federal role in assuring that all Americans have access to health care and health care insurance—even if it involves an increase in taxes (Kaiser Family Foundation, 2006).[7] Americans also tend to think that health care, like public education, should be provided equally to everyone. Two nationally representative polls conducted by the Henry J. Kaiser Foundation in 2000 and 2004 found that most (84%) of

---

[6] The precise wording of the General Social Survey question is "In general, some people think that it is the responsibility of the government in Washington to see to it that people have help in paying for doctors and hospital bills. Others think that these matters are not the responsibility of the federal government and that people should take care of these things themselves." Respondents are then asked to place themselves on a scale that ranges between 1 and 5, with 5 indicating strong agreement with the sentiment that people should "take care of themselves." The combined tabulations for the 1972–82, 1983–87, 1988–91 and the 1998 survey all show that less than 20% of respondents place themselves above a score of 4 on the question. In contrast, nearly 50% place themselves at the opposite end of the scale, which indicates a strong preference toward a significant role of the federal government in helping persons pay for health care (National Opinion Research Center, 2006).

[7] The three Pew Research Center polls cited in this report, conducted between July of 2003 and July of 2005, show that between 64 and 67% of favor the U.S. government guaranteeing health insurance for all Americans—even if a tax increase is involved. The series of six Kaiser Foundation polls cited in this report, spanning the years between 1992 and 2000, show an average 66% level of support for the idea that the federal government should guarantee health care for "all people" who don't have health insurance.

Americans express general agreement with the idea that everyone should have equal access to health care and that nearly half (48%) believed that access to health care should be a right (Kaiser Family Foundation, 2006). Finally, findings from 14 public opinion polls over the 1980–2000 period show that the level of support among Americans for a plan of national health insurance that is financed by tax dollars typically exceeds 50% (Blendon & Benson, 2001).[8]

Taken at face value, it would seem that the ever-widening gap between the majority of the public's beliefs about equitable access to health care and the increasing millions of Americans without either health care insurance or access to affordable health care would ultimately push the country toward fundamental health care system reform. It clearly has not, in large part because public opinion can best be described as fragmented and ambivalent when it comes to solutions. Among the lessons learned in the wake of the demise of the Clinton plan (to be discussed later in this chapter) is the fact that while most Americans share a moral commitment to the uninsured, this value will not by itself create the impetus for fundamental health care system reform. As stated by Blendon et al. (1994, p. 283), "moral concern by itself will not spur the 85 percent of Americans who have health coverage into action on behalf of the 15 percent who do not." The American public still tends to distrust its government, is resistant to even low-level tax increases, and in particular is resistant to reform strategies that are at all suggestive of diminished health care choice or access (Blendon et al., 1994). Thus, it may be that fundamental health care reform will gain the sustained political traction necessary to build consensus around specific solutions only at the point when a critical mass of the voting public reaches the conclusion that health care system reform is essential to their own interests—as well as consistent with their moral beliefs.

Stakeholder Interests and Competing Agendas for Health Care Reform

In the contemporary rhetoric of public policy, the term *stakeholders* is often employed to refer to the groups and organizations that have a compelling interest in the outcome of any policy-making process. Simply

---

[8] In the 14 public opinion polls conducted by such organizations as the Harvard School of Public Health, the Washington Post, and CBS News, the proportion of those surveyed that favored national health insurance ranged from a low of 46% (March, 1980) to a high of 66% (July, 1992). The average proportion of favorable support for national health insurance across all 14 surveys was 57% (See Blendon & Benson, 2001, Exhibit 1).

stated, these are the groups and organizations that stand to either gain or lose dependent upon what policy alternatives are implemented. It is also the case that some stakeholders have more power in the policy making process than others, sometimes because of legitimate authority but often because of other sources of political capital.[9] Because the interests of stakeholders typically conflict in some areas and converge in others, the policy alternatives that are most likely to be implemented are those that serve the overlapping interests of the most powerful stakeholders. Conversely, the policy alternatives that are least likely to be implemented are those that conflict with these overlapping interests. Thus, the pragmatics of social policy formulation and implementation must involve a rigorous appraisal of the political context of policy making: the identification of the stakeholders, their conflicting and overlapping interests, their overt and latent policy agendas, and the authority and political capital that each stakeholder is able and willing to bring to the policy-making process.

Since health care reform can be defined as any action by the federal government that significantly alters the financing, structure, and delivery of health care services, it is obvious that health care reform has a great many stakeholders. From the consumption side, there are stakeholder groups that are relatively well served by the current health care system and those that are not. Well-served consumer groups include middle income citizens, employees of industries that have relatively generous health care benefits, and persons employed by the federal government. Consumer stakeholders that are not well served by the current health care system include undocumented workers, service industry employees, Native Americans who are geographically isolated from IHS clinics, and both the working and nonworking poor. On the provider side of the health care system, the principal stakeholders include different sectors of the medical profession, the nursing profession and other health care professionals, different sectors of the hospital and nursing home industries, the health care insurance industry, the bioengineering industry, and the pharmaceutical industry. Given the employment-based financial structure of the U.S. health care system, different groups of employers also must be defined as key stakeholders in health care reform—often with very different interests. For example, associations representing the interests of large employers are less likely to oppose mandated employee health insurance benefits than associations representing the interests of small employers.

---

[9] Broadly speaking, political capital refers to possessing the assets needed to influence the decisions of other key actors in any political process. It can involve material things such as campaign funds or the ability to perform favors, as well as nonmaterial assets like scientific credibility or moral authority.

Other key stakeholders in health care reform are state governments. Because Medicaid funding is structured as a shared partnership between states and the federal government, any health care reforms that either expand or contract Medicaid program participation and expenditures have a significant fiscal impact on states. In general, state governments oppose any expansions in Medicaid eligibility or benefits that place a higher burden on states, and favor reform proposals that shift the costs of health care for the poor and the uninsured to the federal government.

The Health Care Reform Agenda of Disenfranchised Versus Enfranchised Health Care Consumers

In the U.S. health care system, one is "enfranchised" or eligible to receive nonstigmatized health care on the basis of health care insurance. For Americans under the age of 65, stable employment in the right kind of job in the right kind of industry are the essential requisites for adequate health insurance coverage. Because Medicaid recipients are subjected to the stigma of public welfare, it cannot be said that Medicaid eligibility or the possession of a Medicaid voucher yields the same level of dignified entitlement to health care as an insurance card. Thus, the disenfranchised health care consumers include those on Medicaid, the marginally employed and the unemployed, and those who work in the low-wage economy. For this group of consumer stakeholders, the disenfranchised, the health care reform agenda involves the dismantlement of the employment-based health insurance in favor of a publicly funded system of universal health insurance coverage. Thus, when California voters were given the opportunity to consider a proposition that would have created a single-payer insurance plan (Proposition 186, in 1994), the health care consumer groups that were the strongest supporters included Hispanics (64%) and the uninsured (58%) (Kaiser Family Foundation, 1994).[10]

Nationally, surveys on health care reform options show that only about 40% of the public favor abandonment of the employment-based health care system in favor of asingle-payer public insurance fund (Blendon & Benson, 2001). Generally, Americans who have health care insurance coverage tend to be satisfied with their current level of access to health care and distrust change (Blendon et al., 2005). For the enfranchised health care consumers, composing the majority of the voting public, the health care reform agenda can be characterized as a general desire to achieve universal health insurance coverage with a minimum

---

[10] Proposition 186 was defeated by a wide margin, in excess of 2:1 (Kaiser Family Foundation, 1994).

of personal sacrifice—either in tax burden or perceived quality of health care.

The Health Care Reform Agenda of the Medical Profession

Throughout most of the last century, the medical profession could be regarded as a single stakeholder group when it came to issues of health care reform. Until the 1960s, the AMA could claim with some legitimacy that it represented the unified voice of the medical profession. Over the past 50 years, however, the medical profession has become far more diverse in its views on health care reform and a much smaller proportion of physicians align themselves with the AMA's historic opposition to compulsory national health insurance. At the apex of the AMA's influence, the model of medical practice was medical free enterprise characterized by the private physician in independent practice. However, the physician labor force is now represented by a high proportion of physicians who work in salaried positions or are dependent upon various forms of publicly funded health care programs for a large share of their practice income. Thus, there are sectors of the medical profession that support the expansion of publicly funded health care programs and other sectors of the medical profession that remain vigorously opposed to any expansion of publicly sponsored health care. It is also true that the modern medical profession is challenged by the "democratization" of medical knowledge, meaning that the consumers of health care have multiple sources of information about prevention, disease management, and treatment alternatives aside from the physician—most notably the Internet (Hernes, 2001). In effect, this means that the medical profession is no longer able to retain the same level of authority over health care policy alternatives that had once exerted, even if it could achieve internal consensus. Finally, physicians no longer wholly equate the bureaucratization of medicine solely with publicly financed health care. Managed care plans sponsored through the private insurance industry burden physicians with mountains of paperwork, are notorious for their interference with the clinical judgments of physicians, and are likely a permanent feature of the employment-based health insurance industry.

Despite these developments, there are cross-cutting interests and "hot button" issues that tend to unite physicians around a common policy agenda. These include:

- The preservation of the medical profession's privileged position in terms of authority, prestige, and the economic rewards of medicine.

- The protection of the doctor–patient relationship, both with respect to confidentiality and with respect to physicians' ability to act in the best interests of their patients.
- A promotion of the purchasing power of health care consumers.
- A promotion of public and private investments in medical science and health care technology.
- Assuring a minimal standard of access to essential health care for all citizens.
- Antagonism toward policies that appear to promote or sanction the overt rationing of health care.[11]

Although this is not an exhaustive list of the political issues that tend to bring physicians together, it can be seen that collectively they reflect themes of both professional altruism and professional self-interest. In this respect, the medical profession is not distinctly different from other socially rewarding professions (e.g., lawyers, dentists, military officers, and university professors). However, in historical terms physicians have been uniquely successful relative to other professions in blurring the lines between professional altruism, scientific authority, and collective self-interest (Hernes, 2001; Starr, 1982). In significant respects the political agenda of the medical profession has always resembled Abraham Maslow's hierarchy of needs (Maslow, 1970),[12] in the sense that the profession has been willing (or at least less opposed) to health care reform initiatives that serve both the public good and the medically disenfranchised only after the profession's more basic concerns around economic sustenance, preservation of authority, and professional autonomy have been satisfied. In historic terms, this was evident in the policy compromises that ultimately produced the inflationary financial structure of Medicare (Starr, 1982). In a contemporary context, this dynamic is evident in the prominence of tort reform on the current political agenda of the medical profession relative to the profession's concerns about endemic disparities in health and access to health care.

---

[11] While physicians, like most Americans, strongly oppose the idea of overtly rationing health care, the reality is that is that the employment-based health insurance system rations health care by race, social class, nativity, and a variety of other nonclinical social characteristics having to do with prestige and power. Historically, the medical profession has supported the latter version of health care rationing in preference to equitable access to health care.

[12] Maslow's famous hierarchy of needs has been broadly applied in education, business, and the health professions to explain human needs and behavioral motivations. In essence, Maslow's theory holds that humans seek to satisfy lower order needs like survival and basic safety before they seek higher order needs like self-actualization and the kinds of more noble ends that yield the supreme achievements of humanity.

The Health Care Reform Agenda of the Hospital Industry

Except for incremental measures that expand health insurance coverage without introducing cost controls, there is no single health care reform agenda or strategy for health care reform that unites the disparate sectors of the hospital industry. In part this is due to the fact that the American Hospital Association, as the most powerful hospital industry organization, is compelled by its membership composition to represent the different interests of all three ownership sectors of the hospital industry (investor owned, voluntary not-for-profit, and public hospitals).[13] Thus, the AHA cannot go too far in endorsing either private market-based solutions (favored by the investor-owned hospitals) or public sector financing solutions (favored by public hospitals and the more progressive members of the voluntary hospital industry sector).[14] There is another, perhaps more cynical, argument that suggests that all three sectors of the hospital industry at least tacitly support the status quo in health care finance because each sector of the hospital industry is well served by the system just as it exists. Investor-owned hospital corporations are able to return healthy profits to their shareholders, the voluntary hospitals also see acceptable returns on equity through their capacities to attract a sufficient proportion of insured patients, and public hospitals risk losing their patient base to the other more prestigious (or less stigmatized) privately owned hospitals should health insurance coverage be greatly expanded (Oliver & Dowell, 1994).[15]

---

[13] Another key hospital industry stakeholder group, although not strictly aligned with any one form of hospital ownership, is comprised of teaching hospitals. The interests of teaching hospitals are principally represented by two organizations, the Association of Academic Health Centers and the Association of American Medical Colleges. The central policy concerns of teaching hospitals include adequate reimbursement for uncompensated care, cost allowances from public programs and private insurance carriers that account for the added costs of these hospitals' teaching function, and support for health care research.

[14] To many of its critics, the AHA is heavily biased toward market-based solutions to health care and is a significant obstacle to more radical reform measures that would promote equitable access to health care for all Americans. This impression was reinforced when the AHA's Vice President of Executive Branch Relations hosted a Bush–Cheney campaign fund raising event in October, 2003 (Tieman & Fong, 2003), despite the AHA's official policy of not becoming involved in presidential elections.

[15] The policy statement of the organization representing public hospitals (the National Association of Public Hospitals and Health Systems) endorses universal health care coverage and continued institutional coverage for the safety-net hospitals and clinics serving a disproportionate share of the poor (National Association of Public Hospitals and Health Systems, 2003). Notably, the organization's policy statement does not specifically endorse a publicly funded single-payer plan as a preferred alternative, which would be more likely to place public hospitals in direct competition with the other sectors of the hospital industry.

Oliver and Dowell (1994) describe an instructive "natural experiment" of hospital industry behavior in the face of various potentially politically viable reform alternatives which occurred in California in the early 1990s. In 1992, when California's population of uninsured had reached one-quarter of the nonelderly, three different health insurance market reform proposals were introduced that for a time gained some political traction among either legislators or voters. The first was a plan that would have radically changed the rules of health insurance underwriting with the intended effect of making health insurance more accessible and affordable, while the second was a health insurance proposal that would have required all employers to provide basic health benefits for all employees and their dependents and absorb 75% of the cost health insurance premiums.[16] The third proposal would have provided a uniform health insurance benefit package paid from payroll taxes and means-based worker contributions, framed by a managed competition restructuring of the insurance industry (Oliver & Dowell, 1994).

As noted by Oliver and Dowell (p. 129), the fragmented ownership structure and internal divisions among California's hospitals precluded the industry from doing much more that "staying on the sidelines" while other groups fought for and against alternative reforms. Where the industry did take a clear stand, it involved opposition to proposals that would have introduced cost controls and insufficient hospital benefit provisions. Given the fact that this occurred at a point when one-quarter of California's working age families were not covered by health insurance, the lesson from the California hospital industry example seems to suggest that the hospital industry is unlikely to support fundamental health care reform to the extent that it involves significant compromise on the part of any particular sector of industry. Yet it fundamental reforms in health care financing by definition must include such compromises. Thus, it seems that the prospects for fundamental health care reform are bleak to the extent that consensus from within the hospital industry is a precondition—at least barring a complete collapse of the mixed private and public insurance system that places all sectors of the industry in jeopardy.

The Health Care Reform Agendas of Disparate Employer Groups

As mentioned previously, employers are divided in their interests where major health care reforms are concerned. Large employers in industries that absorb the expenses of health care insurance premiums in their labor

---

[16] The second alternative is actually a summary of a California state senate bill (S.B. 248) and a ballot initiative (Proposition 166) that were alike in their main provisions. For a more detailed summary, see Oliver and Dowell (1994).

costs are not strongly averse to mandated health care coverage, though on principle large employers are in sympathy with small ones when it comes to resisting government regulation. To the extent that the insurance and tax burdens on large employers are increased by the health care costs of the uninsured, their interests diverge from those of small employers and sectors of the large employer industry that evade health benefit costs. Small employers, in large part represented by the U.S. Chamber of Commerce and the National Restaurant Association, oppose mandated health care insurance coverage for a variety of reasons, some more debatable than others.

Among the most debatable is the contention that the profit margins of small employers are insufficient to absorb the costs of health insurance. Strictly speaking this is true, in that as long as some small employers in a given market can evade the costs of health insurance while others are burdened by them, those that absorb the significant costs of health insurance are less price competitive and more likely to go broke. Conversely though, proponents of mandated insurance coverage argue that universal employer mandates level the pricing playing field for all competitors. However, it must be acknowledged that in some small employer industries with a high degree of price sensitive demand (like the restaurant industry), an across-the-board increase in prices might hurt the industry as a whole. Although the public supports universal health care coverage, it is not at all certain that they are willing to absorb the added costs of health care coverage for such incidental luxuries as a restaurant meal, a new permanent, or a visit to a movie theatre.

A less debatable issue behind the resistance of small employers to health insurance mandates is the fact that small employers, relative to large ones, are enormously disadvantaged when it comes to the costs of health insurance. As discussed in the chapter on health care finance (chapter 3), small employers lack the capacity to self-insure like large ones, have less clout when it comes to negotiating health insurance premium pricing, and, most importantly, tend to draw a labor pool that is more disadvantaged with respect to education, income, and health. The kinds of health insurance reforms that small employers do support involve reforms in the regulation of the health insurance industry that would make health care coverage more affordable for many small employers. For example, the National Restaurant Association strongly endorsed the Health Insurance Modernization and Marketability Act of 2005 (S. 1955), which permits small employers to form cooperative insurance pools and insurance purchase consortiums that cross state lines (National Restaurant Association, 2006).

Where the interests and policy agenda of small employers and large employers from all sectors of the economy (manufacturing, service, union, and nonunion) most clearly converge are reforms that promise to constrain health insurance inflation and lower the costs of insurance premiums. Dominant among these reform measures are forms of health care insurance that place a higher threshold on the consumption of health care, like Health Savings Accounts, that make employees responsible for the first dollar costs of health care. In large part this agenda is driven by the globalization of markets that place U.S. industries at a disadvantage due to relative health insurance benefit costs, and the reemergence of rampant health care inflation after a temporary slowing in the early 1990s. Employers from all sectors of the economy have totally lost faith in the motivation and capacity of providers to reduce health care costs, and are now far more committed to a policy agenda that focuses on the demand side of health care costs—specifically the health utilization behaviors of consumers.

Perhaps the most significant recent development in the domain of employer stakeholders in health care policy has been the emergence of a new large employer business model that seeks aggressively to evade both unionization and health care benefits. In decades past, the dominant strategy of large nonunion employers seeking to avoid collective bargaining agreements involved the co-option of workers through preemptive wage and benefit concessions. In contrast, the Wal-Mart strategy both aggressively fights unionization and also recruits a labor force that is less likely (or able) to demand adequate health care benefits as a condition of employment. The success of this model has enabled Wal-Mart to undercut the pricing of other large retail employers, and it is speculated that this model will ultimately move beyond the retail industry into sectors of the economy that are becoming increasingly vulnerable to global competition (Inglehart, 2006). In the retail sector of the economy, this development has caused some convergence of interests between some traditional large employers that are striving to compete with Wal-Mart and organized labor in the promotion of state level health care policy legislation that would require the largest employers to allocate minimum proportion of their payroll to health care benefits. As of 2006, such so-called Wal-Mart legislation had emerged in at least 14 states, with the Maryland legislature over-riding a gubernatorial veto to pass a law requiring employers with 10,000 or more employees to spend at least 8% of wages on health benefits (Wojcik, 2006).[17]

---

[17] This law has been legally challenged by Wal-Mart and the Retail Industry Leaders Association, in part on the basis of Employee Retirement Income Security Act of 1974 (ERISA), federal legislation which restricts the authority of states to legislate large employer benefits.

The Health Care Reform Agenda of Organized Labor

Today, only roughly one in ten American workers belongs to a labor union, in contrast to 50 years ago when the ratio was one in three (Bowers, 2005). However, the organized labor still speaks for the interests and agendas of the nation's nonmanagerial and nonprofessional workers. Indeed, the historical evidence strongly credits the organized labor movement for creating the governmental and nongovernmental social and health insurance systems that benefit all workers and their families (Rosner & Markowitz, 2003). Perhaps ironically, a significant share of the blame for the failure of national health insurance to take hold in the United States can also be laid at the feet of organized labor. Despite the voicing of at least nominal support for national health insurance at various junctures during the post–World War II era, in reality the leaders of organized labor have often been as committed to a private employment–based health system as the health insurance industry itself. The central reason for this paradox has been the conflict between organized labor's espoused mission of promoting the health and welfare of American workers and their families and the role which health benefits have served as a tool of union recruitment since the Taft–Hartley Act of 1947 (Quadagno, 2004).[18] The historic ambivalence of organized labor toward national health insurance is also reflective of divisions within the labor movement between radicals and moderates, and between the workers of low wage/benefit occupations (e.g., farm and service industry workers) and the more advantaged occupations (manufacturing and construction industry workers). Tragically for national health insurance, in the decades since the labor movement has become more unified in its support of radical health care, reform union membership has declined and the labor movement has lost much of its political clout.

The most interesting development, however, is at least the suggestion of a renascence of the labor movement represented by the ascendance of the Service Employees International Union (SEIU). Currently boasting in excess of 1.8 million members, the SEIU has been growing at a time when other unions struggle to maintain their membership. Because it represents the newly dominant service sector of the economy, the SEIU has in many respects upstaged the venerable AFL-CIO as the leading edge of the American labor movement.[19] Unlike the AFL-CIO,

---

[18] The Taft–Hartley Act greatly constrained the union recruitment activities of union organizers, which left bargaining for fringe benefits a more critical priority of union leadership (Quadagno, 2004).

[19] In 2005 the SEIU broke away from the AFL-CIO, a move which many progressives fear (and many conservatives hope) will ultimately weaken the labor movement. Others adopt a

which is heavily invested in the manufacturing sector of the economy and the survival of specific employers, the SEIU (like the building trades) is occupation-based and therefore much more portable in a dynamic economy where specific employers rapidly come and go (Milkman, 2005). While neither the SEIU or the AFL-CIO have committed to a single-payer federally sponsored health insurance fund as the ultimate solution, both labor organizations support universal health care coverage as an alternative to what each decries as the collapse of the employer-based system. Both labor organizations identify a similar short-term and long-term health care agenda. The short-term agenda highlights issues such as the protection of the existing health care benefits of workers and their families, supporting state and federal legislation that requires large employers to commit a proportion of their payroll to health benefits, and protecting the health care benefits of retired workers. The longer term health care agenda involves the revitalization of a national dialog on universal health care insurance, and the achievement of a political consensus on the mandated features of universal health insurance. As defined by the SEIU, these mandated features include (in addition to universal coverage) lowering the costs of health care, placing an emphasis on prevention, and assuring individual choice of doctors and health plans (SEIU, 2006). Despite the appeal of these policy objectives with labor and the public in general, it should be noted that there is an inherent and difficult to reconcile conflict between the objective to lower the costs of health care and the SEIU's mission to increase the wages and benefits of health care workers.

The Health Care Reform Agenda of the Health Insurance Industry

As described in chapter 2, at critical juncture during the administration of Franklin Roosevelt, the country turned toward a patchwork system of employer-sponsored voluntary health insurance and away from a federally sponsored health care trust fund that would have provided universal health care coverage. The critical force that propelled this choice was the vigorous opposition of the AMA to compulsory government health insurance. In more recent decades, the political clout of the AMA has greatly diminished and the fight has been taken up by AHIP (America's Health Insurance Plans, recently created by the merger of the Health Insurance Association of America and the American Association of Health Plans). AHIP is an organization that both reflects the political

different view, believing that the SEIU's break with the AFL-CIO represents a much needed challenge to American labor's institutional inertia.

conservatism that is the hallmark of the finance and insurance industries and the particular interests that health insurance corporations have in protecting the private insurance market. Despite the not-for-profit roots of the health insurance industry and the original conceptions of health insurance coverage as a quasi-public good, the health insurance industry of today (both in the profit and the not-for-profit sectors) exists as a lucrative corporate enterprise with what many perceive is a pernicious grip on national health care policy.

The transformation of the health insurance industry from a beneficent arrangement between employers, workers, and providers to assure the affordability of health care to an industry largely dedicated to the interests of highly paid executives and shareholders occurred in stages over several decades. Clearly though, by the early 1960s the employment-based health insurance industry had enrolled enough of the labor force to become a major force in American health care policy with a clear stake in opposing publicly sponsored health care insurance (Scofea, 1994). Notably, the health insurance industry did not test its clout in opposition to the Medicare legislation of 1965, in large part because the industry's earlier forays into health insurance for the elderly had not been profitable. Instead, the insurance industry successfully sought to carve out a role for itself as the claims intermediary for the Medicare program and as the underwriter of supplemental insurance or so-called Medigap policies (Quadagno, 2004). Thus, the health insurance industry's core interests are tied to the preservation of the fragmented patchwork of public and private health care financing arrangements that characterize the U.S. health care system's fundamental weaknesses.

Although there are multiple issues of interest to the health insurance industry that can be connected to the rubric of health care reform, the central interests of the industry converge on the general issues of cost control and protecting itself from further significant expansions of publicly financed health care—in particular in the form of a single payer health insurance trust fund that would marginalize the role of private health insurance.[20] The stake that the health insurance industry has in cost control has mostly to do with two overlapping issues: the insurance industry's general interest in tort reform that would place limits on the rewards of malpractice litigation, and the worry that unconstrained health care

---

[20] Should the employment-based health insurance system be entirely supplanted by a single payer plan, under any credible scenario there would still be a significant market for supplemental health insurance to cover policy gaps and attend to the demands of privileged consumers. A single payer system will not by itself create a single tiered health care system.

inflation will lead to the final collapse of employment-based insurance. Should that come to pass, a government takeover of health care financing appears all but inevitable.

Given all this, the private health insurance industry's core interests are best served by encouraging incremental solutions to health care inflation, the growing millions of uninsured, and the related problem of uncompensated care that threatens the health care safety net. The incremental approach both preserves the status quo and, if effectively pursued, keeps more radical reform on the margins of public opinion. In the language of the official AHIP Web site (called "Road Map to Reform," see www.ahip.org) the solution to the health care crisis involves the employment of "targeted strategies to give all Americans access through public and private coverage and through support for the public health infrastructure." In other words, incremental reductions in the millions of uninsured through a mix of public programs and private health insurance, with sufficient attention to preservation of the health care safety net to keep it from collapsing altogether.

As demonstrated by the defeat of the most recent attempt to provide universal health insurance coverage and constrain health care inflation, the so-called Clinton plan, the health insurance industry is at once the most intractable and the most formidable opponent to a federalized program of universal health insurance. The intractability arises from the industry's previously mentioned stake in self-preservation. Its formidable character derives from the funds it has at its disposal to fight unfavorable legislation and its demonstrated capacity to leverage its resources through coalition-building. The demise of the Clinton plan had many contributors, including strategic errors by Clinton himself, but the central force was a coalition funded and organized by the health insurance industry that combined high-level political connections with grassroots campaigning (Quadagno, 2004; Starr, 1995).[21] While the health insurance industry's lobbying organization (the HIAA) initially supported both employer mandates and universal coverage, the HIAA turned against the plan when it became apparent that the plan was vulnerable to well-organized opposition (Starr, 1995). The lesson learned, aside from the power of the health insurance industry to quickly mobilize political capital, is to appreciate the limits to which the core interests of the health care industry are genuinely amenable to political compromises that serve a progressive health care reform agenda.

---

[21] The Health Insurance Association of America's primary coalition partner was the National Federation of Independent Businesses, which represented the opposition of small business owners to the employer mandates of the Clinton plan.

The Health Care Reform Agenda of the Pharmaceutical Industry

The lifeblood of the pharmaceutical industry is innovation and the preservation of profit margins sufficient to keep all types of investors happy.[22] As a result, for this industry, the optimal form of health care reform legislation involves the enactment of provisions that expand the purchasing power of pharmaceutical consumers while both constraining competition and government price controls. The pharmaceutical industry has long recognized that to the extent that health care is financed by the federal government, the government has a larger stake in employing its regulatory power and market clout to limit the profits of the industry.[23] Thus, like the health insurance industry, the pharmaceutical industry has been a vigorous opponent of health care reform that would expand the federal role in the financing of health care (Common Cause, 1992; Quadagno, 2004).

In defense of the pharmaceutical industry's worries, the evidence from Europe indeed suggests that publicly financed health care brings with it lower profits for the pharmaceutical industry and a significant role in the targeting of the research and development (R&D) investment. However, evidence from the European experience does not suggest that either leads to a diminished commitment to research and development or inferior public benefits (Hutton, Borowitz, Oleksy, & Luce, 1994).

The only significant exception to the pharmaceutical industry's general opposition to expanded federal financing of health care was the Medicare drug benefit package passed by Congress in 2003 (the Medicare Modernization Act of 2003), which critics claim was a piece of legislation written by the pharmaceutical industry for the pharmaceutical industry (Kuttner, 2006). As pointed out earlier (see chapter 2), this legislation was the largest expansion of the Medicare program in its 40-year history. In contrast to the Bush administration's initial cost estimate of $400 billion at the time the legislation was proposed, the administration's later cost estimates rose to a taxpayer price tag of $1.2 trillion over 10 years alone (Connolly & Allen, 2005).[24]

---

[22] Small shareholders, institutional investors, and venture capitalists.

[23] The pharmaceutical industry has good reason to be worried about federally financed health care. As a case in point, Veterans Affairs health care system has been very successful in its use of a national drug formulary in terms of influencing physician prescribing–behavior toward the selected drugs, the achievement of sizable price reductions from manufacturers, and in reducing drug expenditures(Huskamp, Epstein, & Blumenthal, 2003).

[24] According to the CMS chief actuary for the Medicare program, his job was threatened when he stated his intent to disclose his own higher estimates of the drug benefit package to Congress (Connolly & Allen, 2005).

Much of the reason for the Medicare Modernization Act's inflationary nature has to do with the concessions this legislation makes to the interests of the pharmaceutical industry. The Medicare Modernization Act at once expands the purchasing power of Medicare program beneficiaries but precludes the federal government from using its formidable pharmaceutical purchasing clout to negotiate favorable drug pricing. Thus the Medicare Modernization Act meets the pharmaceutical industry's two key criteria for optimal health reform legislation: expansion of consumer purchasing power for pharmaceutical consumers without either constraints on the industry's anti-competitive practices or the incursion of government price controls (Iglehart, 2004).[25] The Medicare Modernization Act also provides an enormous boon to the health insurance industry, since the act requires that Medicare Part D pharmaceutical benefits be distributed through insurance products developed by the health insurance industry rather than as a direct benefit payment. Since the enactment of the Medicare Modernization Act, former lobbyists from both the pharmaceutical and the health insurance industries have been appointed to key Bush administration policy positions, thus assuring that the interests of both industries also will continue to be promoted as the Medicare Modernization Act is implemented (Hellander, 2005).[26]

Although the interests of the pharmaceutical industry will continue to be best served by an oppositional stance to universal health care coverage through a national health program, the most visible political agenda of the pharmaceutical industry includes such core issues as patent protection, the preservation of prohibitions against the importation of pharmaceutical products from Canada and elsewhere, making the FDA (Food and Drug Administration) drug approval process less time-consuming and burdensome, securing the retention of the industry's ability to engage in direct advertising, and, more recently, tort reform (PhRMA, 2005). Notably, all of these core issues are connected in one way or the other to the prospects for universal health coverage.

[25] While the industry has claimed that competition is essential to assure the control of costs (Mossinghoff, 1994), the industry employs variety of mechanisms to undermine competitive drug pricing (Stolberg & Gerth, 2000).

[26] As noted by Hellander (p. 275) "more than 100 high-level officials in the Bush administration are now regulating industries they formerly worked for as lobbyists, lawyers, or company executives." One former lobbyist for the Pharmaceutical Research and Manufacturers of America (PhARMA) obtained a high-level position in the Department of Health and Human Services (HHS), where she issued a report praising brand-name drugs and warning against government controls on the pricing of new drugs—the equivalent of government-sanctioned pamphleteering for the drug industry. This former aide also played a key role in squelching of multiple research reports that challenged various drug-company claims.

Stakeholder Interests, Agendas, and Alternative Social Justice Perspectives

It was pointed out in chapter 1 that social justice can generally be defined as a political theory or system of thought used to determine what mutual obligations flow between the individual and society. Also as discussed in chapter 1, the four perspectives on social justice (Libertarian, Marxist, Utilitarian, and Rawlsian) come to very different conclusions about the balance between collective and mutual obligations when applied to the general problem of sufficient and equitable access to health care. When these disparate conclusions about the optimal structure of a just health care policy agenda are examined against interests and political agendas of the various stakeholder groups, there are some clear patterns of convergence and fit. However, no one social justice perspective is perfectly aligned with the political agenda of any one stakeholder group. There are also some very interesting paradoxes.

Libertarian Social Justice and Stakeholder Agendas

The Libertarian perspective, because it places its primary emphasis on limited government, individual self-responsibility, and unencumbered free choice, is most closely aligned with the policy agendas of the health insurance industry, the pharmaceutical industry, small employers, and, to a somewhat more limited extent, the medical profession. Both the health insurance and the pharmaceutical industries are well-served by a concept of social justice that places strong emphasis on self-responsibility, freedom of choice, limited government, and limited attention to the issues of disadvantage and inequality. Although the interests and political agenda of the medical profession were well aligned with the Libertarian perspective throughout much of its history, over the past 4 decades the convergence has been limited to the Libertarian perspective's high tolerance for unequal privileges and rewards and its vigorous defense of free choice over all other considerations. In other areas, most notably the medical profession's consensus that there is a public welfare function that extends to essential health care, the fit between Libertarianism and organized medicine just isn't what it used to be. Finally, it should be acknowledged that strong themes of Libertarianism are heard in the public's preference for free choice and deep distrust of federally sponsored health care.

Utilitarian Social Justice and Stakeholder Agendas

As argued in chapter 1, Utilitarianism is the ethical perspective that is most consistent with a public health analysis of the most advanced and desirable health care systems. That's because both the public health perspective and the Utilitarian perspective converge on the utility principle, that is, the preference for policies that achieve *the maximum good for the maximum number of people* (Rescher, 1966). In the context of health care, this would be generally defined as the systems of health care that would yield the highest levels of average population health.[27] Interestingly enough though, as the interests and political agendas of the health care stakeholders are carefully considered, maximization of the common good (or the optimal achievement of population health) is not prominent on the political agenda of any of the stakeholders mentioned. If the desired good is restated as "access to essential health care" rather than health per se, the Utilitarian perspective converges most on the reform policy priorities voiced by the public and organized labor. However, the historic political behavior of both the public and organized labor has shown that maximization of access to health care takes a far second place to concerns about the preservation of individual preferences for health care when the opponents of health care reform manage to frame universal access and individual choice as an either–or dichotomy.

Marxist Social Justice and Stakeholder Agendas

In contrast to the other theories of social justice, the Marxist perspective is quite forthright in its assertion that in a just society there is a positive right to health care (see discussion in chapter 1).[28] As pointed out in chapter 1, Marx's famous dictum that a postrevolutionary socialist society would assure that "each contributes according to their ability and receives according to their need" strongly suggests themes of equity and commonwealth as core purposes of society (Wolff, 2003). Moreover, application of the classic Marxist perspective to health care would assert that the health care system should be subject to collective ownership.[29] The notion of a

---

[27] However, where the Utilitarian perspective would most depart from the public health perspective is the issue of health disparity. Strictly speaking, utilitarianism is agnostic toward the problem of disparity whereas the public health perspective is deeply concerned with it.

[28] As acknowledged in chapter 1, Marx himself did not consider his political theory to be a theory of social justice. However, generations of scholars since Marx have placed his political theory within the rubric of social justice in that his writings clearly address the mutual obligations of social existence.

[29] There are gradients of socialized medicine, ranging from a common social insurance fund with universal coverage and private ownership of the health care system's productive assets to the classic Marxist approach which would assert complete collective ownership of hospitals, clinics, labs, pharmaceutical factories, and so on. The term "socialized medicine" has been long employed by the opponents of universal health insurance, however organized, to incite a variety of reactionary assumptions and images.

positive right to health care fits most closely with the interests and political agendas of those disenfranchised under the employment-based system of health. Although it may seem that the labor movement should align most with the Marxist perspective on a positive right to health care, the contemporary political agenda of organized labor remains committed to the preservation of the employment-based health care system—a system which has never approached universal health care coverage. Organized labor does not suggest a publicly sponsored health national health insurance plan, let alone even hint at the possibility of public ownership of the health care system. As discussed by Quadagno (2004), this is because organized labor's health care agenda has long been "privatized," in essence committed to private sector alternatives to the financing and delivery of health care as opposed to a public health care system.[30] The privatization of labor's health care agenda has been largely attributed to two interwoven factors. The first is the absence of a strong working-class movement and labor-based political party (Quadagno, p. 26), in contrast to Britain and much of Europe. The second factor is the stunning defeat of organized labor, at the behest of business interests and the conservative movement, during the immediate post–World War II years. The successive political and public relations victories of business interests over organized labor culminated in both the Taft–Hartley Act of 1947 and the subsequent purgings of organized labor's more radical elements (Quadagno, p. 31). Had organized labor been able to retain its unity and been more strategic in its response to the postwar McCarthyism of its opponents, it seems likely that the Truman administration would have had a much stronger ally in its quest to extend the concept of social security to compulsory national health insurance—thus assuring a universal positive right to health care.

Rawlsian Social Justice and Stakeholder Agendas

In chapter 1 it was argued that there are two core arguments for a positive right to health care, which for all practical purposes extends to universal health insurance coverage. To recap, one core argument draws upon the *difference principle*, namely the idea that a necessary precondition for a "just" state of inequality is that the inequality in question "must be

---

[30] One effect of the privatization of the labor movement's health care agenda has been the division of interests between workers in high-wage industries with very generous collective bargaining agreements and workers in low-wage industries with weak to nonexistent benefits. In Paul Starr's (1995) incisive postmortem of the political defeat of the Clinton plan for universal health care, he notes that health care financing proposals that would have entailed taxation of the highest benefit health care plans in order to extent more basic benefits to the many uninsured workers were opposed by organized labor.

of greatest benefit to the least advantaged members of society" (Rawls, 2001. p. 43). Because it is hard to see how sustained disparities in access to adequate health care[31] that might be of greatest benefit to one group of the least advantaged would not quickly produce extremes of disadvantage in others, the *difference principle* implies that disparities in access to basic health care can never be regarded as just.

The second core argument for the general positive right to health care that is embedded in Rawls' theory of justice involves the essential requirement that a just democracy requires *fair equality of opportunity*. (Daniels, 2002) That is, just governance entails the obligation to provide for "the general means necessary to underwrite fair equality of opportunity and our capacity to take advantage of our basic rights and liberties, and thus be normal and fully cooperating members of society over a complete life" (Rawls, 2001, p. 174). As stated by Rawls (2001, p. 174):

> ... provision for medical care, as with primary goods generally, is to meet the needs and requirements of citizens as free and equal. Such care falls under the general means necessary to underwrite fair equality of opportunity and our capacity to take advantage of our basic rights and liberties, and thus to be normal and fully cooperating members of society over a complete life.

Thus the Rawlsian position on a positive right health care, like the Marxist position, speaks to the interests and political agendas of one key group of stakeholders, those currently disenfranchised under the employment-based system of health and also the least powerful politically.[32] As mentioned previously, this group includes those on Medicaid,[33]

---

[31] It is conceded that the definition of adequate health care itself is extremely problematic. Within the Rawlsian framework as it interpreted here and elsewhere (Daniels, 2002), it would be that level of health care access and health care quality essential to assure fair equality of opportunity. Since decades of health care research have shown that significant disparities in standards of health care access and health care quality are replicated in other kinds of social disadvantages, it would seem that just standards for what is regarded is basic in health care cannot be far below the standards that constitute optimal health care for the most privileged.

[32] As discussed in chapter 1, while there are some areas of overlap between Marxist interpretations of social justice and the Rawlsian social justice framework, the perspectives diverge on a number of points. In particular the Rawls theory of justice is predicated on a constitutional democracy and does not espouse collective ownership of productive property.

[33] At various points throughout this book it has been pointed out that Medicaid, since it carries with it the stigma of a public welfare program, does not deliver the same level access into the health care system as a conventional insurance card or even Medicare. Although under some circumstances Medicaid program benefits exceed those provided by the typical insurance private plan, these advantages are more than offset by such other factors as the unwillingness of providers to accept Medicaid vouchers.

the marginally employed and the unemployed, and those who work in the low-wage economy. All other stakeholder groups discussed, while generally espousing the goal of universal access to health care, are at best no more than lukewarm to the idea of an all-inclusive positive right to health care and at worst are motivated and well positioned to oppose it (Blendon & Benson, 2001; Kaiser Family Foundation, 1994; Oliver & Dowell, 1994; Quadagno, 2004; Starr, 1995).

In sum, there is no particular theory of social justice that comes close to reconciling the interests of all stakeholder groups, though there are clear patterns of alignment. In particular, the values of Libertarianism serve the vested interests in the employment-based system of health care access well. Utilitarianism, on the other hand, is clearly subordinate to other considerations in the interests and agendas of all stakeholder groups considered. Finally, for those that are least advantaged under the current system of health care financing, their interests align more with both the Rawlsian and Marxist positions on health care reform. Not surprisingly, this affirms that whatever theory of social justice is used to frame the definition of "just" health care reform, both on philosophical grounds and upon grounds of material self-interest, very basic conflicts will ensue between the various groups of policy stakeholders. Now that these conflicts have been illuminated, the chapter will turn to an examination of the health care reform implications of the social justice perspective that is the philosophical basis of this book—the account of social justice argued by John Rawls.

THE PROGRESSIVE POSITION ON HEALTH CARE REFORM

The origins of Rawls' theory of social justice are embedded in progressive political philosophy, a tradition of political thought that embraces both egalitarianism and the idea that the improvement of the human condition, especially for the poor and the powerless, is central to the purpose of organized society and good governance (Boguslaw, 2000). As is argued here, the progressive position on health care reform embraces two extensions of Rawls' theory of social justice to the principles of socially just health care reform. The first principle, pertaining to a positive right to health care, draws its premise from the argument that Rawls' contention (in his later writings), that the "provision for medical care... falls under the general means necessary to underwrite fair equality of opportunity and our capacity to take advantage of our basic rights and liberties" (Rawls, 2001,

p. 174).[34] The second principle, pertaining to the inherently unjust nature of disparities in health care, is no more and no less than an extension of Rawls' *difference principle* to health care. Thus, the two principles of socially just health care are as follows:

1. There is a positive right of access to adequate essential health care, based upon health care's role as critical determinant of fair equality of opportunity and the capacity to take advantage of basic rights and liberties throughout the life course.
2. Disparities in either health care access or health care quality are presumptively unjust, and defensible only where demonstrably linked to superior benefits for the least advantaged.

The only caveat to the above principles, to be expanded upon in later discussion, is that the two principles do not extend to all types of health care. As will become clear in the discussion that follows, they extend only to the types of health care that qualify as a *primary good*, in that they determine fair equality of opportunity and the capacity to exist as a free and equal member of society.

The Positive Right to Health Care: Basis and Structural Considerations

As discussed elsewhere in the book, there are compelling arguments for a positive right to health care–based on Rawls' *difference principle*. However, I concur with Daniels' (2002) interpretation of Rawls, that the core basis for a positive right to health care rests with health care's role as a key determinant of "the general means necessary to underwrite *fair equality of opportunity* [my italics] and our capacity to take advantage of our basic rights and liberties essential to citizenship" in a democratic society (Rawls, 2001, p. 174). Further, in a market economy that typically defines health care as a commodity that is produced, bought, and sold, the "right to health care" generally translates to coverage by health insurance. As stated by Daniels (2002, p. 9), universal access to health insurance is an essential obligation and not something that is either merely socially desirable or suggestive of paternalism:

> Some economists and philosophers may object that giving special status to health insurance will be "paternalistic" and inefficient as some people prefer to trade income for things other than health care. Our social obligation, however, is to provide institutions (such as social insurance

---

[34] See Daniels (2002) for a more extended version of this argument.

or subsidies to provide private insurance) that protect opportunity, not
to maximize aggregate welfare or achieve efficiency above all else.

However, as acknowledged in chapter 1, there is nothing in Rawls' theory
of justice that establishes prima facie any particular scheme of specific
health care entitlements, health care benefit structures, or for that matter
specific limits on the provision of health care. Also, Rawls' theory does
not appear to give clear preference to either a social insurance model of
health care reform, or reforms that would extend the mixed public/private
model to universal coverage. The discussion that follows will give some
consideration to these core issues.

Entitlements and Health Care Rationing

To the extent that health care competes with other *primary* goods (like
education) that are also critical to the preservation of *fair equality of
opportunity,* provisions for the delineation of entitlements to health care
and the rationing of health care are an essential requirement of justice
(Daniels, 2002). However, on what basis should this be accomplished?
Although Rawls' theory offers no specific prescription, it does provide
some essential insights. In order to grasp these insights, some digression
into the distinction Rawls makes between *distributive justice* and *allocative justice* is necessary. It is also necessary to make a distinction between
forms of health care that can be treated as a *commodity,* and kinds of
health care that have the moral standing of a *primary good.*

In Rawls' theory, *distributive justice* pertains to the principles of justice that regulate the institutions that constitute the basic structure of
society, such that a "fair, efficient, and productive system of social cooperation can be maintained over time" (Rawls, 2001, p. 50). On the other
hand, *allocative justice* pertains to the more immediate questions concerning the fair distribution of a given set of *commodities* in response to
"particular needs, desires and preferences [that] are known to us" (Rawls,
2001, p. 50). Rawls leaves the rules for achieving *allocative justice* un-
specified, because they are presumed to be a product of the background
institutions that compose the basic structure of society as a fair system
of cooperation (Rawls, 2002, p. 51). Thus stated, any given *commodity*
(including many forms of health care) may justly be allocated in unequal
shares, if the rules of allocation are established through cooperatively determined institutional procedures. However, forms of health care that are
clearly determinant of *fair equality of opportunity and the capacity to
take advantage of basic rights and liberties* have a higher moral standing
in Rawls' theory of justice than ordinary *commodities,* and as such are

subject to a higher order of consideration—the order of consideration applied to *primary goods*.[35]

Rationing health care entitlements. The preceding ideas suggest that the first task of a just approach to health care reform is a formidable task that entails both science and political philosophy, namely, the identification of health care services and technologies that, because they function as essential determinants of *fair equality of opportunity*, meet the definition of a *primary good*. Where feasible, such *primary good* health care services and technologies should be provided equitably as a universal health care entitlement. On the other hand, where universal entitlement is not feasible, such health services should be distributed in accordance with Rawls' *difference principle*—which implies that disequities in the provision of health care should be of greatest benefit to the least advantaged (Rawls, 2001, p. 172–173). While it is beyond the scope of this book to delineate the health care services and technologies that might quality as a *primary good*, intuitively they are linked to the health status dimensions of survival and incapacity. For example, as discussed earlier in the book (see chapter 6), there have been recent advances in health status measurements that have yielded population indicators that incorporate both survival and incapacity, notably the DALY or "disability adjusted life year" (Murray & Lopez, 1996). Conceivably, a key criterion for the identification of health care services and technologies given entitlement status would be their established contribution to the maximization of DALYs (disability adjusted life years).

While it is acknowledged that the preceding strategy clearly incorporates the defining principle of the utilitarian approach to social justice (the maximum good to the maximum number of people), it is applied in service of a Rawlsian end. Specifically, provision of the general means necessary to underwrite fair equality of opportunity (Rawls, 2001, p. 174). It is also plausible that other nonutilitarian strategies could be enlisted to identify the most essential health services to fair equality of opportunity, including the selection of health services that are particularly relevant to the exercise of individual political participation.

Another dimension of health care rationing, aside from the determination of a limited set of universal entitlements to health care, involves the

---

[35] Rawls makes the distinction between primary goods and ordinary commodities particularly clear in the following passage: "Primary goods are things needed and required by persons seen in the light of the political conception of persons as citizens who are fully cooperating members of society... These goods are things citizens need as free and equal persons living a complete life; they are not things it is simply rational to want or desire, or to prefer or even to crave" (Rawls, 2001, p. 58).

problem of setting individual limits to entitlement. For example, preservation of fair equality of opportunity might establish the grounds for universal entitlement to kidney dialysis to all persons in need of it, but at what point does any one person's consumption of dialysis services exceed the limits of any individual's claim to a finite social resource? One answer might reside in the intervention's continued relevance to the preservation of any individual's fair equality of opportunity and capacity to take advantage of our basic rights and liberties. That is, entitlement ends at the point where the continuation of dialysis provides no benefit to either because the reality of the individual's overall condition is such there is no hope that he or she will be able to resume the exercise of basic rights and liberties, as in the case of a persistent vegetative state or end stage dementia.[36] Another answer, suggested directly by Rawls, involves the limits to entitlements to health care that are based on application of the *difference principle*, "where further provision would lower the expectations of the least advantaged" (Rawls, 2001, p. 173). This argues that the extent of health care entitlements to one group of disadvantaged must be tempered by their impacts on other group of disadvantaged, the classic contrast being the health care entitlements of fragile aged versus the entitlements available to the children of the working poor.

Rationing Health Care Commodities. Other kinds of health care services and technologies, termed health care commodities because they contribute more to lower order considerations like happiness and life satisfaction (Daniels, 2002), are distributed on a different basis than entitlements. Examples might include such popular health care services and technologies as cosmetic dental care, breast implants, medication for sexual dysfunction, and psychotherapy for the worried well. These too are generally limited health care resources, in the sense that there are a finite number of dental schools, medical residencies for plastic surgeons, and so on. In accordance with Rawls, the rules of allocation for such commodities are established through cooperatively determined institutional procedures and are not addressed directly through principles of justice. Thus for example, a state legislature could decide to extend the medical benefits of public employees to nontrauma related cosmetic surgery, but in most places that would invoke the wrath of taxpayers. Within the employer-based insurance market, it is quite common to craft benefit packages that are replete with commodity class health care services, either

---

[36] Rawls' theory of justice is principally concerned with a political conception of personhood, thus this conclusion is likely to differ from the conclusion that might be arise from moral frameworks tied to a normative (e.g., religious) conception of personhood.

to accede to the demands of a powerful union or woo a desirable pool of job applicants. While you or I might question the social values that are reflected in the range of health care commodities available and the inequities of their allocation, if the requirements of procedural justice are satisfied, Rawls' theory has nothing more to say.[37]

Social Insurance Versus Mixed Private/Public Health Insurance

It was stated previously that Rawls' theory of social justice does appear to give clear preference to either a social insurance model of universal health care entitlement, or reforms that would extend the mixed public/private model to include universal coverage. Beyond establishing a convincing case that Rawls' theory of justice extends to a universal entitlement to health care, Daniels' (2002) interpretation of Rawls is also agnostic on the specific financial structure of universal health care—though his interpretation clearly concedes the legitimacy of private health insurance funds as part of the overall scheme (Daniels, p. 9). In the analysis that follows, it will be argued that Rawls' theory is far more compatible with a model that combines a social insurance fund for universal entitlements with private insurance (for lower order health care benefits) than other main types.

Three Basic Approaches to Universal Health Insurance Coverage

Although there are several approaches to the achievement of universal health care, this analysis will focus on the three major models that have been prominent in the domestic political discourse over the past couple of decades.[38] As it is argued here, Rawls' theory of social justice offers two fundamental considerations that can be employed as the evaluative criteria for the different approaches to universal health care coverage that will be described. The first fundamental consideration entails compatibility with *the positive right to health care* (see earlier discussion on the First Principle). The second fundamental consideration involves

[37] There is one important caveat. Many things that might be identified today as health care commodity might someday evolve to becoming a primary good. For example, if the increasing affordability of laser surgery for ordinary vision correction eventually makes the wearing of eyeglasses a stigmatizing marker of poverty, it is conceivable that laser surgery for vision correction may evolve to a primary good.

[38] Although the idea of a social insurance model of universal entitlements to "basic health care" in combination with a private insurance residual has been bandied about for decades, the version described as Type III in this analysis employs Rawls' theory of social justice to delineate public entitlements from private market health insurance benefits.

compatibility with *the presumptive injustice of disparities in health care access and quality* (see earlier discussion on the Second Principle). A third consideration, perhaps less fundamental but nonetheless embedded in Rawls' theory of justice, is the assumption that forms of health care that are unrelated to *fair equality of opportunity* (and thus falling in the class of *ordinary commodities*) are allocated through cooperatively established institutional mechanisms (Rawls, 2001, p. 50). This third consideration sanctions the legitimacy of a private insurance market to defray out-of-pocket expenditures for forms of health care that are desirable from the standpoint of individual ends but are not essential to fair equality of opportunity.

It is acknowledged that all of the three models of universal health insurance to be considered are based on a federal system of public entitlements, as opposed to models that might entail the expansion of state-level entitlements. While it is possible that a model of universal insurance coverage might evolve that places a primary emphasis on state-level solutions, the historic state-level variations in the voluntary entitlements of Medicaid would suggest this is the most unlikely of all scenarios in the absence of a strong federal imperative.

Type I Employment-Based Health Insurance/Public Fund Residual

Description

This is the current model, which relies upon employment as the primary mechanism through which health insurance coverage is negotiated and purchased. Those not in the labor force for reasons of age or permanent disablement are covered in large part by the Medicare social insurance fund, whereas some low-income earners and the poor are covered by Medicaid. Universal coverage could plausibly be accomplished through a number of mechanisms: expansion of the Medicaid program, employer mandates to provide insurance, means-based individual mandates to purchase insurance, and means-based subsidies for the purchase of private insurance

---

Evaluation

Because Type I is no more than an extension of the current system of health care finance, it is burdened with its well-established shortcomings in assuring adequate basic health care. As discussed in previous chapters, differences in health care access and health care quality are in part a function of differences in the quality of health insurance, and the same finding extends to public programs like Medicare and Medicaid. Stratification in the scope and quality of benefits in the employment-based health insurance system inherently replicates occupational stratification, and for this reason it is reasonable to conclude that the employment-based system of health insurance (even if extended to universal coverage) is inherently incompatible with both fundamental considerations of just health care reform. This same argument applies to policy solutions that would achieve universal coverage through the expansion of Medicaid, because as a means-tested public program fraught with stigma, Medicaid will always impose barriers to enrollment and genuine parity in entitlement (Stuber & Kronebusch, 2004).

Type II Comprehensive Universal Social Insurance Fund

Description

This model entails a universal trust fund with a comprehensive array of entitlements covering all forms of health care that are deemed either essential or at least highly desirable by a sufficient share of the voting public. Although akin to Medicare in its tax structure and array of entitlements, unlike Medicare neither age nor disablement would be criteria for inclusion, and the range of the health care entitlements would be sufficient to preclude the necessity of supplemental private health insurance.

Evaluation

This model is akin to the social insurance model of Norway, which aside from permitting nominal user fees for ambulatory health care services, provides publicly funded health care for all its citizens (OECD, 2001). Because this model provides for a positive right to health care that is devoid of disparities in its entitlements, it is compatible with both fundamental considerations of just health care reform. However, the weakness of this model is that it does not translate well to a large and culturally heterogeneous society with an aggressive health care marketing industry and a high level of variation in tastes for nonessential health care. A small, prosperous, and culturally homogeneous nation like Norway is less burdened with the distinction between essential health care entitlements and tastes for nonessential health care that have been fueled by mass advertising. In the United States, achieving political consensus on a stable array of nonessential health care entitlements would be extraordinary difficult, likely unfair in its distribution of tax burdens, and in the long run fiscally unsustainable (refer to the Medicare Modernization Act of 2003 for an excellent but regrettable exemplar). The dilemmas entailed by this model illustrate one reason why Rawls made it so abundantly clear that his two principles of justice are meant to apply to the distribution of *primary goods,* as opposed to the things that are "simply rational to want or desire, or to prefer or even to crave" (Rawls, 2001, p. 58).

Type III Limited Entitlement Universal Social Insurance Fund/Private Insurance Residual

Description

Unlike a universal trust fund with comprehensive benefits, this model provides a limited array of *primary goods* health care entitlements through a universal trust fund, specifically those "that are deemed essential to fair equality of opportunity and each individual's capacity to take advantage of the basic rights and liberties essential to citizenship" (paraphrased from Rawls, 2001, p. 174). The distribution of these primary good health care entitlements will be based upon the two principles of justice, modified from Rawls (2001, pp. 42–43) to read as follows:

1. Each person has the same claim to a full adequate scheme of equal basic health care entitlements, which scheme is compatible with the same scheme of entitlements for all; and
2. Disparities in either access to health care entitlements, or in the quality of health care entitlements provided, are presumptively unjust and defensible only where they are demonstrably linked to superior health care benefits for the least advantaged.

Health care benefits that are of lower order, in that they provide coverage for health care services and technologies that attend to individual ends like happiness, life satisfaction, and subjective quality of life rather than fair equality of opportunity, are treated as ordinary commodities obtained through either voluntary health insurance or out-of-pocket purchase.

Evaluation

This model of universal health insurance is framed very directly from John Rawls' most recent and final treatise on social justice, published posthumously as *Justice as Fairness: A Restatement* in 2001 (Harvard University Press). The model is consistent with the central tenets of Rawls' theory of justice in the following respects: it justifies a limited array of health care as *primary goods* on the basis of their status as determinates of fair equality of opportunity, it places distribution of these limited entitlements under the purview of Rawls' two principles of justice, it makes a clear distinction between the health care services and technologies that are treated as primary goods and those that have the lower order standing of ordinary commodities, and it relegates the latter to the rules of exchange within a legitimized social institution (the free market health care economy).[39] The fundamental challenge is the ability to identify the particular health care services and technologies that are directly determinate of fair equality of opportunity and as such qualify as a *primary good* health care entitlement. As previously mentioned, this is a formidable process that will entail both the social and life sciences. There are also very challenging problems having to do with the slippery slope of health care that is made to become highly desirable from a consumer marketing perspective and its power to confer significant social and political advantage—thus ultimately transforming it to a *primary good*. Even in this system, two-tiered health care is not avoided.

However, in the final analysis this model (in contrast to *Type I Employment Based Health Insurance/Public Fund Residual*) places lower order health care benefits in the residual category rather than the persons, groups, and populations that are "lower order" in the prevailing scheme of health care financing.

THE POLITICS OF PROMOTING A POSITIVE RIGHT TO HEALTH CARE: LESSONS FROM THE HEALTH SECURITY ACT

When considering the prospects and alternative strategies for major policy reforms, it is always prudent to glean the lessons available from prior failures. The obvious historical touchstone in the case of health care reform is the rise and fall of the so-called Clinton Health Care Plan that occurred in the early 1990s.[40] There is no better source for this than Paul Starr's authoritative postmortem essay, "What Happened to Health Care

---

[39] As stated by Rawls (2001, p. 50), "within the framework of background justice set up by the basic structure, individuals and associations may do as they wish insofar as the rules of institutions permit." The universal entitlement to essential or *primary good* health care has already been addressed through the universal health care trust fund, defined in this model as a component of "the framework of background justice."

[40] Known more formally as the Health Security Act of 1993.

Reform?" published in *The American Prospect* within a few months of the Clinton Plan's political collapse in the fall of 1994.

Starr, a sociologist and renowned scholar of health care policy, had been one of a small group of principal authors of the Clinton Plan and a senior advisor on health care policy to the Clinton Administration. In fact, the Clinton Plan's essential structure and the arguments in support of it were published in a book written by Starr in 1992, one year before the Clinton Plan was formally proposed to Congress.[41] The essence of the Clinton Plan was the achievement of universal health insurance coverage through a combination of insurance purchasing mandates, premium subsidies to low-income workers, the establishment of health insurance purchasing cooperatives, a standard health insurance benefit package sanction by a national board, and "managed competition" between insurance plans as a mechanism to control costs (Congressional Budget Office, 1994; Starr, 1995).

In terms of the previously described models of health care reform, the Clinton Plan was a version of *Type I Employment Based Health Insurance/Public Fund Residual*. Strategically, the plan offered the universal health care coverage sought by liberals, the private market mechanisms favored by conservatives, a range of choice over health plans for consumers, and for the powerful health insurance industry it offered an alternative to decimation at the hands of the other possible path to health care reform— a publicly funded single-payer plan.

As described in Starr's (1995) analysis, it seems as if the Clinton administration and its allies had somehow snatched defeat from the jaws of victory. In 1993, just 1 year prior to the Clinton Plan's formal death announcement, nearly all of the traditional enemies of universal health insurance coverage had endorsed both the necessity of reform and the need for a universal plan of compulsory health insurance—including the AMA, the Health Insurance Association of America, the U.S. Chamber of Commerce, and even Senate Minority Leader Robert Dole.[42] As he traces what happened between the season of health care reform promise and the season of defeat, Starr identifies an array of factors that pertain to presidential political miscalculations, wasted time, failed compromises, policy complexity, public relations, contextual shifts, and of course the formidable determination and resources of the opposition. However, at the core of Starr's postmortem analysis on the Clinton plan's demise is the failure to create and sustain unity of resolve among the reform's

---

[41] Published as *The Logic of Health Care Reform* (Knoxville, TN: Whittle Direct Books, 1992).

[42] Although Dole is now a champion of Medicare's new Drug benefit entitlement, in 1965 he was among 116 congressmen that voted against the original Medicare program.

supporters (Starr, 1995, p. 27). What follows is a brief summary of Starr's observations that appear to offer the most compelling political lessons for future reform.[43] Those highlighted include presidential miscalculation, policy complexity, contextual shifts, and the failure to create and sustain unity among supporters.

Presidential Miscalculations

While many analyses of the demise of the Clinton plan suggest that Clinton's fundamental miscalculations are embedded in the design of an overly complex reform package that confused the public, the larger error entails inattention to the political calendar and the role of momentum. In fall of 1993 the opposition to compulsory health insurance was in disarray and strongly sensed the need for compromise. However, by the time the Clinton Plan was being fully considered by Congress in the summer of 1994, the opposition had been given the opportunity to regroup, back away earlier compromises, and identify the strategy needed to sink reform. While it might be said that some of the collateral political events that damaged the prospects for reform may not have plausibly been anticipated (in particular the infamous and protracted Whitewater scandal),[44] the reality is that the political momentum for major legislation always tends to be short-lived and the political agenda of every presidency is perennially under the sword of the next erupting scandal.

A second miscalculation involved a critical failure on the part of Clinton to vigorously explain and defend the specific components of his proposal to key members of Congress. As Starr explains it, "[t]he administration had gone to the trouble of writing a bill and then left it like a foundling on the doorstep of Congress" (Starr, 1995, p. 26). A third miscalculation (not specifically cited by Starr but nonetheless relevant) is that Clinton seems to have allowed the opposition to define the terms of the debate as the battle over the public's perception of health care reform escalated in the spring and summer of 1994. Tragically for the prospects

[43] While this summary is focused on Starr's analysis, it is selective about which of Starr's observations are viewed most relevant.

[44] The Whitewater scandal refers to and investigation into allegations the William and Hillary Clinton had engaged in fraudulent real estate transactions in years prior to Bill Clinton's first presidential campaign. No grounds for prosecution were ever established, despite an extensive investigation by Independent Counsel Kenneth Starr. Starr was able to expand the investigation into Bill Clinton's personal conduct with White House intern Monica Lewinsky, an investigation which ultimately provided the grounds for Clinton's subsequent impeachment.

of universal entitlement to essential health care, Clinton allowed the central message of health security to become obfuscated by disingenuous oppositional rhetoric.

Policy Complexity

There is a fundamental paradox of reform that involves the restructuring of the political economy of basic institutions like education, the federal tax structure, and health care; to the extent that it genuinely attends to the complex trade-offs inherent in policy and the competing interests of stakeholders, it defies comprehensible public explanation. Contrary to the views of many of its critics, the Clinton Plan was not overly complex in its basic strategy, so much as it was overtly cumbersome to explain and justify to the American public. The lesson here seems to be that where complexity cannot be avoided, even more attention needs to be paid to the challenges of public engagement, problem definition, and comprehension of viable solutions. This is not unachievable where there is a sufficient shared sense of public crisis and a more salient convergence of common interests. While Starr's three pronged prescriptive advice for health care reform (speed, simplicity, and incremental change) is well justified by his analysis of the Clinton plan's political failure, in the next season of reform the ground may have shifted back toward radical solutions.

Contextual Shifts

Major policy initiatives are always subject to the instability of social and economic context. Although Starr's analysis identifies several shifts in the political and economic context of the Clinton Plan's legislative journey, two contextual shifts seemed particularly relevant to the undercutting of the political viability of the Clinton health plan. The first involved the beginnings of an economic resurgence and improving employment prospects, which for many middle-class Americans both alleviated their own worries about the loss of employment-based insurance and caused diminished sense of identity with the poor. The second shift involved the resurgence of the political right, which culminated in the GOP's recapturing of the House of Representatives in the November 1994 elections. While political divisions over health care reform did not play a central role in the GOP victory, the fact of the victory did spell the end to the bipartisan cooperation among moderates that had previously yielded critical compromises on health care reform.

The Imperative of Political Unity Among Policy Supporters

As stated previously, the central kernel of wisdom lies in Starr's observation that it was not so much the determination and resources of the opposition that sunk the Clinton reform effort, so much as it was the failure to achieve and sustain unity among the allies of reform over the political fight's long haul. As noted by Starr (p. 29):

> [The opposition's] influence is easily exaggerated. Several of the key interest groups were actually less hostile to reform than in any prior battle over health insurance since the 1930s. The problem was not so much that the opponents had more resources, but that the supporters [of health care reform] could not mobilize theirs. While the antagonists had great clarity of purpose, the groups backing reform suffered from multiple and complex fractures and were unable to unite.

The lesson in this for the future of health care reform is in some key respects optimistic. While the determination and resources of the vested interests that stand in opposition to reform might be formidable, they are not necessarily decisive where unity of purpose among proponents is achievable. In fact, pursuit of the commonwealth is inherently dependent upon community of purpose.

CONCLUDING COMMENTS—INCREMENTAL OR FUNDAMENTAL REFORM?

The conflict between ideology and political feasibility is as acute in the domain of health care as anywhere in the progressive political landscape. In health care reform, this tension is expressed most immediately in the ongoing debate between incremental strategies and more fundamental approaches to health care reform. If it is accepted that the end goal of health care reform is a structure of health care financing that sustains a positive right to an adequate scheme of essential health care entitlements, then debates between incrementalism and more fundamental reforms are really about strategy and tactics. On the other hand, the history of incrementalism in social policy (health care policy in particular) suggests such debates are more often about minimalist political accommodation and the preservation of inherently unjust institutional arrangements. Given the historically unprecedented retreat from *even incremental strategies* to expand enfranchisement to essential health care, the case for fundamental health care reform is self-evident. However, a compelling case for fundamental health care reform does not by itself propel the nation toward a restructuring of the social contract pertaining to health care—the convergence of other facilitating preconditions is required. The question is, which essential preconditions apply? And further, are they currently in evidence?

The conventional approach to answering these kinds of questions involves the gleaning of insights from historical precedent. While many might consider the large expansions of publicly financed entitlements to health care during the 1960s as the most fruitful historical precedent to examine, the health care coverage expansions of the 1960s emerged in a context of sustained economic prosperity, growing global economic domination, and a growing middle class. The situation as it exists today is in many respects is just the opposite: an economic prosperity that is sustained by unprecedented levels of government borrowing and foreign underwriting of national debt, an enormous and ever expanding trade deficit, a shrinking global market share for U.S. products, and a sustained decline in prosperity for all income classes below the top fifth of all family households (U.S. Census Bureau, 2004). Moreover, the health care entitlement expansions of the 1960s did not involve a fundamental reframing of the social contract as pertains to the link health insurance and economic security—perhaps with the sole exception of the elderly. As disquieting as it might seem, in some key respects the 1930s provide the more apt case for historical precedent—at least in terms of health care policy.

The 1930s are generally known for a collapse of the national economy that left a large share of the labor force jobless and in poverty, certainly not the situation we face today. However, the central thread that underscored the rationale and political viability of social insurance (Social Security) was the broad recognition through shared experience that the basic economic security of the majority of American households could not be left solely to vicissitudes of arbitrary market forces. This is in fact precisely the situation faced by the general public in the context of health care finance and worries about access to essential health care. Despite the rise of neoconservative social policies and a general retreat from public entitlements that has characterized the most recent decades, the evidence is mounting that the hyperbole about market solutions to the problem of adequate health care access is wearing thin with the experiences of a growing share of American households. The employment-based model of health insurance is collapsing and leaving too many working Americans in jeopardy: a shrinking proportion of jobs are likely to provide even basic health care benefits, middle-class households have genuine cause to worry about medically induced bankruptcy, and the link between the rising costs of U.S. health care and U.S. global competitiveness (and ergo the economic security of the typical American household) is made obvious to all workers as health care benefits shrink or disappear. It is also apparent that Medicaid is neither designed nor funded to compensate for such a weakened private insurance system.

Ultimately, there are limits to which American wage earners will trade global competitiveness for access to basic health care, and as those limits are reached fundamental reforms that involve the assurance of universal basic entitlement to health care may become more politically viable than they have been in any recent period is U.S. history. There are also limits to which states are willing to trade funding for critical investments in transportation infrastructure and public education for an ever larger commitment of state dollars toward health care for the poor and the families of the growing numbers uninsured workers. Some harbingers of fundamental change include the resurgence of the labor movement in the industries that represent the largest share of low-wage workers, the emergence of a state level bipartisan reform plan (sponsored by a conservative governor) that imposes basic structural reforms in public subsidies and the employment-based health insurance market to achieve near universal coverage,[45] and perhaps to some extend the extremely low level of public confidence in a presidential administration (that of George W. Bush) that has failed to address the worries that many families from across the political spectrum have about health care.

Notably, the central philosophy of both the Congressional majority and the Bush administration on the health care crisis has emphasized incremental market-based reforms—a philosophy that now yields approval from substantially less than one-third of the public.[46] Although the tipping point for a renewed commitment to more fundamental health care reform that entails universal health insurance coverage is uncertain, current labor market and political trends suggest that incrementalism may have had its day.

---

[45] The Massachusetts Health Care Reform Plan, sponsored and signed into law by Governor Mitt Romney (GOP) in April of 2006. For a summary of the plan and challenging policy issues see http://www.kff.org/uninsured/upload/7494.pdf.

[46] The Pew Research Center survey, conducted in the days immediately following President Bush's 2006 Annual State of the Union Address (January 31, 2006), found that only 28% of the public expressed approval of the Bush administration on health care. This was an even further decline in the health care policy poll ratings from a year previous, which then had been at a very low 36% (The Pew Research Center, 2006). Notably, the central points of Bush's State of the Union Address on health care argued for incremental and voluntary private insurance market solutions and a specific rejection of publicly sponsored health care. While many American's object to the idea of "a government-run health care system" (to quote the language used by President Bush in his address), it is clear that Bush's ideas on incremental private insurance market reforms failed to inspire public confidence.

REFERENCES

Blendon, R. J., & Benson, J. M. (2001). Americans' views on health policy: A fifty-year historical perspective. *Health Affairs, 20*(2), 33–46.

Blendon, R. J., Brodie, M., Altman, D. E., Benson, J. M., & Hamel, E. C. (2005). Voters and health care in the 2004 election. *Health Affairs, W5* 86–96.

Blendon, R. J., Marttila, J., Benson, J. M., Shelter, M. C., Connolly, F. J., & Kiley, T. (1994). The beliefs and values shaping today's health reform debate. *Health Affairs, 13*(1), 274–284.

Boguslaw, R. (2000). Liberalism/conservatism. In E. Borgatta & R. Montgomery (Eds.), *Encyclopedia of sociology* (2nd ed., Vol. 3, pp. 1596–1604). New York: Macmillan References USA.

Bowers, C. (2005, July 25). Big unions break from AFL-CIO. *CBS News.*

Common Cause. (1992). Why the United States does not have a national health program: The medical-industry complex and its pac contributions to Congressional candidates, January 1, 1981, Through June 30, 1991. *International Journal of Health Services, 22*, 619–644.

Congressional Budget Office. (1994). *A preliminary analysis of the Health Security Act as Reported by the Senate Committee on Finance.* Washington, DC: The Congress of the United States, Congressional Budget Office.

Connolly, C., & Allen, M. (2005, February 9). Medicare drug benefit may cost $1.2 trillion estimate dwarfs Bush's original price tag. *Washington Post,* p. A01.

Daniels, N. (2002). Justice, health and health care. In R. Rhodes, M. Battin & A. Silvers (Eds.), *Medicine and Social Justice.* New York: Oxford University Press.

Hellander, I. (2005). A review of the data on the U.S. health sector: Fall 2004. *International Journal of Health Services, 35*(2), 265–289.

Hernes, G. (2001). The medical profession and health care reform—friend or foe? *Social Science & Medicine, 52*(2), 175–177.

Huskamp, H. A., Epstein, A. M., & Blumenthal, D. (2003). The impact of a national prescription drug formulary on prices, market share, and spending: Lessons for Medicare? *Health Affairs, 22*(3), 149–158.

Hutton, J., Borowitz, M., Oleksy, I., & Luce, B. R. (1994). The pharmaceutical industry and health reform: Lessons from Europe *Health Affairs, 13*(3), 98–111.

Iglehart, J. (2004). The new Medicare prescription-drug benefit: A pure power play. *New England Journal of Medicine, 350*(8), 826–833.

Inglehart, J. (2006). U.S. hospitals: Mission versus market. *Health Affairs, 25*(1).

Kaiser Commission on Medicaid and the Uninsured. (2006). *The uninsured: A primer.* Washington DC: Henry J. Kaiser Family Foundation.

Kaiser Family Foundation. (1994). *Statewide Survey of California: Publication No. 1026.* Menlo Park, CA: Henry J. Kaiser Family Foundation.

Kaiser Family Foundation. (2005). *September/October 2005 Health Poll Report Survey.* Washington DC: Henry J. Kaiser Family Foundation.

Kaiser Family Foundation. (2006, October). *Kaiser public opinion spotlight: The uninsured*. Retrieved April 14, 2006, from http://www.kff.org/spotlight/uninsured/6.cfm.

Koch, J. (1998). Political rhetoric and political persuasion: The changing structure of citizens' preferences on health insurance during policy debate. *Public Opinion Quarterly, 62*(2), 209–238.

Kuttner, R. (2006, January 2). *Medicare misery: The new Medicare bill is about to kick in, and what it offers to seniors isn't pretty.* Retrieved April 21, 2006, from http://www.prospect.org/web/page.ww?section=root&name=ViewWeb&articleId=10792.

Maslow, A. (1970). *Motivation and personality [by] Abraham H. Maslow.* New York: Harper Row.

Milkman, R. (2005). The SEIU and the future of US labor. *Labor History, 46*(3), 376–387.

Mossinghoff, G. J. (1994). Health care reform and the pharmaceutical industry. *Health Care Management, 1*(1), 187–196.

Murray, C., & Lopez, A. (Eds.). (1996). *The global burden of disease: A comprehensive assessment of mortality and disability from diseases, injuries and risk factors in 1990 and projected to 2020.* (Vol. 1). Cambridge, MA.: Harvard School of Public Health on behalf of the World Health Organization and the World Bank.

National Association of Public Hospitals and Health Systems. (2003). *Improving access to health care for the uninsured.* Retrieved April 18, 2006, from www.naph.org.

National Opinion Research Center. (2006). *General Social Survey codebook.* Retrieved April 13, 2006, from http://webapp.icpsr.umich.edu/GSS/.

National Restaurant Association. (2006). *News release: National Restaurant Association applauds Senate HELP Committee's passage of legislation to improve small business access to healthcare.* Washington, DC: National Restaurant Association.

OECD. (2001). *Private health insurance in OECD countries: Compilation of national reports.* Paris, France: Organisation for Economic Co-operation and Development.

Oliver, T. R., & Dowell, E. B. (1994). Interest groups and health reform: Lessons from California. *Health Affairs, 13*(2), 123–141.

The Pew Research Center. (2006). *News release, February 1–5 national survey.* Washington, DC: The Pew Research Center for the People and the Press.

PhRMA. (2005). *Press release of keynote address: Putting patients first to keep health care in America the best in the world.* Washington, DC: Pharmaceutical Research and Manufacturers of America.

Quadagno, J. (2004). Why the United States has no national health insurance: Stakeholder mobilization against the welfare state, 1945–1996. *Journal of Health and Social Behavior, 45*(Extra Issue), 25–44.

Rawls, J. (2001). *Justice as fairness.* Cambridge, MA: Harvard University Press.

Rescher, N. (1966). *Distributive justice: A constructive critique of the utilitarian theory of distribution.* New York: Bobbs-Merrill.

Roper, W. L. (1989). Financing health care: A view from the White House. *Health Affairs*, 8(4), 97–102.

Rosner, D., & Markowitz, G. (2003). The struggle over employee benefits: The role of labor in influencing modern health policy. *The Milbank Quarterly*, 81(1), 45–73.

Scofea, L. A. (1994). The development and growth of employer-provided health insurance. *Monthly Labor Review*, 117(3), 3–10.

SEIU. (2006). *It's time for an American solution to our health care crisis.* Retrieved April 20, 2006, from http://www.seiu.org/issues/american_solution.cfm.

Starr, P. (1982). *The social transformation of American medicine.* New York: Basic Books.

Starr, P. (1995). What happened to health care reform. *The American Prospect*, 20, 20–31.

Stolberg, S., & Gerth, J. (2000). How companies stall generics and keep themselves healthy. *New York Times*, pp. A1, A14, A15.

Stuber, J., & Kronebusch, K. (2004). Stigma and other determinants of participation in TANF and Medicaid. *Journal of Policy Analysis and Management*, 23(3), 509–530.

Tieman, J., & Fong, T. (2003). Mixing politics with pleasure. *Modern Healthcare*, 33(40), 6–7.

U.S. Census Bureau. (2004). *Current population survey, annual demographic supplements: Table F-2. Share of aggregate income received by each fifth and top 5 percent of families (All Races): 1947 to 2001.* Washington DC.

Wojcik, J. (2006). More states mulling 'Wal-Mart' legislation. *Business Insurance*, 40(8), 4.

Wolff, J. (2003). Karl Marx: Life and Works. In E. N. Zalta (Ed.), *The Stanford encyclopedia of philosophy.* Palo Alto, CA.

Glossary

Access to Health Care: According to the Institute of Medicine[1] access to health care is generally defined as the ability to engage in timely use of the health care services that achieve the optimal health outcomes. Access to health care involves having the financial resources essential to entering the health care system, getting to the geographic and physical locations where the needed health care is delivered, and finding appropriate providers for the needed care.

Adverse Selection: Adverse selection occurs when individual purchasers of insurance or those selected for inclusion to the insurance pool actually have a level of insurance risk that is significantly in excess of the risk and costs assumed in the calculation of the insurance premium.

Burden of Disease: The prevalence and distribution of diseases, disabilities, and mortality that is carried by the population. The burden of disease that is carried by a population or population subgroup incorporates the susceptibilities and exposures to disease that arise from the interaction of biology and social environment as well as those differences in health that can be attributed to disparities in health care.

Capital-Based Competition: The use of competitive advantages in physical facilities and/or health care technologies to either preserve or expand a health care provider's market share. In contrast to price-based competition, it is inherently inflationary.

Capitation: A system of health care financing that is based on the application of a flat rate of reimbursement over a specified period on a per cap

---

[1] IOM. (1993). *Access to Health Care in America*. Washington, DC: National Academy Press.

(per person) basis, in contrast to reimbursement that is based on fees for specified health services.

Carve-Outs: The selective use of either subcontracting the management and provision of a segment of the benefits package to a specialty provider or making some benefits available on a discounted fee-for-service basis through an external provider contract.

Case Management: Case management has a variety of definitions and approaches, but in health care it generally means the assignment of a care coordination specialist to a patient with a difficult-to-manage disease profile or one that involves high utilization of resources.

Centers for Medicare & Medicaid Services (CMS): The federal agency that administers Medicare, Medicaid, and the State Children's Health Insurance program. CMS, in addition to its administrative functions, is also a prominent source of health services research and statistics.

Community Health Centers (CHCs): A diverse group of not-for-profit and public health care clinics that are federally funded under the provisions of the Public Health Service Act to provide an array of primary health care services to low-income and medically underserved communities.

Community Rating: An insurance fund and premium pricing estimation method that is based on geographic residence, generally by county. This method of insurance pricing is more favorable to persons of low income because their higher risks and insurance costs are averaged in with the lower risks and costs of higher income persons.

Cost-Shifting: The practice through which hospitals and other providers recover losses from uninsured patients through higher charges to insured patients.

Diagnosis Related Groups (DRGs): A DRG is determined at hospital discharge and involves a select array of factors that include the patient's final diagnosis and other case characteristics that have proved to be predictive of hospital care costs (e.g., patient age, sex, type of surgery if any, presence of co-morbid conditions). There are roughly 500 DRGs a patient may be assigned to, depending upon individual case characteristics.

Difference Principle: Central to John Rawls' theory of justice, this principle establishes the very limiting circumstances under which inequalities in wealth, power, and status are just. The difference principle states that "just" social and economic inequalities must satisfy two conditions: first, they are to be attached to offices and positions that are open to all under fair conditions of equality of opportunity: and second, they are to be the greatest benefit to the least-advantaged members of society.

Distributive Justice: A political theory or system of thought that is concerned with the just allocation of limited benefits and resources.

Employer Rating: An insurance fund and premium pricing estimation method that is based on employer characteristics. This method of insurance pricing is unfavorable to persons of low income and education and their employers because their higher insurance costs are not averaged in with persons having more income and education that tend to work for different kinds of employers.

Health Insurance Portability and Accountability Act of 1996 (HIPAA): A comprehensive piece of federal legislation that includes a variety of provisions pertaining to health insurance market reforms intended to promote the affordability and accessibility of health insurance, and other provisions that impose very stringent procedural requirements on providers pertaining to the protection of patient confidentiality.

Health Maintenance Organizations (HMOs): Managed care organizations that provide a comprehensive array of health services through capitated financing.

Independent Practice Associations (IPAs): A structure through which physicians in private practice can join together and negotiate managed care contracts with health insurance plans.

Insurance Pool: A set of individuals assigned to a common insurance fund, assumed to share the average risks and related losses (costs) for the occurrence of the insured events.

Libertarianism: A social and political philosophy that advocates maximum individual freedom and minimum government. At the heart of libertarianism is the idea that societies must be governed, but only to the extent necessary to assure the protection of an explicit set of individual rights. Classic libertarianism holds that government's legitimate functions pertain only to basic protections against foreign or domestic threats to life, property, or the exercise of personal autonomy.

Life Expectancy: The average number of remaining years of life for a person at a given age, given the prevailing pattern of mortality in the population. The most commonly used measure of life expectancy is life expectancy at birth.

Managed Care: Managed care is defined in multiple ways, but it commonly encompasses various activities by health care underwriters to control health care costs, quality, and access.[2]

Long-Term Care: The health, personal care, and related social services provided over a sustained period of time to people who have lost or never developed certain measurable functional abilities.[3] Long-term care policies and services encompass the aged, the developmentally disabled, the chronically ill, and persons disabled by trauma.

Marxism: A social and political theory based on historical materialism, which holds that the particular social arrangements that compose different forms of society (social systems) are determined by the modes of production that are dominant in any given historical epoch. Class exploitation and conflict lie at the heart of the Marxist perspective of the nature of industrialized societies, as well as the belief that the oppressive nature of capitalism will ultimately lead to the revolutionary establishment of socialist states.

Medicaid: Established in 1965 through amendments to the Social Security Act, Medicaid is a means-based program for medical assistance for financially needy persons of all ages. Medicaid is funded jointly by individual states and the federal government through general tax revenues. In contrast to Medicare, Medicaid is not structured as a federalized social insurance fund, does not have consistent eligibility criteria and benefits from state to state, and often incurs both stigma and discrimination from providers.

Medicare: Established in 1965 through amendments to the Social Security Act, Medicare is a federally funded health insurance entitlement program for persons over age 65, persons under age 65 with certain disabilities, and persons with permanent kidney failure requiring dialysis or a kidney transplant. In contrast to Medicaid, which is a means-based program for medical assistance for needy persons, Medicare is structured as a form of social insurance with eligibility based on age and disability criteria.

Moral Hazard: The problem of "moral hazard" arises when the state of being insured for a given event leads the insured person to become less averse to the event occurring—thus altering his or her risk-related

---

[2] Per Baily, M. A. (2003). Managed care organizations and the rationing problem. *The Hastings Center Report, 33*(1), 34–42.

[3] Per Kane, R., Kane, R., & Ladd, R. (1998). *The heart of long term care* (p. 314). New York: Oxford University Press.

behavior. In the context of health insurance, the risk event is an "episode of health care" or use of health care. The fact of having health insurance often makes people less averse to episodes of health care and generally more inclined toward using health care.

National Health Insurance: In classic form, national health insurance entails universal coverage for an comprehensive array of health care services, financed through a tax-based public health insurance fund.

Negative Rights: Negative rights involve constraints on others to not impede our actions and preferences, do something to us, or take something from us. Negative rights, where they apply to the actions of the state or governments, are commonly referred to as "liberty rights."

OECD: The Organisation for Economic Co-Operation and Development (OECD) was founded in 1961, replacing the Organisation for European Economic Co-operation, which had been established in 1948 under the Marshall Plan. The OECD is comprised of 30 member states, each having a democratic form of governance and a market economy.

Point-of-Service (POS) Providers: A form of preferred provider arrangement that permits the health care consumer to choose his or her provider, who may or may not be a part of a preferred provider panel, who then functions as the "gatekeeper" for other health care services related to the episode of care. The consumer may choose another provider for a subsequent episode of care.

Positive Rights: Rights that pertain to what is owed to us or what we can legitimately claim we should be provided. Depending upon the theory of justice applied, positive rights may include such rights as personal safety, basic education, employment opportunity, a just minimum wage, and basic health care.

Preferred Provider Organizations (PPOs): Networks of providers (e.g., physician groups, hospitals, pharmacies) that contract with health insurance underwriters to furnish an array of health care services and products at a discounted price.

Prospective Payment System (PPS): A system of reimbursement implemented in 1983 as amendments to the Social Security Act. It changed the basis of Medicare payments to hospitals from a fee-for-service based system to one based on the patient's assignment to a Diagnosis Related Group (see DRG).

Rawlsian Theoretical Perspective: Viewpoints and positions on issues of social justice that are directly derived from the theoretical works of John Rawls on social justice, in particular his two principles of justice.

Right to Health Care: The right to health care entails a societal obligation to furnish individuals and/or populations with some established array of health care services that may be preventative, curative, or even restorative.[4]

Roemer's Law: A principle of health care policy that states *that supply tends to induce its own demand where a third party guarantees reimbursement of use.*[5] In the context of institutional care like hospitals and nursing homes, this suggests that to the extent that public funds are available to subsidize the costs of care, a market dynamic of "build the beds and they will come" emerges. Roemer's Law is named for its founder, the late Milton Roemer, formerly a Professor of Health Services at UCLA.

Safety Net: The health care system safety net is generally defined as the clinics, hospitals, and individual health care providers that care for a disproportionate share of the poor, the uninsured, those afflicted by stigmatizing health conditions, and persons otherwise isolated from the mainstream health care system.

SES Gradient: In the context of social epidemiology and health care policy, the SES gradient refers to the linear relationship that prevails worldwide between socioeconomic status (income, education, and occupation) and health. Higher SES demonstrates a positive linear relationship to health and longevity, even within very affluent populations and income groups.

Single-Payer System: A system of health care financing that provides for payment of health care services through a single organization, most typically as an essential function of government and through a public fund supported by tax revenues.

Social Epidemiology: A scientific discipline that has, as its primary and explicit concern, the investigation of the *social* determinants of population distributions of health, disease, and wellbeing.

Social Health Maintenance Organization (S/HMO): A comprehensive community-based long-term care program that integrates medical care and social supports under a model of capitated financing. Typical S/HMO benefits include case management, personal in-home support services,

---

[4] Per Hessler, K., & Buchanan, A. (2002). Specifying the content of the human right to health care. In R. Rhodes, M. Battin & A. Silvers (Eds.), *Medicine and social justice*. New York: Oxford University.

[5] Per Roemer, M. I. (1961). Bed supply and hospital utilization: a natural experiment. *Hospitals, 35*, 36–42.

adult day care, respite care (including short-term nursing home care), and coverage for pharmaceuticals.

Social Justice: A philosophical construct that refers to a political theory or system of thought used to determine what mutual obligations flow between the individual and society. A theory of social justice identifies what society as a whole owes to its individual members and, in turn, what individual members owe to society.

Stakeholders: Groups and organizations that have a compelling interest in the outcome of any policy-making process. In essence, the groups and organizations that stand to either gain or lose, dependent upon what policy alternatives are implemented.

Two-Tiered System of Health Care: Two-tiered systems of health care entail disparities in the organization of health care wherein there is one system of health care for the segment of the population with adequate health care insurance coverage, and another for those dependent upon either inadequate public subsidies for health care or "charity care" from the limited number of health care providers willing to provide it.

Uncompensated Care: Care that is provided both without payment and without obligation to pay for persons unable to afford it, and bad debt—which represents a provider's decision to write-off fees for health care that are deemed uncollectible. Both forms of uncompensated care compose a significant source of the financing for health care delivered to the poor and the uninsured.

U.S. Public Health Service (PHS): Originally founded in 1798 as the Marine Hospital Service, the PHS exists as a function of the Department of Health and Human Services. The central mission of the PHS and its eight major divisions entails the protection and advancement of the public's health.

Utilitarianism: A theory of distributive justice, often extended to a social and political philosophy, that is founded upon the *principle of utility*: the idea that utility (whatever is valued as a good thing) should be distributed in accordance with whichever scheme yields the maximum good to the maximum number of people.

Utilization Review: The auditing of clinical records for the purposes of identifying care delivery by providers that fails to meet explicit standards of care established by the insurance underwriter.

Voluntary Health Insurance: Health insurance plans that are funded from purchasers that include individuals, private and public employers, employment industry purchasing cooperatives, beneficent societies, and labor unions. The term "voluntary" refers to the voluntary nature of participation in the insurance plan, in contrast to the compulsory nature of a tax-based public health insurance fund (see national health insurance).

Index

Access to health care
  defined, 236, 335
  disparities in, 236–239
Adult Day Centers, 198
African Americans, health care disparities, 237
Aged, growth of population and long term care, 214
Agency for Healthcare Research and Quality (AHRQ) *2004 National Health Care Disparities Report*, discussion of findings, 249
Allopathic medicine, 42
Almshouses, 35
Ambulatory Care Facilities, 159–160
American Hospital Association (AHA)
  evolvement of Blue Cross plans, 48
  reform interests and agenda, 302–303
American Medical Association (AMA)
  history, 39–44
  oppositon National Health Insurance, 47–49, 59
Americans with Disabilities Act (ADA), 81
Anesthesia, 37
Antiseptic Techniques, 36
Aristotle, 8

Balanced Budget Act of 1997, 80
Blue Cross and Blue Shield Plans, origins, 48–49
Burden of disease, 225, 335
Bush, George H, 294

Bush, George W.
  retrenchment agenda, 85
  reform agenda, 294
  health care policy issue, public opinion, 331

Capital-based competition, 64, 335
Carve-outs, 116, 336
Case Management, 116, 200–201, 336
Catastrophic Coverage Act of 1987, 82
Certificate of Need legislation, 74
Centers for Disease Control and Prevention, 137
Centers for Medicare & Medicaid Services, 336
Charity Hospital of New Orleans, 186–187
Children's Bureau, 55
Clinton, Willianm J.
  Clinton Plan(Health Security Act), 294, 325–329
Community Health Centers (CHC's), 136
Consequentionalist theory, 9
Consolidated Omnibus Budget Reconciliation Act of 1985 (COBRA), 119

Daniels, Norman
  Rawls and right to health care, 25, 317–319
Dependency ratio, defined, 209
Deficit Reduction Act of 2005, 84
Defined Contribution Plans, 118
DALY (Disability Adjusted Life Year), 225
Dispensaries, 46

343

Index

Consumer Voice and Choice in Long-Term Care

Suzanne R. Kunkel, PhD
Valerie Wellin, Editors

Consumer voice and choice is a relatively new concept in the area of long-term care decision-making. It provides the opportunity for consumers to give input and make decisions about the quality of and satisfaction with their services. However, these changes have created a need for more fundamental changes in the long-term health care system at large. Among these changes are a commitment to a new model of service delivery; continued assistance by program administrators, clinical and social service personnel, and other direct-care workers to make sure consumers continue their active role in assessment of programs and services; and support by policy makers and agency leaders.

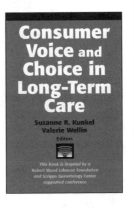

Partial Contents:

Part I: Consumer Choice • Older Consumers and Decision Making • Choice and the Institutionalized Elderly • A Description of Racial/Ethnic Differences Regarding Consumer Directed Community Long-Term Care • Integrating Occupational Health and Safety into the United States' Personal Assistance Services Workforce Agenda

Part II: Consumer Voice • The Consumer/Provider Relationship as Care Quality Mediator • Resident Satisfaction with Independent Living Facilities in Continuing Care Retirement Communities

Part III: Policy Issues, and Moral & Legal Challenges • Gifts or Poison? The Cultural Context of Using Public Funds to Pay Family Caregivers • Response to Quality • When Consumer Direction Fails

2006 · 480pp · hardcover · 0-8261-0210-7

11 West 42nd Street, New York, NY 10036-8002 • Fax: 212-941-7842
Order Toll-Free: 877-687-7476 • Order On-line: www.springerpub.com

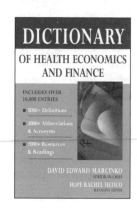

Jonas and Kovner's Healthcare Delivery in the United States 8th Edition

Anthony R. Kovner, PhD
James R. Knickman, PhD

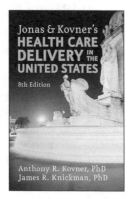

How do we understand and also assess the health care of America? Where is health care provided? What are the characteristics of those institutions that provide it? Over the short term, how are changes in health care provisions affecting the health of the population, the cost of care, and access to care?

"This book properly focuses attention on the challenges of the delivery of health care: how to achieve quality, efficiency, value, fairness, and universal access."

—**Steven Schroeder,** Former President
Chief Executive Officer, Robert Wood Johnson Foundation
Professor of Public Health, University of California, Berkeley

Partial Contents:

Part I: Perspectives • Introduction: The State of Health Care Delivery in the United States • Measurement • Financing for Health Care • Public Health: Policy, Practice, and Perceptions • The Role of Government in Health Care • Comparative Analysis of Health Systems in Wealthy Nations

Part II: Providing Health Care • Acute Care • Chronic Care • Long Term Care • Health-Related Behaviors • Pharmaceuticals and Medical Devices • The Health Care Workforce • Information Management

Part III: System Performance • Governance, Management, and Accountability• The Complexity of Healthcare Quality• Access • Cost Containment

Part IV: Futures • Futures in Health Care • Appendix A: Glossary, A.R. Kovner • Appendix B: A Guide to Sources of Data• Appendix C: A Listing of Useful Health Care Websites • Author Index • Subject Index

2005 · 753pp · softcover · 0-8261-2088-1

**11 West 42nd Street, New York, NY 10036-8002 • Fax: 212-941-7842
Order Toll-Free: 877-687-7476 • Order On-line: www.springerpub.com**

Dictionary of Health Insurance and Managed Care

Edward Marcinko, MBA, CFP, CMP, Editor-in-Chief
Hope Rachel Hetico, RN, MHA, CPHQ, CMP
Operations Editor

To keep up with the ever-changing field of health care, we must learn new and re-learn old terminology in order to correctly apply it to practice. By bringing together the most up-to-date abbreviations, acronyms, definitions, and terms in the health care industry, the *Dictionary* offers a wealth of essential information that will help you understand the ever-changing policies and practices in health insurance and managed care today.

DICTIONARY
OF HEALTH INSURANCE
AND MANAGED CARE

3-IN-1 REFERENCE
INCLUDING:
- 5000+ Definitions
- 3000+ Abbreviations & Acronyms
- 2000+ Resources, Readings and Nomenclature Derivatives

DAVID EDWARD MARCINKO
EDITOR-IN-CHIEF
HOPE RACHEL HETICO
OPERATIONS EDITOR

Special Features:
- Over 10,000 entries
- Detailed terminology covering new HIPAA regulations
- New terminology
- List of confusing definitions
- Simple examples
- Expanded definitions of older terminology still in use

Partial Contents:
- Foreword
- Preface
- Acknowledgments
- Dedication
- Instructions for Use
- Abbreviations and Acronyms
- Terminology: A-Z
- Appendix: Textbook References and Readings

2006 · 360pp · softcover · 0-8261-4944-4

11 West 42nd Street, New York, NY 10036-8002 • Fax: 212-941-7842
Order Toll-Free: 877-687-7476 • Order On-line: www.springerpub.com